ORGAN DONATION AND TRANSPLANTATION – PUBLIC POLICY AND CLINICAL PERSPECTIVES

Edited by **Gurch Randhawa**

Organ Donation and Transplantation – Public Policy and Clinical Perspectives
Edited by Gurch Randhawa

Published by InTech

Janeza Trdine 9, 51000 Rijeka, Croatia

Publishing Process Manager Anja Filipovic

Technical Editor Teodora Smiljanic

Cover Designer InTech Design Team

Additional hard copies can be obtained from orders@intechopen.com

Organ Donation and Transplantation – Public Policy and Clinical Perspectives,
Edited by Gurch Randhawa
p. cm.
ISBN 978-953-51-0039-3

For EU product safety concerns:
IN TECH d.o.o., Prolaz Marije Krucifikse Kozulić 3, 51000 Rijeka, Croatia,
info@intechopen.com or visit our website at intechopen.com.

Meet the editor

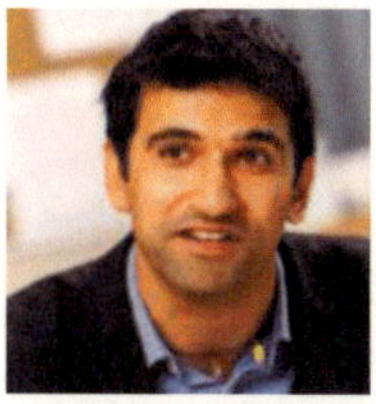

Professor Gurch is Professor of Diversity in Public Health and Director of the Institute for Health Research at the University of Bedfordshire, UK. He has an extensive research track-record related to social, cultural and religious issues in organ donation and transplantation. He is Co-Chair of the European Working Party on Organ Donation & Public Issues. He was a Member of the UK's NICE Guidelines Development Group on Organ Donation and a Member of the UK Department of Health's Organ Donation Taskforce. Currently he is a Member of the UK Donation Ethics Committee; and a Non-Executive Director of the Human Tissue Authority.

Contents

Preface

Advances in medical technology have offered the hope of life to patients who would have otherwise had to face the prospect of death. This is especially so, in the area of transplantation where it is possible to replace organs such as the heart, kidney, liver, lung, and pancreas.

Transplantation has succeeded in prolonging the lives of those fortunate enough to have received the gift of a body organ. What was once a rare and risky procedure for the privileged few has now become a well established routine treatment and a positive option for those with organ failure. Alongside this life-saving development, there lies another sadder side to the story - there are not enough organs to meet the ever increasing demand. One can only begin to understand the emotions of the patients who wake up each day, knowing that a transplant is the only realistic option for a healthy and prolonged life, but are in the agonising situation of waiting for a suitable organ to become available. This principally involves waiting for someone else to die and their loved one's consent for the organs to be used for transplantation. The sad fact is that this situation is relatively common and transplant patients continue to wait while the waiting lists consequently grow longer day by day. This does not only place increasing emotional and physical burden among the waiting patients and families but heaps a great financial burden upon health services.

Thus we are in a unique position in the forum of transplantation as opposed to other areas of health care; the expertise and financial resources exist but the organs for transplant do not.

This book attempts to provide an analysis and overview of public policy developments and clinical developments that will hopefully ensure an increased availability of organs and greater graft survival. Medical, policy, and academic experts from around the world, who are at the forefront of their respective fields, have contributed chapters to the book.

Gurch Randhawa
Professor of Diversity in Public Health &
Director of the Institute for Health Research
University of Bedfordshire
UK

Part 1

Public Policy Issues in Organ Donation and Transplantation

1

Transplant Inequalities – A United Kingdom Perspective

Gurch Randhawa
Institute for Health Research, University of Bedfordshire, UK

1. Introduction

The UK's Organ Donation Taskforce brought policy and resource focus to tackling transplant-related inequalities. In its first report, they stated, 'There is an urgent requirement to identify and implement the most effective methods through which organ donation and the "gift of life" can be promoted to the general public, and specifically to the BME (Black and minority ethnic) population. Research should be commissioned through Department of Health Research and Development funding' (Department of Health 2008a). The Taskforce's second report stated that 'The Taskforce strongly recommends that the Programme Delivery Board builds on the foundations of the interviews with faith and belief groups…., to ensure that the valuable dialogue that was established is maintained' (Department of Health 2008b).

These recommendations were in response to the plethora of evidence that highlights the variation in - demand for, access to, and waiting times for - transplant services in the UK. These variations impact upon minority ethnic communities in particular. The solutions to rectifying this situation are complex and require a holistic approach that considers both the short-term requirement to increase the number of organ donors from minority ethnic groups, and the longer term focus to decrease the number of minority ethnic patients requiring a transplant, via preventative strategies.

2. Background

South Asians (those originating from the Indian subcontinent - India, Sri Lanka, Pakistan and Bangladesh) and African-Caribbean communities have a high prevalence of Type 2 diabetes (Riste *et al.*, 2001; Forouhi *et al.*, 2006; Roderick *et al.*, 2011). A further complication is that diabetic nephropathy is the major cause of end-stage renal failure (ESRF) in South Asian and African-Caribbean patients receiving renal replacement therapy (RRT), either by dialysis or transplantation (Roderick *et al.*, 2011). Furthermore, South Asians with diabetes are at much greater risk of developing ESRF compared to 'White' Caucasians (Riste *et al.*, 2001; Forouhi *et al.*, 2006; Roderick *et al.*, 1996). Thus, not only are South Asians and African-Caribbeans more prone to diabetes than Whites, they are more likely to develop ESRF as a consequence.

Importantly, the South Asian and African-Caribbean populations in the UK are relatively young compared to the White population. Since the prevalence of ESRF increases with age, this has major implications for the future need for RRT and highlights the urgent need for preventive measures (Randhawa 1998). The incidence of ESRF has significant consequences for both local and national NHS resources.

Kidney transplantation is the preferred mode of RRT for eligible patients with end-stage renal failure. There are currently approximately 8,000 people on the transplant waiting list in the UK - the majority waiting for kidney transplants, but substantial numbers also waiting for heart, lung, and liver transplants. However, a closer examination of the national waiting list reveals that some minority ethnic groups are greater represented than others. For example:

- 1 in 5 people waiting for a transplant are from the African-Caribbean or South Asian communities (Table 1).

Ethnicity	Organ awaited															*Total*	
	Kidney		**Pancreas**		**K & P**		**Heart**		**Lung**		**Heart/ lung**		**Liver**		**Multi-organ**		
	N	%	**N**	%	**N**	%	**N**	%	**N**	%	**N**	%	**N**	%	**N**	*N*	%
White	6802	74.7	77	92.8	346	93.3	90	90.9	222	96.1	10	83.3	277	82.7	24	7848	76.5
Asian	1360	14.9	2	2.4	18	4.9	5	5.1	2	0.9	2	16.7	37	11	0	1426	13.9
Black	700	7.7	2	2.4	3	0.8	1	1	5	2.2	0	0	6	1.8	0	717	7.0
Chinese	97	1.1	0	0	1	0.3	1	1	0	0	0	0	2	0.6	0	101	1.0
Mixed	19	0.2	0	0	0	0	0	0	0	0	0	0	0	0	0	19	0.2
Other	125	1.4	2	2.4	3	0.8	2	2	2	0.9	0	0	11	3.3	0	145	1.4
Not rec.	6	0.1	0	0	0	0	0	0	0	0	0	0	2	0.6	0	8	0.1
Total	*9109*		*83*		*371*		*99*		*231*		*12*		*335*		*24*	*10264*	

Source: NHS Blood & Transplant, 2009

Table 1. Patients listed (active or suspended) for an organ transplant in the UK as at 31st December 2008, by ethnic origin and organ

- 14% of people waiting for a kidney transplant are South Asian and over 7% are African-Caribbean (Table 2), even though they compromise only 4% and 2% respectively of the general population.

Age (yrs)	Ethnic origin							Total
	White	Asian	Black	Chinese	Mixed	Other	Not rec.	
0-9	0.5%	0.9%	0.4%	0.0%	5.3%	0.0%	0.0%	0.6%
10-19	1.2%	2.3%	1.4%	1.0%	5.3%	0.0%	0.0%	1.4%
20-29	6.2%	7.4%	4.4%	4.1%	10.5	7.8%	0.0%	6.3%
30-39	11.7%	13.1%	16.6%	9.2%	21.1%	18.0%	16.7%	12.3%
40-49	22.7%	20.8%	34.3%	17.4%	21.1%	28.1%	66.7%	23.3%
50-59	25.0%	31.1%	23.0%	40.8%	21.1%	25.0%	0.0%	25.9%
60-69	24.6%	19.4%	15.7%	21.4%	10.5%	15.6%	16.7%	23.0%
70-79	7.9%	4.9%	4.0%	6.1%	5.3%	5.5%	0.0%	7.1%
80+	0.1%	0.1%	0.1%	0.0%	0.0%	0.0%	0.0%	0.1%
Total	***7166***	***1378***	***703***	***98***	***19***	***128***	***6***	***9498***
Total %	***75.5%***	***14.5%***	***7.4%***	***1.0%***	***0.2%***	***1.4%***	***0.0%***	
Pop %	92.1%	4.0%	2.0%	0.4%	1.1%	0.4%		

Source: NHS Blood & Transplant, 2009

Table 2. % registered (inc suspended) on list for a kidney (inc. kidney/pancreas) transplant in UK as at 31 December 2008, by age decade and ethnic origin

- South Asian people are also more likely to need a liver transplant. While 4% of the UK population are South Asian, Asian people comprise over 10% of the liver transplant list (Table 3). This is because viral hepatitis - hepatitis B & C - that can lead to liver damage and liver failure is more prevalent in the South Asian population.

Age (yrs)	Ethnic origin						Total
	White	Asian	Black	Chinese	Mixed	Other	
0-9	14	1	0	0	0	0	15
10-19	8	1	0	0	0	1	10
20-29	15	3	1	0	0	3	22
30-39	21	1	1	0	0	1	24
40-49	55	11	0	0	0	2	68
50-59	109	16	4	0	0	2	131
60-69	75	4	0	2	0	3	84
70-79	1	0	0	0	0	1	2
Total	***298***	***37***	***6***	***2***	***0***	***13***	***356***
Total %	***83.7%***	***10.4%***	***1.7%***	***0.6%***	***0.0%***	***3.7%***	
Pop %	92.1%	4.0%	2.0%	0.4%	1.1%	0.4%	

Source: NHS Blood & Transplant, 2009

Table 3. Number registered on list for a liver transplant in UK as at 31 December 2008, by age decade and ethnic origin

- Just 1% of people registered on the Organ Donor Register are South Asian and 0.3% of people registered are African-Caribbean
- 1.2% of people who donate kidneys after their death are South Asian and 0.7% are African-Caribbean (Table 4).

Donor type	**Ethnic origin**						***Total***
	White	**Asian**	**Black**	**Chinese**	**Mixed**	**Other**	
Deceased	2135	33	19	4	11	5	2207
%	96.7%	1.5%	0.9%	0.2%	0.5%	0.2%	
Living	2103	142	93	11	8	42	2399
%	87.7%	5.9%	3.9%	0.5%	0.3%	1.8%	

Source: NHS Blood & Transplant, 2009

Table 4. Kidney donors in UK, Jan 04 – 2006-2008, by donor type and ethnic origin

- South Asian and African-Caribbean people wait on average twice as long as White persons for a kidney transplant. White patients wait on average 722 days, Asian patients wait 1496 days and Black people wait 1389 days (Table 5).

Ethnic origin	**Average wait median (days)**
White	722
Asian	1496
Black	1389
Other	948

* based on registrations in 1998-2000
Source: NHS Blood & Transplant, 2009

Table 5. Time actively registered on list for kidney transplant, UK*

- 1 in 8 people who died waiting for a transplant in 2006 were of African-Caribbean or South Asian origin (Table 6)

Ethnic origin	*Kidney*	*Pancreas*	*K/P*	*Heart*	*Lungs*	*H/L*	*Liver*	*TOTAL*	*%*
White	212	-	9	24	50	7	81	**383**	*85.5*
Asian	34	-	-	3	-	-	8	**45**	***10.0***
Black	10	-	-	1	-	-	1	**12**	***2.7***
Chinese	3	-	-	-	-	-	-	**3**	***0.7***
Mixed	1	-	-	-	-	1	-	**2**	***0.4***
Other	1	-	-	1	-	-	1	**3**	***0.7***
TOTAL	*261*	-	*9*	*29*	*50*	*8*	*91*	***448***	

Source: UK Transplant, 2007

Table 6. Patients dying in 2006 whilst list for a transplant

3. Improving access to services

Research evidence has consistently demonstrated that the quality of diabetes and renal care, patient compliance, and knowledge of diabetes and its complications is lower among South Asians and African-Caribbeans (Gholap et al, 2011; Randhawa et al, 2010a; Wilkinson et al, 2011a). The UK's Department of Health has responded to this evidence by publishing a series of standard-setting documents that seek to influence public health interventions and clinical practice by highlighting the health inequalities that exist and encouraging the early identification and treatment of 'at-risk' populations. For example, The Diabetes National Service Framework (NSF) highlights the importance of improving access to services, in particular to meet the needs of minority ethnic groups (Department of Health 2002). The document also stresses the need to develop tailored education programmes to tackle issues such as diet, exercise, obesity, and treatment adherence. In a similar vein, this theme is continued within the Renal Services NSF, which also recognises the need to develop culturally-competent education programmes for the diverse renal patient population (Department of Health 2004). Within primary care, the Quality and Outcomes Framework (QOF) introduced standards for monitoring diabetes and kidney disease in 2006. These standards sought to ensure 'at-risk' patients were assessed and treated much sooner within primary care than was previously the case. A recent audit of these policy initiatives suggests that clinical practice may be improving (Wilkinson et al, 2011b).

4. Improving transplantation rates

A range of studies have documented that a lack of awareness concerning organ donation and transplantation among minority ethnic communities is the over-riding reason for the lack of donors from these communities. This tragically translates into higher refusal rates among non-white families (69%) compared to white-families (35%) in hospitals (Barber et al, 2006; Department of Health, 2008a; Perera and Mamode, 2010).

4.1 Increasing awareness of the need for organ donors among the African-Caribbean and South Asian communities

It is interesting to note, that once minority ethnic communities are engaged with the issue of organ donation, they are keen to lend their support and encourage their communities to sign up as organ donors (Exley et al 1996, Darr and Randhawa 1999, Hayward and Madill 2003, Alkhawari, Stimson and Warrens 2005, Davis and Randhawa, 2006, Morgan et al 2006).

Religion has also been a key influencer in the decision to donate organs or not (Randhawa et al 2010b, Hayward and Madill 2003, Alkhawari, Stimson and Warrens 2005, Davis and Randhawa 2006). Although religious interpretations are not explicit in their reference to organ donation as religious scriptures were written prior to the development of transplantation, most interpretations are broadly supportive of organ donation. However, there are some differences in opinion among some religious scholars and consequently it is imperative to support these scholars in developing an informed debate amongst their peers to reach some consensus. Subsequent to this, there is a need to identify how best to encourage religious 'stakeholders' to engage with their local community concerning the issue of organ donation and transplantation.

In an effort to increase knowledge and awareness of organ donation among minority ethnic communities there have been a series of BME organ donor campaigns led by NHS Blood & Transplant since 2009. These campaigns have included a series of community-based events taking place in areas of high BME-population density, supported with a range of educational materials (including religious leaflets, posters, podcasts, etc). It is too soon to comment on the success of these campaigns.

5. Looking to the future

It is clear that black and minority ethnic groups are disproportionately affected by renal health problems both in terms of access to appropriate services, a higher prevalence of renal complications, a reduced likelihood of a transplant, and longer waiting times on the transplant waiting list. Solutions are multi-faceted requiring a focus on the prevention of long-term conditions as well as the need to transplant patients with organ failure.

Meaningful public engagement is critical to developing tailored community education programmes that can focus both on the need to prevent and manage long-term conditions, and also focus on the need for increased organ donors from all ethnic backgrounds. This is a difficult challenge as many of these communities live within the most deprived (and hard-to-engage) communities in the UK. Not only should we engage the public with the discourse of 'disease prevention' as well as 'organ donation', but there is a need to identify whether the social class of a patient and/or their family influences *live* donation, as this may have implications for current reimbursement arrangements. This issue may have particular relevance to minority ethnic groups who experience the greatest levels of deprivation in the UK.

It has been suggested previously by commentators that religion acts as a prohibitor to organ donation among the South Asian population, but empirical research seems to suggest otherwise. The position of one's religion towards donation is used by individuals as a helpful guide in reaching their decision as to whether to donate or not (Randhawa et al, 2010b). The introduction of community-based information programmes need to be evaluated to assess whether this impacts upon the number of African-Caribbeans and South Asians on the Organ Donor Register. Indeed, all public organ donor campaigns should be formally evaluated to identify which members of the public benefit from such campaigns and to identify which members of the public are still not being reached. Moreover, research should be commissioned to identify how best to unravel public concerns that are 'cultural' as opposed to 'religious' (Randhawa et al, 2010c).

The Potential Donor Audit (an audit developed to identify the true potential for organ donation from dead donors, together with the reasons for non-donation) has highlighted the higher refusal rate for non-White potential donors compared with White potential donors (Barber et al, 2006). It is essential to ensure staff at the front line charged with approaching families for donor requests, known as Specialist Nurses for Organ Donation (SNODs), are provided with relevant training to ensure they are able to meet the needs of families from a range of ethnic and faith backgrounds.

6. Conclusion

Inequalities in renal and transplant services are well documented in the research literature and policymakers have sought to ensure that clinical guidance and public education campaigns are attuned to addressing the inequalities gap. Policy documents such as the Diabetes NSF, Renal Services NSF and QOF are heralded as landmark documents as they offer the prospect of national minimum standards for clinical care and the identification and treatment of 'at-risk' populations. The development of community-based organ donor campaigns are a recent development in the UK and have the potential to offer a more meaningful route to public engagement.

Whilst this paper has been confined to the narrow focus of ethnicity. It is worth noting that this is the case because of the availability of transplant-related data in the UK. It is likely, that similar to other areas of healthcare, that issues such as social class, gender, age, ethnicity, religion, gender, and education have a complex inter-relationship on renal health and transplantation. Therefore, it is imperative that such information is routinely collated and analysed to inform policy and practice.

7. References

Alkhawari, F., Stimson, G., Warrens, A. (2005) 'Attitudes towards transplantation in UK Muslim Indo-Asians in West London', *American Journal of Transplantation*, 5, 1326-1331.

Barber K, Falvey S, Hamilton C, Collett D, Rudge C. (2006) Potential for organ donation in the United Kingdom: audit of intensive care records. *BMJ*. 332(7550):1124-7.

Darr, A., Randhawa, G. (1999) 'Public opinion and perception of organ donation and transplantation among Asian communities: An exploratory study in Luton, UK', *International Journal of Health Promotion & Education*, 37, 68-74.

Davis, C., Randhawa, G. (2006) 'The influence of religion on organ donation among the Black Caribbean and Black African population - a pilot study in the UK', *Ethnicity & Disease*, 16, 281-5.

Department of Health (2008a) Organs for Transplants: A report from the Organ Donation Taskforce. London, Department of Health, 2008, at 48.

Department of Health (2008b) The potential impact of an opt-out system for organ donation in the UK - An independent report from the Organ Donation Taskforce, London, Department of Health, 2008, at 30.

Department of Health (2004) National Service Framework for Renal Services, London: Department of Health, 2004.

Department of Health (2002) National Service Framework for Diabetes: Standards, London: Department of Health, 2002.

Exley, C., Sim, J., Reid, N., Jackson, S., West, N. (1996) 'Attitudes and beliefs within the Sikh community regarding organ donation: A pilot study', *Social Science and Medicine*, 43 (1996), 23-8.

Forouhi NG, Merrick D, Goyder E, et al. (2006) Diabetes prevalence in England, 2001 - estimates from an epidemiological model. *Diabet Med.*23(2):189–197.

Gholap N, Davies M, Patel K, Sattar N, Khunti K.(2011) Type 2 diabetes and cardiovascular disease in South Asians. Prim Care Diabetes, 5(1):45-56.

Hayward, C., Madill, A. (2003) 'The meanings of organ donation: Muslims of Pakistani origin and white English nationals living in North England', *Social Science & Medicine*, 57, 389-401.

Morgan, M., Hooper, R., Mayblin, M., Jones, R. (2006) 'Attitudes to kidney donation and registering as a donor among ethnic groups in the UK', *Journal of Public Health,* 28, 226-234.

Parera S and Mamode N (2010) South Asian patients awaiting organ transplantation in the UK. Nephrology Dialysis and Transplantation, 26, 1380-4.

Randhawa G, Jetha C, Gill B, Paramasivan S, Lightstone E, Waqar M (2010a) Understanding kidney disease and perceptions of kidney services among South Asians in West London: focus group study. *British Journal of Renal Medicine*. 15, 23-28.

Randhawa G, Brocklehurst A, Pateman R, Kinsella S, Parry V (2010b) 'Opting-in or Opting-out?' The views of the UK's Faith leaders in relation to organ donation. *Journal of Health Policy*. 96, 36-44.

Randhawa G, Brocklehurst A, Pateman R, Kinsella S, Parry V (2010c) Utilising faith communities in the UK to promote the organ donation debate: The views of UK faith leaders. *Journal of Diversity in Health and Social Care*, 7, 57-64.

Randhawa, G. (1997) 'Enhancing the health professional's role in requesting transplant organs', *British Journal of Nursing*, 6, 429-434.

Randhawa, G. (1998) 'The impending kidney transplant crisis for the Asian population in the UK', *Public Health*,112, 265-8.

Riste L, Khan F, Cruickshank K.(2001) High prevalence of type 2 diabetes in all ethnic groups, including Europeans, in a British inner city: relative poverty, history, inactivity, or 21st century Europe? *Diabetes Care*.24(8):1377–1383.

Roderick P, Hollinshead J, O'Donoghue D, Matthews B, Beard C, Parker S, Snook M (2011) Health inequalities and chronic kidney disease in adults. London, NHS Kidney Care.

Roderick, P., Raleigh, V., Hallam, L., Mallick, N. (1996) 'The need and demand for renal replacement therapy amongst ethnic minorities in England', *Journal of Epidemiology and Community Health*, 50, 334-9.

Wilkinson, E., Randhawa, G., Farrington, K., Feehally, J., Choi, P., Lightstone, L. (2011a) Lack of awareness of kidney complications despite familiarity with diabetes - a multi-ethnic qualitative study. *Journal of Renal Care*, 37, 2-11.

Wilkinson E, Randhawa, G, Roderick P, Rehman T, Abubacker T (2011b) The impact of quality improvement initiatives on diabetes care among South Asian people. *Diabetes & Primary Care*, 13, 90-98.

2

An Examination of Organ Donation in the News: A Content Analysis From 2005-2010 of the Barriers to Becoming an Organ Donor

Brian L. Quick[1], Nicole R. LaVoie[1] and Anne M. Stone[2]
[1]*University of Illinois at Urbana-Champaign*
[2]*Portland State University*
USA

1. Introduction

Presently, more than 111,000 people are waiting for an organ transplant (United Network for Organ Sharing, 2011). Given the impact that this shortage has on individuals, families, and society, research examining factors influencing the decision to become an organ donor is imperative. A report indicate that most Americans learn more about organ donation from television than any other source (Conesa, Zambudio, Ramirez, Canteras, Rodriguez, & Parrilla, 2004). Thus, an important first step is determining what content is covered, as well as how organ donation is depicted, on television news. As part of a larger study on campaign strategies for improving organ donation rates, we examined television news coverage of organ donation across ABC, CBS, CNBC, CNN, FOX, and MSNBC from January 2005 through December 2010. In order to better understand the potential impact these news stories may have on viewers, we employed the Health Belief Model (HBM; Rosenstock, 1974). The following describes the utility of the HBM for analyzing the content of organ donation news transcripts. Drawing from the agenda setting literature, which suggests that the media shapes not only what people think about but also how they think about it, (McCombs & Shaw, 1972) we assert that examining news content provides a meaningful context to better understand why people generally have favorable attitudes toward organ donation and still do not take the step to register to become an organ donor.

2. Utility of Health Belief Model for examining news coverage

Examining news coverage related to organ donation provides a context for understanding why people may not become organ donors despite research suggesting people are favorable to organ donation (Gallup, 2005). The Health Belief Model offers a useful theoretical lens with which organ donation researchers may explain and predict this behavior. This is clearly an important goal for scholars and practitioners charged with creating successful organ donation campaigns. The following outlines the core assumptions of the HBM as described by Rosenstock.

The Health Belief Model (HBM) is a value-expectancy theory developed to explain and predict why people participate in efforts to prevent or detect disease (Rosenstock, 1974). It is important to note that of the various health behavior theories, the HBM is particularly well suited to framing interventions for infrequent behaviors, like organ donation. Six main concepts serve as the foundation for the HBM: perceived susceptibility, perceived severity, perceived benefits, perceived barriers, cues to action, and self-efficacy (Glanz & Bishop, 2010). First, perceived susceptibility to a health threat, or how likely people feel they are to develop a certain condition, must be assessed. Second, the perceived severity of health threat (i.e., how serious the condition would be) is considered. Few studies examine the perceived severity of the organ shortage. For example, one study suggests that high school students are unaware of the organ shortage (Quick, LaVoie, Scott, Morgan & Bosch, in press). Third, perceived self-efficacy, which is also described as people's confidence in their ability to successfully perform behaviors to prevent a threat, plays an important role in whether or not a person joins an organ donor registry (Anker, Feeley, & Kim, 2010; Siegel, Alvaro, Lac, Crano, & Dominick, 2008). Recent research by Anker and colleagues (2010) suggests that self-efficacy mediates the attitude-behavior relationship within the context of organ donation.

The fourth key feature of the HBM concerns perceived barriers. Perceived barriers are factors that would prevent a person from taking the preventive action. Morgan and colleagues (Morgan, Miller, Arasaratnam, 2003; Morgan, Stephenson, Harrison, Afifi, & Long, 2008) discovered various barriers preventing individuals from joining an organ donor registry including what they called noncognitive factors, such as medical mistrust, the jinx factor, and the ick factor. Fifth, the HBM examines the role of perceived benefits of performing a specific task. Benefits refer to the positive consequences of performing healthy behaviors or, conversely, not performing unhealthy acts. Parisi and Katz's (1986) work suggests that individuals often join an organ donation registry because they want to be a hero by saving or improving the lives of others (Parisi & Katz, 1986; Quick et al., in press). Finally, cues to action are the strategies that allow a person to feel that they can act. Research shows that various media such as newspaper (Feeley & Vincent, 2007), television dramas (Morgan, Harrison, Chewning, DiCorcia, & Davis, 2007) and television news (Quick, Kim, & Meyer, 2009) can serve as integral sources of organ donation information for individuals. These sources may provide consumers with cues to action or with inaccurate information. With respect to the current chapter, television coverage serves as an external cue to prompt viewers to join a registry. Each of these concepts is important in predicting whether or not an individual is likely to engage in a behavior. In short, the HBM suggests that if a person believes they are at risk, the associated consequences of that risk are substantial, and there is something the individual can do to prevent that negative effect, he/she will act, especially following exposure to an internal or external persuasive cue such as a news story.

The current investigation examines television news coverage under the guidance of the HBM. Horton and Horton (1990) suggested that it was important for researchers to acknowledge other variables in organ donation studies instead of relying on a "simple assessment of awareness, attitudes, and behaviors" (p. 791). Scholars have since sought to address this limitation by addressing general benefits and barriers to organ donation (Horton & Horton, 1991), the role of communication with families (Afifi, et al., 2006; Morgan, et al., 2005), as well as the influence of sociocultural factors on organ donation (Kim, Elliot, & Hyde, 2004).

Despite literature that has examined media coverage of organ donation (Feeley & Vincent, 2007; Morgan, Harrison, Chewning, Davis, & DiCorcia, 2007; Quick, Kim, & Meyer, 2009), no research to the authors' knowledge has accounted for the ability of news media to shape perceptions of organ donation using the HBM as a theoretical lens. As such, the following research questions draw from the HBM to describe the content of news articles.

A major tenet of the HBM is that the need for changing a health behavior is communicated (Rosenstock, 1974). Moreover, according to the HBM, individuals weigh the benefits and barriers prior to making a decision and are likely to engage in a behavior only if the rewards outweigh the drawbacks. Assuming the threat is clearly communicated, if one is aware and confident that he/she can perform the recommended behavior, and the benefits outweigh the barriers, HBM researchers would expect that individual to perform the advocated behavior. In the spirit of better understanding television news coverage with respect to the organ shortage, the process of joining an organ donor registry, along with the benefits and barriers to registering as an organ donor, we advance the following research questions:

RQ1: Do television news coverage of organ donation communicate the severity of the organ shortage?
RQ2: Is more attention devoted to the benefits or barriers of organ donation?
RQ3: Does television news transcripts communicate to the audience about how to join the organ donor registry?
RQ4: Do television news transcripts endorse joining an organ donation registry?

3. Method

3.1 Sample and procedure

This study examined television news coverage of organ donation from January 2005 through December 2010. Television news transcripts were collected using Lexis Nexis. A total of 743 stories were selected and analyzed from ABC (n = 161), CBS (n = 126), CNBC (n = 2), CNN (n = 402), FOX (n = 30), and MSNBC (n = 22). Each news transcript was the unit of analysis for the present investigation. Certainly, many of these storied appeared in various forms across these networks. We were interested in reviewing all transcripts that mentioned organ donation and for this reason we employed a broad search term to garner a wide range of news transcripts. Our interest in analyzing stories that explicitly discussed organ donation or the transplantation process led us to use search terms that would find these statements in the text of the article. Following previous research we used "organ don! or organ transplant!" as key terms (Quick, et al., 2009).

After the news transcripts were identified and retrieved, a codebook was developed by the authors using the core assumptions outlined by Rosenstock (1966) in the HBM. Then, following extensive training, two coders independently coded 10% (n = 100) of the news transcripts (Lacy & Riffe, 1996; Lombard, Snyder-Duch, & Bracken, 2002). After establishing respectable intercoder reliabilities across the coded categories, the authors worked through their disagreements and then proceeded to code the remaining news transcripts. Reliability between the trained coders was established with a Brennan & Prediger's kappa for each category (Brennan & Prediger, 1981). We selected to employ Brennan and Prediger's kappa over Cohen's kappa because the chance agreement term in Cohen's kappa increases with increasing levels of marginal agreement. In other words, coders are penalized for achieving high rates of marginal agreement. Brennan and Prediger's kappa corrects for this by disregarding the marginal altogether and assumes chance agreement is determined solely by the number of categories in the coding scheme.

3.2 Categories

The categories investigated in this study emerged from a careful review of literature on the benefits and barriers of organ donation (Feeley, 2007; Feeley & Vincent, 2007; Morgan, et al., 2007; Quick, et al., 2009) and the core assumptions of the HBM (Glanz & Bishop, 2010).

3.2.1 Perceived susceptibility and severity

Because the shortage of organs in the United States (severity) is directly related to the need for organ donation (susceptibility) we collapsed these two constructs of the HBM. Specifically, we coded whether or not news coverage communicated the organ shortage (SA = .97, $K_{B\ \&\ P}$ = .94), and more specifically, we coded whether the stories provided statistical evidence (SA = .99, $K_{B\ \&\ P}$ = .98) such as the number of (a) individuals waiting for an organ transplant (SA = .98, $K_{B\ \&\ P}$ = .96), (b) individuals that die each day waiting for a transplant (SA = .98, $K_{B\ \&\ P}$ = .96), and (c) individuals that die annually waiting for a transplant (SA = 1.0, $K_{B\ \&\ P}$ = 1.0). Additionally, we coded narrative evidence (SA = .96, $K_{B\ \&\ P}$ = .92) from the vantage point of an organ donor (SA = .97, $K_{B\ \&\ P}$ = .94), organ recipient (SA = .95, $K_{B\ \&\ P}$ = .90), or a person on a waiting list (SA = .98, $K_{B\ \&\ P}$ = .96).

3.2.2 Perceived benefits

News stories framing organ donors as good people (heroes) (SA = .98, $K_{B\ \&\ P}$ = .96) or simply presented successful stories about organ donors (SA = .97, $K_{B\ \&\ P}$ = .94) or recipients (SA = .96, $K_{B\ \&\ P}$ = .92) were coded to understand how television news programs describes the benefits of organ donation.

3.2.3 Perceived barriers

Literature on organ donation has identified a number of barriers to organ donation (Morgan et al., 2008; Stephenson, Morgan, Roberts-Perez, Harrison, Afifi, & Long 2008; Salim et al., 2010; Siminoff, Burant, & Ibrahim, 2006). We coded for seventeen barriers to organ donation. These barriers are broadly categorized in terms of their relation to barriers to a person becoming a donor and barriers to a person agreeing to receive a donation. Barriers for those considering organ donation include: religious barriers (SA = .99, $K_{B\ \&\ P}$ = .98), superstitions (SA = 1.0, $K_{B\ \&\ P}$ = 1.0), unable to have an open-casket funeral (SA = 1.0, $K_{B\ \&\ P}$ = 1.0), potential for organs to be purchased on the black market (SA = 1.0, $K_{B\ \&\ P}$ = 1.0), the doctor will take all organs (SA = .97, $K_{B\ \&\ P}$ = .94), the doctor will not try to save the donor's life (SA = .99, $K_{B\ \&\ P}$ = .98), the rich and famous get organs first (SA = .96, $K_{B\ \&\ P}$ = .92), the donor recipient or family may learn the donor's identity (SA = 1.0, $K_{B\ \&\ P}$ = 1.0), fear of body being mutilated (SA = .99, $K_{B\ \&\ P}$ = .98), undeserving or ungrateful recipients (SA = .99, $K_{B\ \&\ P}$ = .98), and cultural barriers (SA = .99, $K_{B\ \&\ P}$ = .98). Organ recipients may face barriers including: financial costs to the family (SA = 1.0, $K_{B\ \&\ P}$ = 1.0), funeral delays (SA = 1.0, $K_{B\ \&\ P}$ = 1.0), organ rejection (SA = .99, $K_{B\ \&\ P}$ = .98), and problems with side effects from medication (SA = 1.0, $K_{B\ \&\ P}$ = 1.0).

3.2.4 Cues to action

We coded cues to action by noting if the coverage encouraged the audience to become an organ donor (SA = .99, $K_{B\ \&\ P}$ = .98). We also looked for whether or not a celebrity endorsement was used (SA = 1.0, $K_{B\ \&\ P}$ = 1.0).

3.2.5 Self-efficacy

Finally, we coded for whether or not news coverage communicated how audience members could become an organ donor (SA = .99, $K_{B\ \&\ P}$ = .98). If the article did communicate how to become a donor, we noted the method advocated [e.g., driver's license (SA = .99, $K_{B\ \&\ P}$ = .98), donor card (SA = 1.0, $K_{B\ \&\ P}$ = 1.0), website registry (SA = 1.0, $K_{B\ \&\ P}$ = 1.0), talk to family (SA = 1.0, $K_{B\ \&\ P}$ = 1.0), and/or talk to friends (SA = 1.0, $K_{B\ \&\ P}$ = 1.0)].

3.3 Data analysis strategy

For the current study, chi-square goodness-of-fit statistics were used to determine if the major categories differed in frequency. For many of the categories, the options were nonindependent because a news transcript can and often contained multiple categories. Therefore, Cochran's Q tests were run to demonstrate global differences whenever there were more than two related coded variables. Following a statistical significant Cochran's Q, McNemar tests were conducted to specify where statistically significant differences occurred. In order to reduce the likelihood of committing a type I error, Bonferroni corrections were made to reduce the likelihood of falsely rejecting the null hypothesis.

4. Results

4.1 Television news coverage organ shortage

The first research question examined how much attention was devoted to the organ shortage across the six networks. Results indicate that a minority of news stories cited the organ shortage (n = 153). Of those stories mentioning the organ shortage, the majority used statistical evidence to support the need for additional potential donors (n = 110). Of the statistical evidence cited, a Cohran Q test revealed statistical differences in how much attention was devoted to the number of individuals waiting for an organ transplant and the number of individuals that die daily and annually waiting for an organ transplant, $Q(2, N = 743) = 57.68$, $p < .001$. Specifically, McNemar tests showed that more attention was given to the number of individuals on a waiting list (n = 84) compared with considerably less attention given to the number of deaths daily (n = 30) and annually (n = 28) due to the organ shortage at $p < .001$. The McNemar test showed no statistical difference between attention given to the number of deaths daily and annually, $p = .07$.

In addition to documenting the organ shortage by sharing statistical evidence, several news stories used narratives to communicate the organ shortage (n = 142). Of the narratives present, statistical differences emerged between stories told from various vantage points, $Q(2, N = 743) = 63.13$, $p < .001$. McNemar tests showed more stories were aired from the vantage point of an organ recipient (n = 250) than stories from the vantage point of a donor (n = 58) or person on a waiting list for an organ transplant (n = 25), $p < .001$. Additionally, tests revealed a statistical difference between news stories shown from the vantage point of a donor compared with those shown about individual(s) on a waiting list.

It is also worth noting that several news stories specifically mentioned organs in particular with kidneys receiving the most attention (n = 266), followed by hearts (n = 140), livers (n = 115), lungs (n = 56), pancreases (n = 20), and intestines (n = 10), Q(4, N = 743) = 366.79, p < .001. Clearly, the majority of news attention is devoted to talking about kidney transplants which is not surprising considering the majority of organs transplanted are kidneys.

4.2 Television news coverage of benefits and barriers to organ donation

RQ2 asked about the amount of coverage to the benefits and barriers of registering to become an organ donor. With respect to the benefits of organ donation, our results found frequent coverage portraying organ donors as heroes (n = 174). In addition to framing organ donors as heroes, several news stories told successful stories about organ donation from the vantage point of the donor (n = 144) and recipient (n = 250), with statistical differences emerging between the them, Q(1, N = 743) = 81.42, p < .001.

With respect to barriers, differences were found across these television networks, Q(12, N = 743) = 131.28, p < .001. The McNemar tests revealed greater attention to potential for organs to be purchased on the black market (n = 27), the rich and famous get organs first (n = 25), organ rejection (n = 18), and the doctor will not try to save the donors life (n = 17) than cultural barriers (n = 7), fear of body being mutilated (n = 5), religious barriers (n = 4), the doctor will take all organs (n = 4), problems with side effects from medication (n = 4), financial costs to family (n = 1), delay funeral (n = 1), and undeserving or ungrateful recipients (n = 1) at $p \leq .05$. No coverage was given to superstitions regarding bad luck following registering as an organ donor, unable to have an open-casket funeral, or fear that the donor recipient or family may learn the donor's identity.

4.3 Television news coverage of joining the organ donor registry

The third research question examined how much television news coverage is devoted to informing viewers about how to become an organ donor. The results suggest very limited attention is devoted to informing viewers of ways to join the registry (n = 45). Of the most common ways to enroll in a statewide registry, our findings suggest variability in the amount of coverage regarding the various ways to join, Q(5, N = 743) = 40.44, p < .001. McNemar tests showed that attention given to indicating one's wish on an organ donor card (n = 18), driver's license (n = 17), and talking with family (n = 13) was significantly more likely to be mentioned than the organ donation registry (n = 3), telephone hotline (n = 1), and talking with a friend (n = 1). No statistical differences emerged between an organ donor card, driver's license, and talking with family. Additionally, no differences were observed between attention to the organ donation registry, telephone hotline, and talking with a friend about intentions to be an organ donor.

4.4 Television news coverage of endorsing organ donation registry

The final research question assessed whether television news transcripts endorse organ donation. Not surprisingly, our results revealed that news stories rarely encourage viewers to join an organ donor registry. (n = 25), χ^2 (1, N = 743) = 646.37, p < .001. Similarly, infrequently did these stories feature a celebrity endorsing organ donation (n = 52), χ^2 (1, N = 743) = 549.56, $p < .001$

5. Discussion

Individuals learn about organ donation from various sources, and these sources present this information with various degrees of accuracy. More and more, communication campaigns promoting organ and tissue donation have become effective mechanisms to enhance organ donor registrations across college campuses (Feeley, Anker, Watkins, Rivera, Tag, & Volpe, 2009), driver's license facilities (Harrison et al., 2010; Harrison, Morgan, King, & Williams, 2011), and in the workplace (Morgan, Harrison, Chewning, Di Corcia, & Davis, 2010). As these efforts have certainly played a pivotal role in educating individuals about the importance of organ donation, individuals still learn much about organ donation from newspapers (Feeley & Vincent, 2007), television dramas (Morgan et al., 2007), and news programs (Quick et al., 2009). The current study sought to reveal how recent news coverage on television depicts organ donation with respect to the organ shortage, the benefits and barriers to donation, the process of registering as an organ donor, and the overall estimate of news industries' endorsement of organ donation. We also gave attention to whether there was celebrity support for this issue. We discuss our findings with an eye for how they may shape public perception about organ donation.

The first research question inquired about attention given to the organ shortage in the United States. Previous research suggests modest attention is given to educating individuals about the organ shortage in newspapers (Feeley & Vincent, 2007) and television news (Quick et al., 2009). Our report is consistent with these studies in that approximately one in five stories explicitly mentioned the need for more organ donors. With respect to evidence used to back their claim, more news stories used narrative evidence than statistical evidence. More specifically, the majority of stories relying on narratives used stories from the vantage point of organ recipients as opposed to donors or persons on a waiting list for a transplant. With an emphasis on the positive outcomes of organ donation, it is likely viewers will be able to see the benefits arising from organ donation. However, by not highlighting stories about people who find themselves on a waiting list, viewers may not grasp the reality that people die each day due to the organ shortage. Presenting viewers with a realistic understanding of the organ shortage is critical if we want to begin seeing decreases in the number of people waiting for a transplant. Although used less than narratives, statistics were, with some regularity, presented to convey the number of people awaiting an organ transplant, as well as the number of individuals dying daily and annually due to the organ shortage. In their analysis of ABC, CBS, and NBC news transcripts, Quick and colleagues (2009) found that less than 5% of stories cited statistical evidence to support the need for more organ donors. The good news is that since their study, we found statistical evidence is used three times more often on television news programs (15%) across ABC, CBS, CNBC, CNN, FOX, and MSNBC. Fortunately, individuals are exposed to these statistics because organ donation campaigns continue to do a good job of emphasizing the need for more organ donors (Feeley et al., 2009; Harrison et al., 2010; Morgan et al., 2002).

The framing of organ donation remains a critical concern among organ donation researchers and practitioners alike. As Morgan and colleagues (2007) have found, television dramas run a successful counter-campaign (Harrison et al., 2008) by featuring plots around various organ donation myths (e.g., doctor will not try to save an organ donors life). Thus, it is important to determine whether television news coverage is adding to this counter-campaign. A shortcoming of Quick and colleagues (2009) study was their inattention to coverage of various barriers preventing individuals from joining organ donation registries. The current study sought to extend their work by explicitly examining various barriers (e.g., medical mistrust). Our results revealed that television news rarely gives attention to barriers to organ donation. Specifically, of the four most commonly aired barriers including the black market, the rich and famous get organs first, organ rejection, and the doctor will not try to save the donors life, none of these barriers appeared in more than 5% of the news programs. This can be perceived as good or bad depending on how one interprets this finding. It is good in that television news is not perpetuating these barriers by devoting a fair amount of attention to them. Alternatively, given the fact that television dramas reinforce many of these barriers with regularity (Morgan et al., 2007), news programs have an opportunity to debunk many of these beliefs. This could be a missed opportunity to reduce the organ shortage because we know from recent reports that medical mistrust remains a key barrier to registering as an organ donor (Morgan et al., 2008; Salim et al., 2010; Siminoff et al., 2006).

Conversely, television news continues to emphasize the benefits of organ donation by producing successful stories from the vantage point of organ recipients and organ donors. Of the stories observed, one in three told a story of an organ recipient, one in four depicted organ donors as heroes, and one in five told a story of an organ donor. A recent study by Quick and colleagues (in press) discovered that high school students preferred promotional materials depicting organ donors as heroes. Certainly, if their study is generalizable to the broader public, then television news is providing a beneficial service by highlighting the benefits of organ donation and by portraying donors as heroes that save and significantly improve the quality of life for many individuals.

A concern noted in earlier studies examining television news coverage of organ donation was the inadequate attention regarding ways to register as an organ donor (Quick et al., 2009). They found that approximately 7% of stories informed individuals on how to register as an organ donor, with the majority of stories mentioning a driver's license and donor card as the most common methods for registry. Our findings are similar in that a mere 6% of stories explicitly stated how to register to become an organ donor. Again, indicating one's wish on a driver's license or donor card remain the most common ways to register as depicted in television news programs. Sadly, little attention is devoted to organ donation registrations online. To date, most states have an organ donation registration that ensures individuals' intentions to be organ donors are followed. Illinois was the first state to introduce a First-Person consent organ donor registry. Since then, most states have adopted a similar registry and as a result, more lives are saved and significantly improved due to organ transplantation.

A goal of journalism is to remain objective. For this reason, it is not surprising that few stories explicitly endorse organ donation. In our study, less than 4% of stories promote organ donation. Surprisingly, less than 10% of studies devoted attention to celebrity endorsements of organ donation. Relying on celebrity endorsements creates a double-edge sword. On one hand, celebrities attract attention and have the potential to raise awareness about the organ shortage and the importance of registering to become an organ donor. However, celebrity endorsement of organ donation can at the same time play into fears regarding beliefs that the rich and famous can purchase their way to the top of organ transplant waiting lists. Future research should investigate the persuasive appeal of celebrity endorsements in organ and tissue donation with various demographics.

6. Conclusion

Overall, our findings suggest that there has been some improvement in the depiction of organ donation news stories since prior studies. Specifically, using narratives to highlight the positive aspects of donation, as well as the increase in statistical evidence to underscore the need for donors, may persuade some viewers to consider the registry. Further, the minimal attention given to organ donation myths and the representation of donors as heroes, both are findings that should have a positive effect on donor registration rates. However, there is still much left to be desired with respect to the framing and depiction of organ donation stories in the news. For example, more stories regarding waiting recipients might enhance the perceived severity of the shortage, and more stories featuring those who donated their organs might help to debunk donation myths or frame donations as heroic and selfless acts.

The depiction of organ donation in the news certainly needs continued attention and further investigation. Because prior studies have found that entertainment television often purports organ donation myths (Morgan et al., 2007), television news may play an important role in balancing those depictions and viewer perceptions regarding donation. Further, news is often perceived to be "accurate" and "realistic" by viewers, but television dramas are considered to be more entertaining. Thus, future research should examine whether television viewers give more weight to organ donation news stories or to entertainment television with respect to their beliefs, attitudes, and behaviors regarding donation. Finally, with the increase in media channels (e.g. internet), it is possible that people may not watch traditional news programming as much as they once did. Further, with the rapidly growing number of television stations, people may be more selective in what source, whether it is television or internet, they choose from which to derive their news. Therefore, future studies should examine a wider selection of news sources, as well as determine whether selective exposure to news sources and/or type of news source has any effect on the depiction or perception of organ donation.

In short, television news plays an important role in presenting what viewers see as "reality," and, thus, may have a substantial impact on how organ donation is depicted and how viewers perceive the issue. Although news outlets are supposed to remain "neutral," it is possible that organ donation campaigns may find an additional resource for promotion through these outlets. By presenting factual stories, news stations remain neutral, but by highlighting specific angles of those stories and featuring information on how to donate, they may help to increase organ donation rates. The findings of this study generally signal some hope for organ donation advocates with respect to television news coverage. However, there are certainly areas that need to be addressed and improved upon in order for the news media to depict and promote organ donation in a way that could potentially make a significant impact.

7. Acknowledgements

The authors acknowledge Andy Herren for his many hours of coding television news transcripts. The authors would also like to acknowledge Health Resources Services Administration's Division of Transplantation (HRSA/DoT), United States Department of Health and Human Services for funding this project, grant #R39OT15493-02. The contents of this publication are solely the responsibility of the authors and do not necessarily represent the views of HRSA/DoT.

8. References

Afifi, W. A., Morgan, S., Stephenson, M. T., Morse, C., Harrison, T., Reichart, T., et al. (2006). Examining the decision to talk with family about organ donation: Applying the theory of motivated information management. *Communication Monographs,* Vol. 73, pp. 188-215, ISSN: 0363-7751

Anker, A. E., Feeley, T. H., & Kim, H. (2010). Examining the attitude-behavior relationship in prosocial donation domains. *Journal of Applied Social Psychology,* Vol. 40, pp. 1293-1324, ISSN: 0021-9029

Brennan, R. L., & Prediger, D. J. (1981). Coefficient kappa: Some uses, misuses, and alternatives. *Educational and Psychological Measurement,* Vol. 41, pp. 687-699, ISSN: 0013-1644

Conesa, C., Zambudio, A. R., Ramírez, P., Canteras, M., Rodriguez, M. M., & Parrilla, P. (2004). Influence of different sources of information on attitude toward organ donation: A factor analysis. *Transplantation Proceedings,* Vol. 36, pp. 1245-1248, ISSN: 0041-1345

Feeley, T. H. (2007). College students' knowledge, attitudes, and behaviors regarding organ donation: An integrated review of the literature. *Journal of Applied Social Psychology,* Vol. 37, pp. 243-271, ISSN: 0021-9029

Feeley, T. H., Anker, A. E., Watkins, B., Rivera, J., Tag, N., & Volpe, L. (2009). A peer-to-peer campaign to promote organ donation among racially diverse college students in New York City. *Journal of the National Medical Association,* Vol. 101, pp. 1154-1162, ISSN: 0027-9684

Feeley, T., & Vincent, D. (2007). How organ donation is represented in newspaper articles in the United States. *Health Communication,* Vol. 21, pp. 125-131, ISSN: 1523-0236

Gallup Organization (2005). 2005 National Survey of Organ and Tissue Donation Attitudes and Behaviors. Conducted and Prepared by the Gallup Organization for Division of Transplantation Health Resources and Services Administration. Retrieved October 15, 2010 from http://organdonor.gov/survey2005/organ_donation.shtm

Glanz, K., & Bishop, D. B. (2010). The role of behavioral science theory in development and implementation of public health interventions. *The Annual Review of Public Health,* Vol. 31, pp. 399-418, ISSN: 0163-7525

Harrison, T. R., Morgan, S. E., & Chewning, L. V. (2008). The challenges of social marketing of organ donation: News and entertainment coverage of donation and transplantation. *Health Marketing Quarterly,* Vol. 25, pp. 33-65, ISSN: 0735-9683

Harrison, T. R., Morgan, S. E., King, A. J., DiCorcia, M. J., Williams, E. A., Ivic, R. K., & Hopeck, P. (2010). Promoting the Michigan Organ Donor Registry: Evaluating the impact of a multifaceted intervention utilizing media priming and communication design. *Health Communication,* Vol. 25, pp. 700 - 708, ISSN 1523-0236

Harrison, T. R., Morgan, S. E., King, A. J., & Williams, E. A. (2011). Saving lives branch by branch: The effectiveness of driver licensing bureau campaigns to promote organ donor registry sign-ups to African Americans in Michigan. *Journal of Health Communication,* Vol. 16, No. 8, pp. 805 - 819, ISSN 1081-0730

Horton, R. L., & Horton, P. J. (1990). Knowledge regarding organ donation: Identifying and overcoming barriers to organ donation. *Social Science and Medicine,* Vol. 31, pp. 791-800, ISSN: 0277-9536

Horton, R. L., & Horton, P. J. (1991). A model of willingness to become a potential organ donor. *Social Science and Medicine,* Vol. 33, No. 9, pp. 1037-1051, ISSN: 0277-9536

Kim, J. R., Elliot, D., & Hyde, C. (2004). The influence of sociocultural factors on organ donation and transplantation in Korea: Findings from key informant interviews. *Journal of Transcultural Nursing,* Vol. 15, pp. 147-154, ISSN: 1043-6596

Lacy, S., & Riffe, D. (1996). Sampling error and selecting intercoder reliability samples for nominal content categories: Sins of omission and commission in mass communication quantitative research. *Journalism and Mass Communication Quarterly,* Vol. 73, pp. 969-973, ISSN: 1077-6990

Lombard, M., Snyder-Duch, J., & Bracken, C. C. (2002). Content analysis in mass communication: Assessment and reporting intercoder reliability. *Human Communication Research,* Vol. 28, pp. 587-604, ISSN: 0360-3989

McCombs, M. E., & Shaw, D. L. (1972). The agenda-setting function of mass media. *Public Opinion Quarterly,* Vol. 36, pp. 176-187, ISSN: 0033-362X

Morgan, S. E., Harrison, T., Afifi, W. A., Long, S. D., Stephenson, M. T., & Reichart, T. (2005). Family discussions about organ donation: How the media is used to justify opinions and influence others about donation decisions. *Clinical Transplantation,* Vol. 19, No. 5, pp. 674-682, ISSN: 0902-0063

Morgan, S. E., Harrison, T., Chewning, L., Davis, L., & DiCorcia, M. (2007). Entertainment (mis)education: The framing of organ donation in entertainment television. *Health Communication,* Vol. 22, pp. 143-151, ISSN: 1523-0236

Morgan, S. E., Harrison, T., Chewning, L., DiCorcia, M., & Davis, L. (2010). The effectiveness of high- and low-intensity worksite campaigns to promote organ donation: The worksite Organ Donation Promotion Project. *Communication Monographs,* Vol. 77, pp. 341 - 356, ISSN 0363-7751

Morgan, S. E., & Miller, J. K. (2001). Beyond the organ donor card: The effect of knowledge, attitudes, and values on willingness to communicate about organ donation to family members. *Health Communication,* Vol. 14, pp. 121-134, ISSN: 1523-0236

Morgan, S. E., Miller, J. K., & Arasaratnam, L. A. (2003). Similarities and differences between African Americans' and European Americans' attitudes, knowledge, and willingness to communicate about organ donation. *Journal of Applied Social Psychology,* Vol. 33, pp. 693-715, ISSN: 0021-9029

Morgan, S. E., Stephenson, M. T., Harrison, T. R., Afifi, W. A., & Long, S. D. (2008). Facts versus 'feelings': How rational is the decision to become an organ donor? *Journal of Health Psychology,* Vol. 13, pp. 644-658, ISSN: 1359-1053

Parisi, N., & Katz, I. (1986). Attitudes toward posthumous organ donation and commitment to donate. *Social Science and Medicine,* Vol. 5, pp. 565-580, ISSN: 0277-9536

Quick, B. L., Kim, D. K., & Meyer, K. (2009). A 15-year review of ABC, CBS, and NBC new coverage of organ donation: Implications for organ donation campaigns. *Health Communication,* Vol. 24, pp. 137-145, ISSN: 1523-0236

Quick, B. L., Lavoie, N. R., Scott, A. M., Morgan, S. E., & Bosch, D. (in press). Perceptions about organ donation among African American, Hispanic, and White high school students. *Qualitative Health Research*, ISSN: 1049-7323

Rosenstock, I. M. (1974). Historical origins of the health belief model. *Health Education Monographs,* Vol. 2, pp. 328-335, ISSN: 0073-1455

Salim, A., Berry, C., Ley, E. J., Schulman, D., Desai, C., Navarro, S., et al. (2010). The impact of race on organ donation rates in southern California. *Journal of the American College of Surgeons,* Vol. *211*, pp. 596-600, ISSN: 1072-7515

Siegel, J. T., Alvaro, E. M., Lac, A., Crano, W. D., & Dominick, A. (2008). Intentions of becoming a living organ donor among Hispanics: A theory-based approach exploring differences between living and nonliving organ donation. *Journal of Health Communication,* Vol. 13, pp. 80-99, ISSN: 1081-0730

Siminoff, L. A., Burant, C. J., & Ibrahim, S. A. (2006). Racial disparities in preferences and perceptions regarding organ donation. *Journal of General Internal Medicine,* Vol. 21, pp. 995-1000, ISSN: 0884-8734

Stephenson, M. T., Morgan, S. E., Roberts-Perez, S., Harrison, T., Afifi, W., & Long, S. D. (2008). The role of religiosity, religious norms, subjective norms, and bodily integrity in signing an organ donor card. *Health Communication,* Vol. 23, pp. 436-447, ISSN: 1523-0236

United Network for Organ Sharing. (2011). Data retrieved on August 17, 2011, from http://www.unos.org

3

European Living Donation and Public Health (EULID Project)

Martí Manyalich et al.*
Hospital Clínic de Barcelona
Spain

1. Introduction

Donation from alive people has been growing strongly in the recent years, thanks to the advance in the field of organ transplantation and its success as a treatment to procure quality-adjusted life years for many patients with end-stage diseases. The choice of transplantation from a living donor (LD) offers some advantages compared to that for a deceased donor. However, it also carries disadvantages related to donor risks in terms of health and safety, and there are several controversial ethical aspects to be taken into account.

There is no specific pronouncement of the European Union in relation to standards to quality and safety for the living donor process, and there is a great heterogeneity among European Countries legislation, ethical concern, and protection systems and donor´s data registries on the topic. The EULID project aims to establish European common standard framework regarding living donor issues to guarantee their health and safety thorough common practices and regulation.

2. What is EULID project?

2.1 General description of the project

The European Living Donation (EULID) project's (http://www.eulivingdonor.eu/) was cofounded by the Public Health Executive Agency (PHEA), acting under the powers delegated by the European Commission.

Twelve partners from eleven European Countries have worked cooperatively from April 2007-September 2009, the promoter has been the Hospital Clínic de Barcelona, Barcelona, Spain and partners have been: ANT Fundatia Pentru Transplant, Bucharest, Romania; Centro Hospitalar do Porto, Porto, Portugal; Hôpital Necker, Paris, France; Institute for LifeLong Learning, Barcelona, Spain; ISS-Centro Nazionali Trapianti, Rome, Italy; Paraskevaidion Surgical and Transplant Center, Nicosia, Cyprus; Poltransplant, Warsaw,

* Assumpta Ricart, Ana Menjívar, Chloë Ballesté, David Paredes, Leonídio Días, Christian Hiesse, Dorota Lewandowska, George Kyriakides, Pål-Dag Line, Ingela Fehrman-Ekholm, Danica Asvec, Alessandro Nanni Costa, Andy Maxwell and Rosana Turcu
Hospital Clínic de Barcelona, España.

Poland; Rikshospitalet, Oslo, Norway; Sahlgrenska University Hospital, Göteborg, Sweden; Slovenija Transplant, Ljubljana, Slovenia; UK Transplant, Bristol, United Kingdom.

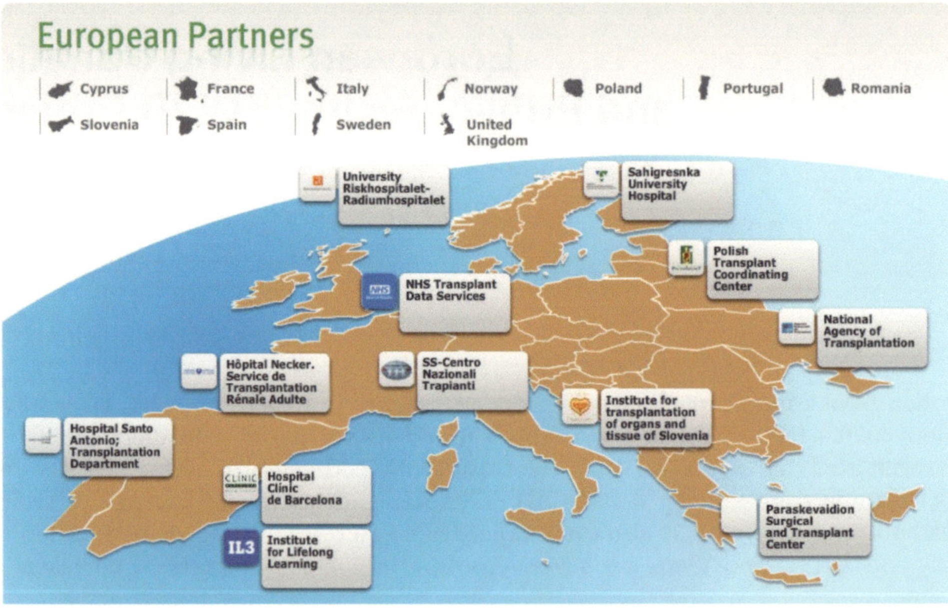

Fig. 1. EULID partners

The main objective was to analyze the current situation among European Union Countries and to contribute establishing common standards regarding legal, ethical, protection and registration practices for organ Living Donors in order to guarantee them the best health and safety scenarios.

2.2 Specific objectives of the project

- To analyze and compare the different European countries legal and ethical frameworks on living donors health and safety in order to establish European legal and ethical recommendations in relation to organ living donors health and safety/on the issue.
- To analyze and compare legislated and non-legislated protection practices on organ living donors health and safety employed in European countries in order to establish European recommendations in relation to living donors health and safety protection practices/on the issue.
- To establish and validate an e-registry database model on organ living donors data that allows having a common European database registry and common national registries on the issue.
- To establish recommendation on a European framework on legal and ethical aspects, protection practices and database registries related to organ living donors in order to guarantee them the best health and safety scenarios in the European Union.
- To disseminate the European action framework/common standards on organ living donors health, safety and protection among professionals and public opinion/general public.

3. Ethical concerns regarding donation of organs from living donors in eleven European countries

3.1 General aspects of living donation ethics

In most issues in medicine in Western countries the two main universal traditions of bioethics are *deontology* and *utilitarianism.* These traditions strongly influence the culture of healthcare professionals and the resolution of codes of practice, regulations and legislations.

Both traditions, while often conflicting, bring different perspectives to ethical controversies, such as those arising in the field of living donation. It is widely accepted that the Beauchamp and Childress' principals' seeks a compromise between general moral theories, and it is accepted as forming the bedrock of medical ethics. They advocate four prima facie principles: 1. *Beneficence* (doing well); 2. *Non-maleficence* (avoiding harm); 3. Respect for *autonomy*; 4. *Justice* (fairness). Depending on the context and on whether a deontological or utilitarian approach is favored, a trade-off between principles must be negotiated or achieved. Issues relating to beneficence and non-maleficence lie in the domain of the doctor-patient relationship, and refer more to the deontological tradition. Issues with respect to autonomy and justice apply more to groups of patients rather to individuals and interact more widely with the law, social policy and culture. In the field of living organ donation, all four principles should be given consideration in the different ethical concerns and questions arising.

3.2 Ethical concerns relating to the principles of non-maleficence and beneficence

3.2.1 The principle of subsidiarity

In EU countries having efficient or growing cadaveric donation programs, it is essential that living donation must be an add-on to cadaveric donation, and that promotion of living donation by governments ensure that cadaveric donation is not hampered and is developed to its maximal potential.

Given the only thing that can prevent the promotion of living donation is the risk that implies for the donor, it is essential to keep priority to cadaveric donation. Thus it appears to the EULID participants that the principle of subsidiarity should be maintained, particularly in the case of non-renal living donation.

3.2.2 Benefits for the donor

For the EULID project participants, it should be reemphasized that the benefit for the donor, particularly during the evaluation process of the risk/benefit for the donor, cannot be other than moral, including for unrelated donors (anonymous volunteers and donors involved in cross-over donation programs).

3.2.3 The living donor with higher risk

For the EULID participants, there is a consensus to avoid donation in candidates with higher risk than "standard", including the short-term (peri-operative mortality and morbidity), and the long term (organ failure) risks related to the organ removal. Whatever the donor-recipient relationship, the same medical criteria according to current recommendations should be applied for the evaluation of the risk in the donor and the definition of contraindications for donation.

3.2.4 Living donation within the context of emergency

For the EULID participants, there is a consensus to recommend that in the situation of liver transplantation in emergency, cadaveric donation should be considered rather than living donation.

3.3 Ethical concerns relating to the principle of autonomy

3.3.1 Restriction of the donor's autonomy

In Europe, it is widely accepted that protection of the potential living donors by legislation and regulations implies restrictions of the donor's autonomy, which is, in the present case, overruled by the principle of non-maleficence. For the EULID participants, there is a consensus for limiting the autonomy of potential living donors by establishing or maintaining legislations or regulations restricting living donation, in order to ensure the protection of the donors, and to prevent organ trafficking and commercialism.

3.3.2 Process of the informed consent and of the assessment of the donor's autonomy

The ethical practice of medicine requires appropriate informed consent for medical procedures. In the case of living donation, informed consent is particularly important since the donor does not receive any medical benefit from the procedure itself, and undertake the possibility of medical risks.

For the EULID participants, there is a consensus for assessing the autonomy of potential organ donors in European Countries by common procedural safeguards including:

- An extensive specific information process of the potential donor who should be capable of understanding the information presented in the consent process;
- The involvement of healthcare professional(s) having appropriate experience and not involved in the organ removal or subsequent transplantation procedure;
- The formal collection of the consent, either in written form or before an official body;
- A reflection period after medical acceptance and decision to donate.

3.3.3 Living donation in non competent minor donors

The United States Live Organ Donor Consensus Group had argued that minors younger than 18 years could ethically serve as live solid organ donors in exceptional circumstances. The Amsterdam forum on the care of the living kidney donor stated the general agreement that minors less than 18 years of age should not be used as living kidney donors. In Europe, the Additional Protocol to the convention on human rights and biomedicine stipulates in Article 14, Paragraph 1 "No organ or tissue removal may be carried out on a person who does not have the capacity to consent"

There is a consensus for EULID participants to exclude non-competent minors less than 18 years of age from consideration for potential organ donation in any circumstances.

3.4 Ethical concerns relating to the principle of justice

Justice is a very important principle in the ethics of transplantation where Demand far exceeds Supply. It applies primarily to the allocation of organs from cadaveric donors, requiring in that context a rank-ordering system with some ethical justification for the method chosen. However, the moral demand for justice has several implications for living donation and transplantation.

3.4.1 Gender inequities in living donor transplantation

The international data presented to the Amsterdam forum on the care of the living kidney donor revealed that approximately 65% of live kidney donors have been women and approximately 65% of recipients have been men. It was agreed that these data on gender imbalance display an excessive disparity, perhaps reflecting a psychological submission of women or discrimination of women in many Countries, including Western Countries. Several strategies have been proposed in order to eliminate gender disparity in transplantation: publish center-specific data, increase education, establish gender-specific support groups, eliminate institutional and provider gender-bias, and promote gender-specific research.

There is a consensus for EULID participants for considering that gender inequities in living donor transplantation should be addressed by promoting targeted strategies at the level of centers and of transplantation agencies.

3.4.2 Impact of donor programs on cadaveric donation

There is a balance in the relationship between cadaveric transplantation and living donor transplantation. There is a consensus for EULID participants for considering that the promotion of living donation must be conducted as a contribution to increase the availability of organs for recipients, and must not undermine the efforts for promoting and developing cadaveric donation.

3.5 Organ trafficking, transplant tourism and commercialism of organs

Numerous reports have highlighted trafficking in human beings who are used as sources of organs from poor people in developing countries, within the context of the global shortage of organs. In 2004, the WHO called on member states "to take measures to protect the poorest and vulnerable groups form transplant tourism and the sale of tissues and organs, including attention to the wider problem of international trafficking in human tissues and organs" (WHA 57.18).

There is a consensus for EULID participants for considering that the general prohibition on organ commercialism by international and national laws should be strictly maintained. Purchasing or offering to purchase organs for transplantation or their sales by living persons should be banned. Laws should ensure that any gifts or rewards are not, in fact, disguised forms of payment for donated organs. Incentives in the form of "rewards" with monetary values that can be transferred to third parties, tax reduction or healthcare payment reductions are not different from monetary payments. This does not, however, preclude the reimbursement of reasonable and verifiable expenses incurred by the donor, including loss of income, or paying the costs of recovering organs for transplantation.

3.6 Ethical issues on donor-recipient relationship

3.6.1 Directed donors (genetically and non-genetically related)

From the very beginning there seems to exist a great consensus about genetically-related donors. However this form of transplant is not free from possible coercion. Indeed familiar ties may impose a greater pressure to donate than between friends who may be freer to take an autonomous decision.

There is a consensus for EULID participants for considering that the directed donation of organs from living donors to family members or persons with a pre-existing emotional relationship should be permitted. However, a clear policy that defines the pre-existing emotional relationships that are acceptable must be developed, and the final rule, which technically permits any directed donation of living donor organs to a named person, should be amended to be consistent with this policy.

3.6.2 Directed unrelated donors

This form of donation is more based on emotions than in an equitable allocation system. Also to promote one's cause takes money, so wealthier individuals will enjoy greater success in contacting prospective donors. It is also possible that some intended donors aspire to donate according to race, ethnic, religious or other pattern of preference. Some argue that it's necessary to respect the autonomy of these potential donors and that the utility and the benefit of these procedures would consist in increasing the availability of organs and the quality of life and survival of receptors.

There is a consensus for EULID participants for considering that solicitation of living donors and the directed donation that results may involve unethical and illegal practices that place recipients and donors at risk and should be rejected by the transplantation community. The solicitation of organs from living donors potentially circumvents the principles of justice and utility on which organ-allocation policies are based. Solicitation is not accepted by European Union and by all the transplant societies.

3.6.3 Unrelated non directed donors (NDD)

Non-directed altruistic donors can donate to an unknown patient in the cadaveric list or enter in a paired kidney exchange programme (domino paired exchange for example).

Also of concern is the issue of anonymity. By principle, to avoid the possibility of future coercion over the recipient, it is important to maintain the identification of the donor and the recipient anonymous. After the transplant if both wish to meet or correspond it's better to promote a thorough discussion about the risks and benefits of such a meeting or communication.

There is a consensus for EULID participants for considering that to avoid the possibility of future coercion over the recipient, it is important to maintain anonymity. It is also important the participation of an independent donor advocate promoting the knowledge of the risks and the assessment of the conformity of the evaluation. The registry under the control of health authorities detailing the medical and psychological follow-up is also essential.

3.6.4 Paired exchange programs (and other similar programs)

Resulting from the scarcity of cadaveric organs for transplant some forms of living donor programmes have been implemented. Regrettably not all living related donors are compatible with their intended receptors. As a consequence there are some exchange programs under development that deserve some ethical reflections.

In general, in a paired exchange program the donor who wants to benefit his incompatible (ABO or cross match positive) but related partner (emotionally or genetically) when he is giving to the receptor of other pair is helping also the receptor of the other pair, while he achieves its principal aim that is to help his partner. This is no doubt a fair and equitable distribution of benefits. Also the utility of this action is unquestionable because it allows for two patients to be transplanted and removed from the general waiting list, consequently increasing the likelihood of other patients to be transplanted and therefore improving their access to a deceased donor pool.

But a paired exchange programme puts other generic problems, like those with group O patients. Group O candidates have longer waiting times for transplantation. Also in a living paired exchange programme they are in difficulty because they can be transplanted in a conventional way only if his or her A or B blood type donor can donate to an A or B receptor who is cross-matched positive with his or her O related intended donor. In an unconventional paired donation the blood type O donor 2 will be asked to be more altruistic because he has the possibility to donate to his related donor and he is being requested to make his gift to an unrelated one.

There is a consensus for EULID participants for considering that paired exchange can be accepted when the anonymity is guaranteed and there is an independent body dependent from health authority for the regulation and organization of the process.

In the case that one patient could not receive the kidney beyond the point of no return; there is a consensus for EULID participants that the patient should have priority for a future transplant with a kidney from the cadaveric pool.

4. Legislation concerns regarding donation of organs from living donors in eleven European countries

4.1 Activities undertaken

It was analyzed through a survey among partners the living donor low in partner's countries. If there is specific legislation about living donor, which aspects it regulates, accreditation system for programs for extraction of organs from living donors. This survey gave knowledge about the current situation regarding this issue. All partners answered the survey and all results were analyzed. A report was developed after the analysis, making possible to detect the key points in legislation practice.

4.2 Report on the legislation regarding donation and transplantation

The report is designed to illustrate the state of the art of legislative and regulatory approaches in the field of living donation (LD) and transplantation of organs among 11 EULID project partner European Countries.

The general legislative and regulatory layout in the field of living donation and transplantation, including the sanctions and penalties applied in case of major violation (i.e. procurement in persons without obtaining consent or in person enable to consent, organ trafficking, organ sale or purchase, and transplant tourism).

The legislated or regulated enactments on donor- recipient relationship, including paired/pooled donation and unrelated directed and no directed donation.

The legislated or regulated procedures on the organizational aspects of living donation: the evaluation of the donor, the information for the donor and the consent of the donor, and the provisions surrounding the post donation follow-up and the protection of the living donors, including the existing LD follow-up registries.

4.3 Existing legislation and regulation on financial, economical and social concerns regarding the living organ donor

4.3.1 World Health Organization (WHO)

The United Nations specialized agency for health, has adopted in the World Health Assembly in 1991 the Guiding Principles for human organ transplants (Resolution WHA 40.13) which have had a great influence on professional code and legislations. These principles emphasized voluntary donation, non commercialization and the preference for deceased donors over living donors and for genetically related donors over non related donors on 22 May 2004, the 57th World Health Assembly adopted the Resolution WHA 57.18 concerning human organ and tissue transplantation, recommending notably the extension of the use of living donors, in addition to deceased donors, and to take measures to protect the poorest and vulnerable groups from "transplant tourism" and the sale of tissues and organs, including attention to the wider problem of international trafficking in human tissues and organs.

4.3.2 The Council of Europe

In Europe, an important source of rules concerning the issue of living organ donation and transplantation are the documents of the Council of Europe (COE):

- The Convention for the protection of Human Rights and the dignity of the human being with regard to the application of biology: Convention on Human Rights and Biomedicine (Oviedo Convention) was adopted on April 4th 1997 and came into force on December 1st 1999(CETS NO.:164). It is the first legally- binding supranational text designed to preserve human rights and dignity from the misappropriate use of medical advances. Specific provisions of this convention apply notably to the procurement of organs from living persons, the prohibition of financial gain, and sanction.
- The Additional Protocol to the Convention for the protection of the Human Rights and Biomedicine was adopted in Strasbourg on January 24th 2002, and came into force on May 1st 2006. It applies the principles of the Oviedo Convention on human rights and Biomedicine to the field of organ transplantation, covering all concerns of living donation.

4.3.3 The European Union

The Commission is planning to respond to the main policy challenges in relation to organ donation and transplantation: ensure quality and safety of organs, enhancing the efficiency and accessibility of transplantation system in the UE Member States and increase organ availability and fight organ trafficking.

The communication entails 2 mechanism of action:

- an action plan for strengthened coordination between Member States and;
- an EU legal instrument on quality and safety of organ donation and transplantation.

The action plan will be based on the identification and development of common objectives, agreed quantitative and qualitative indicators and benchmarks, regular reporting, and identification and exchange of best practices. The envisioned EU legal instrument will complement the cooperation approach taken under the action plan by providing an appropriate and flexible European legal framework.

4.3.4 Specific national regulations

It is of importance to note that due to the fact of the great differences on legal frameworks, culture values and geographical, historical and sociological backgrounds of the different countries involved, even if all countries have developed specific parliamentary acts addressing living donation concerns, it is found a huge heterogeneity between legislative contents. Some Countries i.e. Sweden, Norway and Cyprus have developed only a minimal set of legal dispositions, while contrastingly in other Countries such in France, hard legislation (i.e. parliamentary acts) encompass all detailed provisions addressing to the LD procurement and donation activities, which are in other countries considered in regulations or such in Scandinavian Countries , in guidelines or codes of practice. The consequence of this heterogeneity is that each procedure and concern on LD activities may be regulated, according to the Country, by the low, by binding or not binding regulations elaborated by the health authority or the national transplant authority, or by guidelines and codes of practice elaborated by professionals.

4.4 Procedures of authorization for living donation and transplantation activities

In 10 partners countries, the activities of LD procurement and transplantation are legally submitted to an authorization given by health authority to the transplantation centres, usually the national transplant authority. The only exception is Norway, country in which for historical and geographical rationales there is only one transplantation team within the country and not having set a national transplant Authority.

In the majority of Countries requiring administrative approval for LD activities (7 on 10 countries), the authorization is specifically given for LD activities (procurement and/or transplantation), while in Portugal and Slovenia the authorization includes both cadaver and living donor procurement activities. In Cyprus, donation should be performed in an approved medical institution.

4.5 Procedures of prior approval for living donation surgery in a given donor

In Slovenia, Cyprus, Norway and Spain it is not required to get an administrative approval before performing surgery in a given living donor. In Portugal, Italy, Romania and France the authorization should be requested by the transplant team and given by an ad hoc committee (in France the approval is not required if the donor is the father or the mother of the recipient). In Sweden, Poland and United Kingdom the transplant Authority gives the authorization. In Italy a magistrate is also involved in this procedure.

4.6 Registration of the donor prior to living donation surgery

Prior registration of living donors at national or regional level to the national transplant authority is required by legislation or regulation in 6 countries. Registration is recorded at the level of the transplant team hospital in Portugal and Cyprus. In Sweden, Norway and UK, there is no mandatory registration of the donors.

4.7 Non-resident donor policies

Non-resident donors (from European and/or non-European countries) are authorized to donate in all partners countries except in Cyprus. In Italy, Slovenia and Norway procurement of organs in living non-residents is possible only if the recipient is resident.

4.8 Living donor committees/commissions (Localization, dependence, members and role)

All the partners countries except Cyprus have committee/commissions involved in the process of donation. In Sweden, Norway, Poland, Portugal, Spain and Romania the committee is established at the hospital level. In Italy, Slovenia, UK and France it is set up at the regional or the national level.

The living donor commission may function as an independent and dedicated structure or as in Spain, Poland, Portugal and Slovenia the commission is included in a generic committee (e.g. ethical committee). The commission is generally dependent from the transplantation authority or from the Ministry of Health, but in Italy it is independent and in Spain it is depending from the hospital/university.

The attributions of the committees are markedly different between participating countries. In the majority of countries the main duty assigned to the committee is to give an authorization for donation. Also a large majority of commissions does have the task to evaluate the donor-recipient relationship, as well the evaluation of donor suitability. Only a minority of committees plays a role in the information for the donors, directly or by verifying the content and the understanding of information given by the transplant physician.

According to their different attributions, the composition of the committees is also very heterogeneous between the participating countries.

A large majority of commissions includes in their members psychologists or psychiatrists as well. Often, also ethicists are included. In 7 countries the commissions includes physicians, who are transplant physicians in 4 countries. The presence of transplant team representative physicians is allowed only in Norway and UK. In addition, commission may include jurists (3 countries), administrative staff (in 3 countries), social workers (Slovenia, Norway and Spain) and nurses (Spain).

Of note, an advocate of the donor is required by most professional recommendations and by the resolution CM/Res (2008)6 of the Council of Europe. The advocate of the donor is defined as "a professional having appropriate experience and who is not involved in the organ removal or subsequent transplantation procedure". Such advocate of the donor only incorporated in the commission of 2 countries: UK and Poland. In the UK the advocate is entitled "independent assessor", is specifically trained, and operates at the level of the hospital transplantation centre under the authority of the human tissue authority (HTA) committee for living donors. Its role, defined in the procedure guidance, is to assess potential donors, by way of an interview, to ascertain if the requirements of the low (Human Tissue Act) have been met. He must than complete and submit a report to the Authority, detailing weather the requirements have been met, and provide a recommendation regarding the donation (that is, weather the donation should be approved or not approved by the Authority). In Spain, the independent physician who is responsible to deliver information for the donors may be also considered as having some tasks attributed to the advocate of the donor.

Direct audition of the donor by the living donor committee is performed in all partner countries except in Slovenia and in UK, where this task is committed to the independent assessor. The audition is facultative in Spain, requested by the committee if necessary.

In case of refusal of the authorization by the committee, an appeal procedure is allowed in Norway, Poland and in UK. Other countries do not make provision of an appeal procedure.

The chart fig.2 summarize the main Legal and Regulatory dispositions on donation procedures in the partners countries.

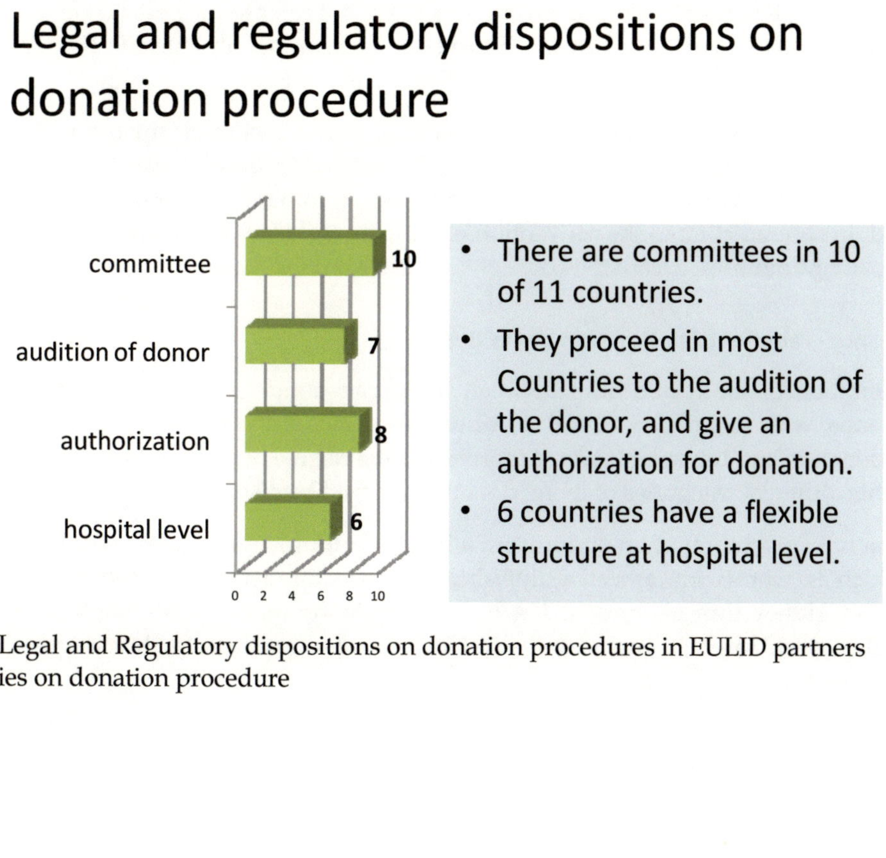

Fig. 2. Legal and Regulatory dispositions on donation procedures in EULID partners countries on donation procedure

4.9 Sanctions and penalties in case of violation of ethical and legal dispositions regarding living donation and transplantation

The convention of Human Rights and Biomedicine, and the additional protocol to the convention of Transplantation of Organs and Tissues of Human origin stipulate that "parties shall provide for appropriate sanctions to be applied in the event of infringement of the provisions contained in the convention and the protocol:

- The prohibition of financial gain or comparable advantage from the human body and its parts, and the prohibition of advertising the need for, or availability or organs or tissues, with the view to offering or seeking financial gain or comparable advantage.
- The prohibition of organ and tissue trafficking.
- The prohibition of organ removal of a person who does not have the capacity to consent, including minors and persons who have a mental disorder. An organ may be removed from a living donor only after the person concerned has given free, informed and specific consent to it in written form or before an official body. The person concerned may freely withdraw consent at any time".

The convention on Actions against Trafficking in human Beings contains also important provisions addressing to the criminalization of trafficking in human being, the criminalization of the use of services of a victim, and effective, proportionate and dissuasive sanctions and measures in case of criminal offences that shall be adopted by each party.

Organ commercialism and organ trafficking are submitted to penal prosecutions and sanctions in all EULID partners countries, except in Cyprus and Spain. In Spain transplantation low does not prescribe any sanctions, but refer to the penal code which does not consider such cases specifically. Transplant tourism is only specifically. Transplant tourism is only specifically considered in the Penal Code of France.

The procurement of organs in persons unable to consent, including minors and mentally disabled is condemned and submitted to penal sanctions in most of partners countries. In Cyprus, Italy and Poland however, the procurement in minors/or mentally disabled is not referred, in contradiction to the convention on Human rights and Biomedicine signed by all participating Countries, except the UK.

4.10 Donor- recipient relationship definition

The definition of the relationship between the organ donor and its recipient may be of importance, with regards to ethical, legal and also medical concerns surrounding living organ donation and transplantation. According to the degree of relation between donor and recipients, different categories of living donations should be distinguished:

- The transplantation of an organ from a living donor to a genetically related recipient, which is worldwide a well established practice for decades in the case of living donor kidney transplantation. The donor may be brother or sister, mother or father, child, grandparent, cousin of the 1st degree or cousin of further degrees of the recipient.

- The transplantation of an organ from a living donor to a non-genetically, related recipient. Another proposed terminology for such donors is "emotionally related donors". The donor may be a spouse, a legally-registered or non-registered partner or a friend of the recipient. This category comprises also the legally-related donors, including adoptive parents and partners of parents of recipients.
- The transplantation of an organ from a non-related donor within the context of non-directed living kidney donation. The donor has no established close personal relationship with the recipient. These include:
  - The anonymous volunteers also named truly altruist donors, or "good Samaritan" donors.
  - Kidney donors involved in a "paired kidney exchange" or a "pooled kidney exchange" donation program for ABO-Type or tissue-type incompatibility donor-recipient pairs.

A majority of the countries participating in EULID project have established legislations or regulation addressing the donor-recipient relationship. Three countries, Cyprus, Norway and Portugal do not have any regulatory or legal limitation in the donor-recipient relationship, but in fact unrelated living donor (non-directed and directed) transplantation is not actually performed in these countries. In Romania only, there is no regulatory or legal limitation in the donor-recipient relationship. It is specified that, in case of donation of minor, a magistrate register is consent.

4.11 Information, evaluation, consent and follow-up of the donors

4.11.1 Information for the donor

As started by the Additional protocol to the Convention on Human Rights and Biomedicine in the Article 12, Chapter III "the donor, and where appropriate, the person or body providing authorization, shall beforehand be given appropriate information as to the purpose and nature of the removal as well as on its consequences and risks".

In most of partners countries, legislation of regulations require that information for the organ donors should be given by the persons or bodies independent from the transplant team. In Cyprus, Italy, Poland, Portugal, Slovenia, Spain and the UK, the information process involves an independent physician (in UK it is the "independent assessor"). In France, the donor committee should by the law deliver information during the interview of the donor before the members of the commission.

In Norway, Romania and Sweden, there is no regulation on this concern, and information for donors is usually delivered by individuals from the transplant team.

4.11.2 Evaluation of risks for the donor

The evaluation of risks for the donor is a crucial phase in the process of donation, which is used in the estimation of the risk-benefit ratio of the organ procurement for a given donor within the context of a transplantation which is indented in a given recipient. It results in a statement on the suitability or non-suitability of the possible donor. The evaluation of risks includes the evaluation of the medical risks related to the organ removal and to surgical and anaesthetic procedures, as well the psychological and social risks.

As started by the Additional Protocol to the Convection on Human Rights and Biomedicine in the Article 10, Chapter III "Before organ removal, appropriate medical investigations and interventions shall be carried out to evaluate and reduce physical and psychological risk to the health of the donor".

The evaluation of the risk for the donor is regulated in most partners countries. Independent donor committees are involved in Italy, France, Poland, Portugal, Spain and the UK. In Spain and Slovenia, the evaluation process involves an independent medical team. The evaluation of the donor is not regulated in Norway, Romania and Sweden.

Psychological assessment is required by regulations only in Romania, Slovenia and the UK.

4.11.3 Consent of the donor

As stated by the Additional Protocol to the Convention on Human Rights and Biomedicine in the Article 13, Chapter III "An organ or tissue may be removed from a living donor only after the person concerned has given free, informed and specific consent to it either in written form or before an official body. The person may freely withdraw consent at any time".

The partner countries have in the legislation or in regulations provisions addressing the question of living donor consent. However, procedures for registering the donor consent differ notably according the country. The consent is collected in written form by a regional Court Magistrate in France, Italy and Spain and in Romania for minors. The donor commission is responsible in Romania and in the UK. An independent physician is involved in Poland and in Portugal (physician under the control of the hospital director), and in Slovenia it is the transplant Authority. In Cyprus and Norway, legislation requires also a written consent.

In Sweden there is no regulatory provision for the registration of the donor consent.

4.11.4 Follow-up of a donor

In Portugal, Romania, Sweden and Norway there is no regulatory provision concerning the medical follow-up of the donor. In the other 7 partner countries, legal or regulatory provisions address to the medical donor follow-up, but not specifically to the psychological follow-up.

On May 2008, a living donor follow-up National Registry is established in Italy, Poland, France, Sweden, Norway (at hospital level) and United Kingdom, but not in Spain, Slovenia, Cyprus, Portugal and Romania.

If a donor requires a transplantation following organ donation because of terminal organ failure, partner countries have not incorporated prioritization in their allocation systems, except in Cyprus when priority is given to the previous donor to receive a national cadaver donor kidney and in Norway where in case of liver failure the liver donor is put in emergency position for receiving a cadaver donor liver procured in Scandia transplant OSO area. In fact, all donors with liver failure following donation are incorporated in most countries in a "super-urgent" category for liver allocation for patient with acute liver failure.

5. Protection concerns regarding donation of organs from living donors in eleven European Countries

5.1 Evaluation of the potential risks for the living donors

5.1.1 General considerations of donor risks

In every living donation setting, the basic principle is that an organ or part of an organ is removed from a healthy individual in order to be transplanted into a needing recipient. The donor and the recipient are usually connected in some way, either genetically (related donation) or emotionally (unrelated donation). Before the surgical procedure, a donor evaluation process is needed to ensure that the potential donor is physically and mentally fit for the procedure, that no contraindications to surgery exists and to rule out any coercion, unethical or financial bindings between donor and recipient. All potential donors with proper motivation, and that have received thorough information are aware that inherent risk are involved in living donor transplantation. After the donation the donor will need a recovery period before his or her preoperative function is restored, and there is a need for follow up both in the short term postoperative course as well as in the long term, to ensure that possible negative events linked to the donation is detected and treated properly. In order to ensure an evidence based practice in living organ donation, data on donor and recipient outcomes should be registered in a systematically manner to allow scientific evaluation of quality and risk of the procedures.

Our current knowledge of the outcome and risks of living donation are based on the practice that has been performed during the last 4 decades in different centres around the world. Of particular importance is the selection criterion that has been utilized. It has been a more or less universal rule, that the donor is healthy, with no signs of disease. Thus, the assessment of risks in this report is based on this assumption. This implies, that the donor evaluation must be focused at identifying individuals that have the lowest possible risk for undesirable outcomes, further underlining the importance of selection in the evaluation process as the fundament of risk management in living donor.

The risks involved in living donation can be divided into the following broad categories, independent of the particular organ donated (table 1):

Risk category	Related factors in donation process
Physical	Invasive tests, donor surgery, post operative complications, organ function short and long term
Psychological	Donor-recipient relationship, recipient outcome, donor postoperative recovery and function, quality of donor evaluation and follow up
Social	Work capacity, family situation, type of work, donor social activities
Economical	Cost associated with donation and follow up, insurance status, sick-leave regulations,

Table 1. Risks involved in living donation

For didactic purposes, it is meaningful to present the risk factors in such a manner, but in clinical practice it is important to recognize that a complication or negative event in conjunction with the donation might influence any number of the above mentioned risk dimensions.

- Physical risks: The risk of physical complications is related to donor age, general health status and previous history as well as the organ donated. In order to be able to describe complications to the donor surgery, and hence risk in a consistent manner.
- Psychological risk: Several studies indicate that coercion between donor and recipient might be a major risk factor for the mental well being of the donor, and any other motivation that altruistic reasons may have a similar risk of psychological side effects. During the evaluation process, findings that contraindicate donation can be uncovered. Moreover, the motivation of the donor might be altered by the evaluation process itself.
- Social risk: The social risk with regards to role in the family, ability to live unrestricted and have the same work situation is low in most cases. Persons with physically demanding jobs might be particularly at risk in the event of complications to donor surgery. If it can be anticipated that there is an increased risk that the donor cannot lead the same social life after the donor operation as he did previously, the particular subject should be rejected as a donor.
- Economic risk: Several of the non physical factors related to donor risk, are dependent on organizational and legal aspects in the country where the living donation is performed. Social insurance regulations such as the right to paid sick leave and reimbursement of expenses related to travel and limitation in the rights to have life insurance etc., will have an obvious impact on the economical risks associated with living donation. It is also apparent that economic risk factors will influence both the social as well as the psychological risk of a donation.

5.2 Donor protection

The main protection systems for the living donor, regardless of organ are:

1. Careful donor evaluation and selection
2. Use of independent donor advocate
3. Limiting of living donor transplantation to high volume centres
4. Database systems for registration of all donation related morbidity and mortality
5. Perioperative, short term and long term donor follow-up regimens in centres performing this kind of transplantations

None of the above mentioned systems are to EULID team knowledge legislated in Europe or other parts of the world.

Legislative mechanisms that are important in donor protection are:

1. Right to free health care
2. Right to reimbursement of donation related costs
3. Right to sick leave until full recovery after donation, irrespective of length
4. Patient damage insurance systems, providing patients that experience major complications or serious disability with financial coverage.

The legislation regarding the above mentioned factors varies greatly among the European states, as well as how the health system is organized.

5.3 Social insurance and protecting systems for the living donor

Every country has its own systems concerning general social security. Usually the social insurance systems cover everyone that lives and works in that country. It provides financial protection for families, children, for persons with a disability and in connection with work injury, illness and old age. Being a member within European Union, the social insurance benefits in other EU member states, also are available at a certain extent. The living donors should be covered within the systems and our recommendations are given separately.

Social insurance aims to provide security at every stage of life. Throughout the 20th century reforms were gradually introduced and there is still room for improvements and equal rules within EU.

Regarding authorization of sick pay this is made by a physician or the physician of the Social Insurance Office. This seems to be a general rule for all countries.

The employer usually pays for sick leave during the first 2 weeks and then the official authority pays for the remaining period. The amount of payment varies from 60-100% of income, generally 80%.

How long it is possible to be on sick pay varies from 3-18 months in the different countries. Usually some sort of rehabilitation is required and starts usually 6-12 months after start of sick leave and the social insurance usually takes part in this. The rehabilitation is a co-work between different areas. Health care is responsible for medical treatment, the employer for work-related measures and the municipality for social measures.

Pension age varies between 60 and 70 years in different countries and five countries have different ages for males and females according to our survey.

Firing due to sick leave should not be possible but a 3/10 countries have this possibility.

If social-medical insurance is public such a system is easier to regulate. All the partners countries except one have a public system.

5.4 Informative leaflet

5.4.1 General considerations of the informative leaflet

The leaflet developed in the EULID project was translated in 12 languages. It has two different parts with information; one focused on the future kidney Living Donors and the other on the future liver Living Donors.

5.4.2 Contents of the living donor informative leaflet

- Information about the reasons for transplantation and the options to become a donor.
- Donor investigations and selection procedure.
- Surgical approach, normal intercourse and adverse events.
- Psychosocial support and rules for the donors in the evaluating process and after donation period.
- Long-term follow-up.

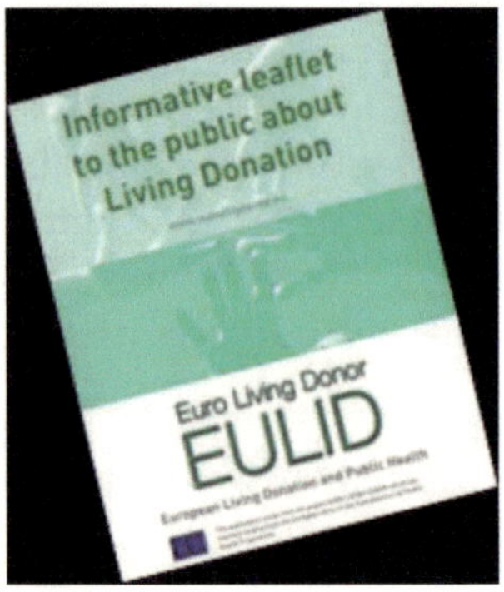

Fig. 3. EULID informative leaflet

6. Living donor registration practices

6.1 Living donor registry

6.1.1 Development of living donor registry

The donation of an organ by a living person to save or transform the life of another is a wonderful act and it is deeply embedded within European law that this should be an altruistic act and consequently it is illegal to trade in human organs or to advertise the buying or selling of human organs. Living donation is complex at the social level with many factors coming to bear upon the decision to donate and the experience of the donor both pre and post donation. The scarcity of organs for use in transplantation and the complexity around the decision to donate and the concerns it may create for the donor and recipient requires that living donation be supported through the creation of an evidence base. The evidence base is required to show that living donation is safe both in the short and long term and that each donation takes place in the form of an altruistic gift and without financial inducement. It is intended that the EULID database and web portal will support the objective to create such an evidence base and so we have started by looking at the donor registration process within the countries participating in the EULID project. The survey has been at a high level to begin to create a picture of the general approach within the EULID project group. The partners of the project created a survey aiming to collect data about the following issues:

- The existence of legal requirements to collect data on living donation
- The existence of a responsible body that holds the data about living donation
- The status of the responsible body
- The type of data reported
- The reporting process

The survey form was sent to a named contact in each EULID Project participating country in order that they could research and report on their national situation. The results were as below:

- Eight countries report that they have a national authority with responsibility for authorising living donation in their country. Two countries, Norway and Sweden report that no such body currently exists in their country and one country did not answer.

- Ten countries report that data about all living donation is collected and held centrally in their country and one country did not answer.
- Five countries report that the data that is collected is at a summary level recording just activity while five countries report that data is reported at the case level. One country did not answer.
- Is there a legal requirement to supply the data?
- In seven countries there is a legal requirement for data on living donation to be reported and in the four remaining countries reporting takes place on a voluntary basis.
- Seven countries report that a transplant coordinator or other member of the transplant team, for example surgeon or physician is responsible for data reporting. In one country responsibility rests with a statistician and in three countries there exists the concept of an Authorised or Responsible person identified to make the reporting.
- Six respondents feel that full reporting is achieved in their country and four respondents feel that reporting in their countries is not fully complete. One country felt unable to express an opinion.
- Seven countries report a system of auditing is in place to monitor reporting compliance and four countries report that no such system is in place in their country.
- In seven countries the data is held by a State body, for example a ministry or other state body such as the NHS in the UK. In four countries the data is held by a body outside of the state such as a university or registry
- All countries record which organ had been donated.
- Eight counties record the nationality of the donor and three do not.
- Nine countries record the country in which the donor is resident and two do not.
- Nine countries record the relationship between the donor and the recipient and one does not.
- Ten countries record the nationality of the recipient and one does not.
- Ten countries record the country in which the recipient is resident and one does not.
- Eight countries record clinical data about the donor, for example complications and survival and three do not.

6.1.2 Data to be collected in the living donor registry database

6.1.2.1 Concept and features of the database

The database is central to the collection of data about living donation and is supplied in a generic format so that it can be used in every country. It is designed to serve the health care professionals who hold the data about living donation activity in their country and who are able to enter this in to the database through a clear and easy to use frontend which can be accessed through the web once the user is set up with an account and access authorized. Additionally the data in the database will be available with "open-access" to the general public who can access data about living donation activity in their country and other countries who contribute data to the database. Through this approach we hope to encourage full participation in the supply of data and to provide the general public with a valuable information resource. We feel that for living donation this possibility is currently unique in concept as we are not aware of any similar facility available with direct access for the general public and healthcare professionals.

Ease of use was an essential prerequisite to encouraging participation and the regular entry of data in to the database. Ease of use is also essential to ensure time efficiency for busy health care professionals and to support data accuracy. This requirement has been achieved through a clear and logical screen layout, the use of "pick-lists" and real time validation to support the accuracy of data entry. To establish the database it was important to gain a clear understanding of its purpose in order to ensure that the data collected is closely relevant to the purpose of the database and to avoid the burden of collecting data which may not be used. The data is required primarily to support the monitoring of donation activity along with ensuring the safety of the process and high level outcome but it is not intended that the database support any detailed clinical analysis.

The database is founded on a 3 level model. All participants are required to contribute at the "Obligatory" data level, with additional data items categorized as "recommended" and "excellence" being optional.

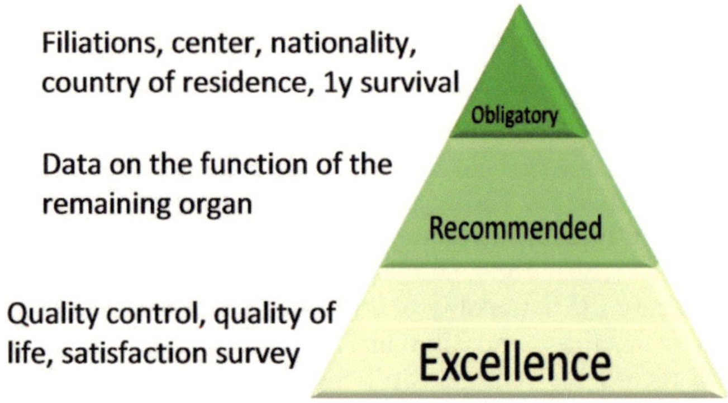

Fig. 4. Registry model data

Donor confidentiality is maintained within the database concept by ensuring that each donor record is anonym on entry to the database and issued with a unique number.

The website (www.eulivingdonor.eu) has the capability to be used in different languages and is currently presented in both English and Spanish. The language selection is driven by the browser's configuration. The default language will be English.

Information is displayed on the screen without the need to scroll and information is grouped logically on the screen to aid use with the main element highlighted with a black frame. All pages are protected by session control access.

6.1.2.2 Data items to be collected

Basic data for both living kidney and liver donors (Donor Registration)

- First initial of donor given name
- First initial of donor family name
- Gender
- Year of birth
- Donor country of residence
- Nationality or recipient
- Recipient country of residence
- Relationship of donor to the recipient
- Type of donation

- Organ donated
- Date of donation
- Centre for donation
- Centre for follow-up
- Post operative outcome

This pop-up menu will guide the registering centre to choose alive or death. In case of death, the date of death has to be filled out. This data are necessary to have an idea of the general evolution and outcomes of living donation performed in the EU. Secondly it can bench mark every center to the average result in the EU for every type of donation.

6.2 Summary and recommendations about the strategy to monitor living donors

Based on the preliminary retrospective data input, the EULID database registry has already proven to be a valuable tool for evaluation and comparing trends and quantitative and qualitative data on living donation for both kidney and liver. The high frequency of missing data in both kidney and liver donor subjects, stresses the need of the implementation of an international European database registry in order to evaluate and stratify political, social and clinical regulations and policies. Out of demographic data trends, the registry was able to highlight valuable information on donor and recipient residency, relationship and allocation.

In the interest of monitoring both donor and recipient flow within EU member states as well as the type of allocation, these data registries are extremely important. These factors stress the fact that when trends on European levels should be reported and monitored, a central registry system should be implemented in every EU member state, in order to provide quantitative and qualitative peers to every clinical living donor program within every EU member state, but on top to be able to provide necessary information on a permanent basis to EU health care boards and politicians.

Recommendations about the strategy to monitor Living Donors

- Registration of all living donor cases is mandatory for the purpose of traceability, safety and transparency of activity and outcome of living donor procedures performed within all EU member states.
- Collection of living donor data has to be done through an established central database system, accessible by appropriately authorized persons.
- Data on identification, countries of residency, nationality, type of donation, health care institutions and outcome are obligatory to register, with protection of the donor's proper privacy. An official point of contact has to be made to the embassy of donor's country of residence.
- A regulatory audit is mandatory and data should be both monitored on a national as well as institutional level.

6.3 Living donor satisfaction survey

6.3.1 General aspects

Living donation is a strategy to face the shortage of organs for transplantation, but it requires the protection and follow-up of the donor. The evaluation of donor's satisfaction and the impact of the donation, are key issues to guarantee the quality of the procedure.

The goal of this study is to assess the degree of living donors' satisfaction with donation and the impact of living donation on donor quality of life.

A living donor follow-up questionnaire including 54 questions has been created according to the Delphi's method, assaying the following donation related aspects: decision making, information received, stress, impact.

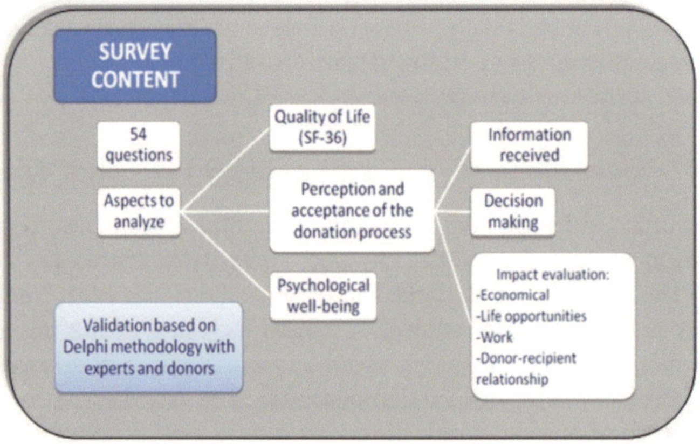

Fig. 5. Living donor satisfaction survey content

6.3.2 Methodology

We have set up a questionnaire on the basis of the ones already available at the Hospital Clínic of Barcelona and reviewed it in terms of content and language. The survey has been designed to explore the following aspects: 1. Perception and acceptance of the donation process, information received, decision making and potential impact of donation on the donor life-style, the ability to obtain future insurability, employment, financial barriers or difficulties donors may face in the donor-recipient relationships. With the support of the Department of Sociology of the University of Barcelona.

The questionnaire, applying a Likert scale from 1 to 4 (Strongly agree, agree, disagree and strongly disagree), has been designed as an agile and easy to use tool for assessment, ordering the questions according to the natural course of the donation process. The original questionnaire has been developed in Spanish, translated to English and from English to each partner country's language.

Delphi technique has been used to develop the survey which has been assessed by 13 experts, all actively working in living donation as nephrologists, urologists, general surgeons and transplant coordinators. Pilot test was performed on 10 living donors and the following aspects related to decision making and survey behavior were observed: type of reactions, degree of comprehension, spontaneity in answering multiple-choice questions, signs of exhaustion, quandaries and comments. Survey acceptability was high (all participants consented to participate) and questions were clearly understood.

The EULID project targeted living donors at 6 to 18 months after donation as it was considered that donors´ satisfaction < 6 months after donation refers mainly to the surgical procedure while assessment > 18 months after donation does not clearly reveal the decision making and surgical procedure related aspects.

7. Conclusion

The EULID project seeks to contribute to a European consensus that could lead to best practices and to elaborate recommendations that will help to establish a protection framework for living organ donors' health and safety through laws and regulations in the labour, social, medical, and psychological fields. In the same way, the consensus and elaboration of common registries and the recommendations of their application are important improvements to be implemented in the living organ donor field.

8. Acknowledgment

The authors would like to express their gratitude to all participants in all the different stages of the project, especially to the respective representatives from each partners centre for their great support and professional help.

A very special thanks goes out to Dr. Francis L. Delmonico, Director of Medical Affairs for The Transplantation Society, Advisor of the World Health Organization, Professor of Surgery at Harvard Medical School, Medical Director of the New England Organ Bank in Newton, Massachusetts, and to Dr. José O. Medina-Pestana, Professor of Medicine, Federal University of São Paulo Brazil and Head of Renal Transplantation Unit in Hospital do Rim e Hipertensão, São Paulo); for their external advice and scientific evaluation of the project.

Appreciations also go out to Maria López for her assistance and administrative support and to Dr. Entela Kondi for supporting us during the English revision of the materials.

In conclusion a special acknowledgement goes out to all Living Donors who participated in the project, recognizing that the conclusion of this study would not have been possible without their participation.

9. References

The Ethics Committee of the Transplantation Society (2004). *The Consensus Statement of the Amsterdam Forum on the Care of the Live Kidney Donor.* Transplantation 2004; 78(4):491-92.

The Authors for the Live Organ Donor Consensus Group (2000). *Consensus Statement on the Live Organ Donor.* JAMA. 2000; 284:2919-2926.

Barr ML, *et al* (2006). *A report of the Vancouver forum on the care of the live organ donor: Lung, liver, pancreas and intestine. Data and medical guidelines.* Transplantation 2006; 81(10): 1373-1385.

The Declaration of Istanbul on organ trafficking and transplant tourism. Transplantation. 2008 Oct 27; 86(8):1013-8.

Hilhorst MT. (2008) *Living apart together: moral frictions between two coexisting organ transplantation schemes.* J Med Ethics. 2008;34:484-8.

Pruett TL, *et al* (2006). *The ethics statement of the Vancouver forum on the live lung, liver, pancreas and intestine donor.* Transplantation. 2006; 81:1386-7.

Ross LF, Woodle ES. (2000) *Ethical issues in increasing living kidney donations by expanding kidney paired exchange programs.* Transplantation. 2000; 69:1539-43.

World Heath Organization. Guiding principles on human organ transplantation. Lancet. 1991; 337(8755):1470-1.

WHO World Health Organisation [Internet]. Geneva: WHO; c2009. [WHA57.18 Human organ and tissue transplantation]; 2004 May 22 [cited 2009 Oct 6]. Available from http://www.who.int/transplantation/en/A57_R18-en.pdf

Council of Europe-Treaty Office [Internet]. Strasbourg: Council of Europe. Council of Europe-ETS no. 164 Convention for the Protection of Human Rights and Dignity of the Human Being with regard to the Application of Biology and Medicine; 1997 Apr 4 [cited 2009 Oct 6]. Available from http://conventions.coe.int/Treaty/en/Treaties/Html/164.htm

Council of Europe-Treaty Office [Internet]. Strasbourg: Council of Europe. Council of Europe-ETS no. 186 Additional Protocol to the Convention on Human Rights and Biomedicine concerning Transplantation of Organs and Tissues of Human Origin; 2002 Jan 24 [cited 2009 Oct 6]. Available from http://conventions.coe.int/Treaty/EN/Treaties/Html/186.htm

European Parliament [Internet]. Strasbourg: European Parliament. European Parliament resolution of 22 April 2008 on organ donation and transplantation: Policy actions at EU level (2007/2210 (INI)); 2008 Apr 22 [updated 2008 Nov 25; cited 2009 Oct 6]. Available from http://www.europarl.europa.eu/sides/getDoc.do?pubRef=-//EP//TEXT+TA+P6-TA-2008-0130+0+DOC+XML+V0//EN

Clemens KK, *et al* (2006). *Psychosocial Health of Living Kidney Donors: A Systematic Review.* Am J Transplant 2006; 6(12): 2965–77.

Ferriman A. (2008). *Becoming a live kidney donor.* BMJ 2008; 336(4657):1374-6.

Dew MA*Guidelines for the Psychosocial Evaluation of Living Unrelated Kidney Donors in the United States.* Am J Transplant 2007; 7(5): 1047-54.

Johnson EM, *et al* (1999). *Long-term follow-up of living kidney donors: quality of life after donation.* Transplantation 1999; 67(5): 717–721.

Fehrman-Ekholm I, *et al* (2000). *Kidney donors don't regret: Follow-up of 370 donors in Stockholm since 1964.* Transplantation 2000; 69(10): 2067– 71.

Ware JE Jr, Sherbourne CD. (1992). *The MOS 36-item short-form health survey (SF-36). I. Conceptual framework and item selection.* Med Care 1992; 30(6):473-83.

Beavers KL, *et al* (2001). *The Living Donor Experience: Donor Health Assessment and Outcomes After Living Donor Liver Transplantation.* Liver Transpl. 2001;7(11):943-7.

Sharp J, McRae A, McNeill Y. (2010). *Decision making and psychosocial outcomes among living kidney donors: a pilot study.* Prog Transplant. 2010; 20(1):53-7.

Johnson EM, *et al* (1999). *Long-Term Follow-Up of Living Kidney Donors: Quality of Life After Donation.* Transplantation 1999; 67 (5):717-21.

Lumsdaine JA, *et al* (2005). *Higher quality of life in living donor kidney transplantation: prospective cohort study.* Transpl Int 2005; 18(8):975-80.

Miyagi S, *et al* (2005). *Risks of donation and quality of donors' life after living donor liver transplantation.* Transpl Int 2005; 18:47-51.

Goyal M, *et al* (2002). *Economic and health consequences of selling a Kidney in India.* JAMA 2002; 288:1589-1593.

Kessler M. (2008). *Legal and regulatory aspects of living-donor transplantation.* Nephrol Ther. 2008 Feb; 4(1): 49-51.

Gruessner RWG, Benedetti E. (2008). *Living donor organ transplantation.* McGraw-Hill Professional; 2008. ISBN 978-0-07-145549-7. United States of America.

4

Action Taken to Boost Donor Rate in Croatia

Mirela Busic[1] and Arijana Lovrencic-Huzjan[2]
[1]*Ministry of Health and Social Welfare*
[2]*University Departement of Neurology, University Hospital Center «Sestre milosrdnice», Referral Centar for Neurovascular Disorders of The Ministry of Health and Social Welfare*
Croatia

1. Introduction

Over the last 50 years, organ transplantation has become a widely accepted and successful treatment method that has provided the best therapeutic benefit for more than one million people worldwide (Council of Europe Consensus document, 1999). Due to the outstanding results and success of transplant medicine, there has been a dramatic increase in waiting lists after the 1980-ies. At the same time, the number of organs available for transplantation does not nearly match the demand. Organ shortage has led some countries to find an alternative in living donation, but in most European countries, deceased donation is recognised as the most appropriate source of organs for transplantation. Deceased donation is primarily based on donation after brain death. It has been estimated that no more than 1% of deceased persons and no more than 3% of people who die in the hospital fall into this category (Matesanz & Dominguesz-Gil, 2007). Although the number of potential brain-dead donors is limited due to that fact, there is evidence showing that organ shortage is not primarily the result of a lack of suitable donors but, rather, the result of the failure to accurately identify them, obtain the consent, and procure the organs (Matesanz & Miranda, 2002). Partial strategies in many countries have resulted in mild or transient increases in organ donation or even no improvement at all (Hou, 2000). However, several successful models and strategies exist which can serve as guidance to countries attempting to increase their donor rates; the "Spanish Model" is definitely one of the most widely acknowledged. Recently, Croatia has risen to a role model status which other countries might like to follow and replicate. This paper illustrates actions taken in Croatia to increase the donor rate, and highlight the great achievements that recently ranked Croatia among world leaders in organ transplantation and donorship.

2. How does Croatia compare with other countries?

Remarkably, only 10 years ago Croatia was at the tail end of Europe with a (effective) donor rate of only 2.7 per million population (pmp). Over the last ten years the number of donors has multiplied ten times over and the (effective) donor rate has increased from 2.7 to 28 pmp (Fig.1.)

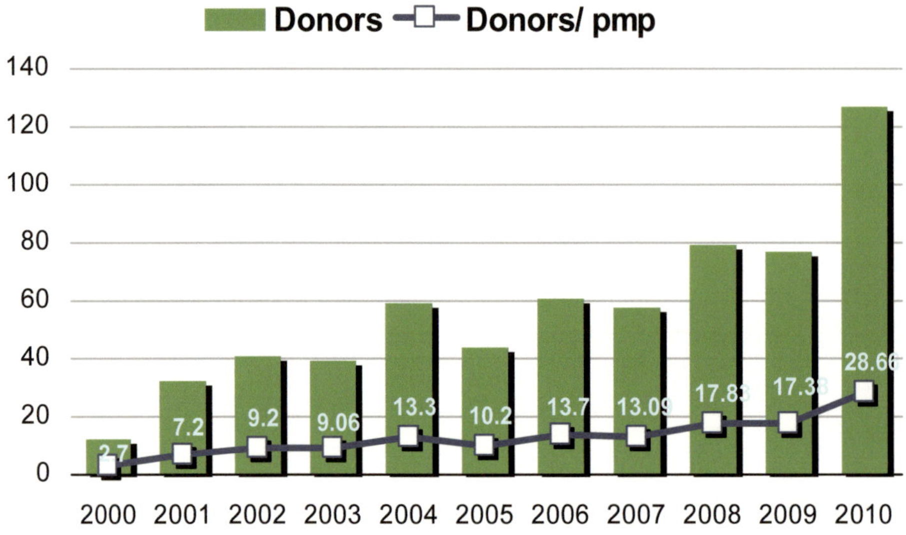

Fig. 1. Number of effective Donors/effective Donors per million in Croatia from 2000 to 2010

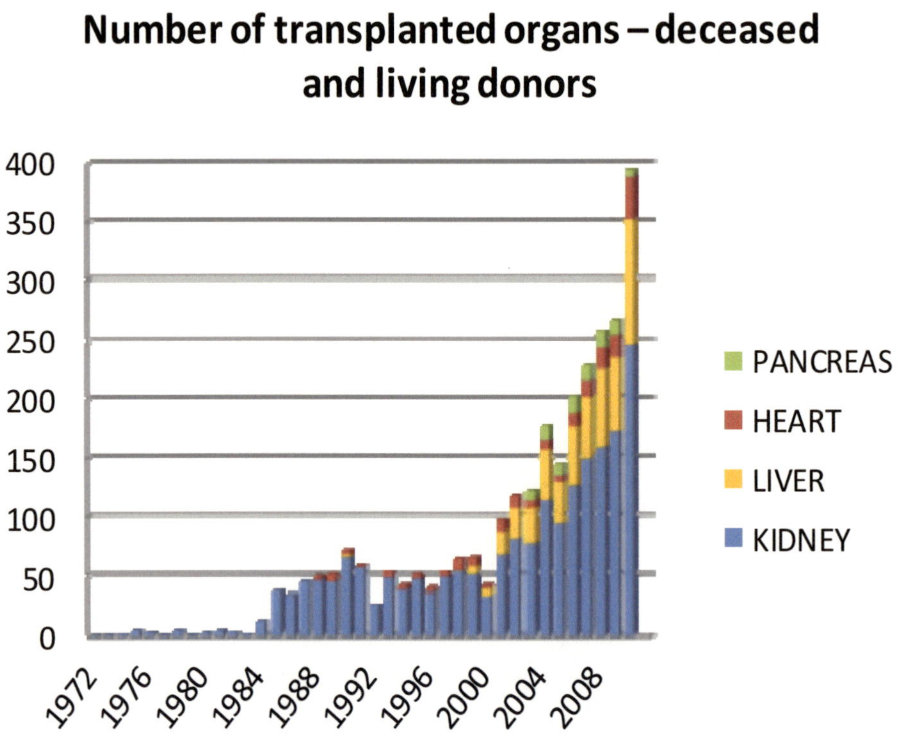

Fig. 2. Total number of transplanted organs in Croatia (1972–2010) from deceased and living donors

While in recent years the number of donors has been stagnating or only slightly increasing by 2% per year on average in Europe, last year Croatia burst its own annual number of donors and overall number of transplantations, increasing both by 64% and 54 % respectively (Fig. 2.), thus positioning Croatia at the top of the world's transplantation scene. Similar success was recorded only in Spain and Portugal, while many other highly developed countries (such as the Netherlands, the United Kingdom, and Norway), which traditionally rely on living and donation after circulatory death (DCD), significantly lagged behind Croatia, both in deceased and overall donor and transplantation rate. More specifically, when comparing the international data for 2010 (The Transplant Newsletter of the Council of Europe, 2011), a wide range of organ donation rates among countries is still observed. The world leader Spain had the highest actual donor rate (32 pmp), followed by Croatia and Portugal (30,2 and 30,1 pmp) (Fig. 3).

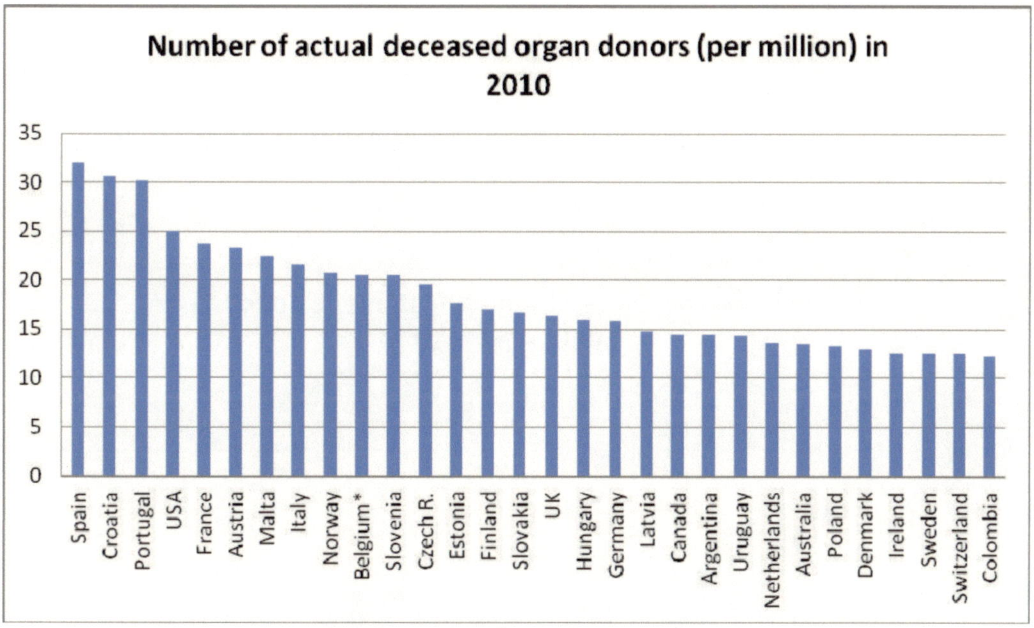

*Source; Newsletter Transplant of the Council of Europe 2011

Fig. 3. Number of deceased organ donors/per million in 2010

The Republic of Croatia ranked first in the world in the number of transplanted kidneys (overall and deceased) (Fig. 4., Fig. 5.), and the number of transplanted livers per million people (Council of Europe, 2010) (Fig. 6.). At the same time, along with Austria, Croatia ranked second in the heart transplant rate (Fig. 7.). If we compare the total transplant rate, Croatia ranked third in the world; only the United States and Austria reported a higher total number of transplantation performed per million populations due to high number of lung transplants (Fig. 8.).

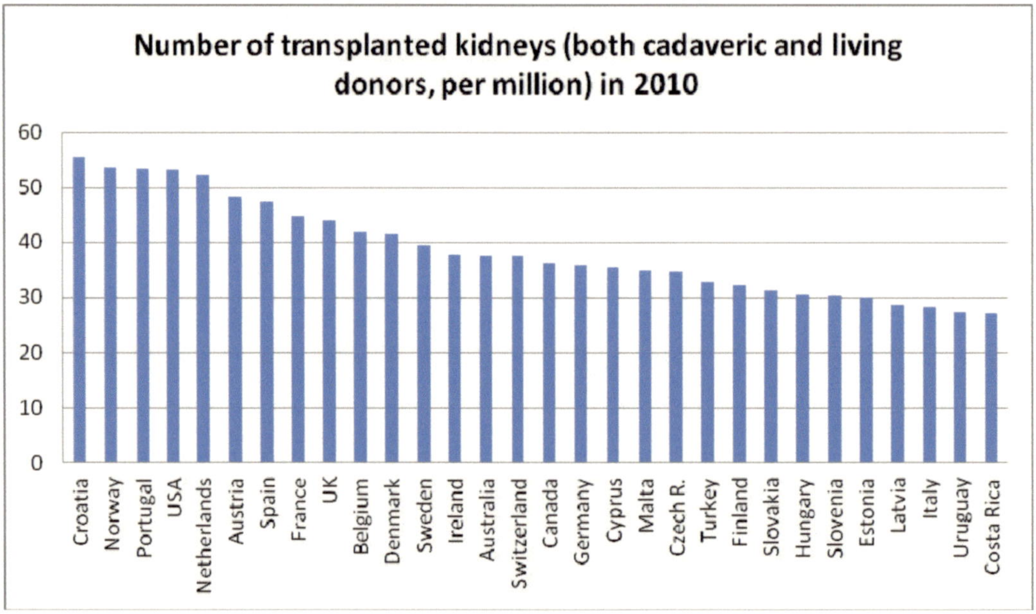

Source: Newsletter Transplant of the Council of Europe 2011

Fig. 4. Number of total transplanted kidneys (cadaveric and living donors) per million in 2010

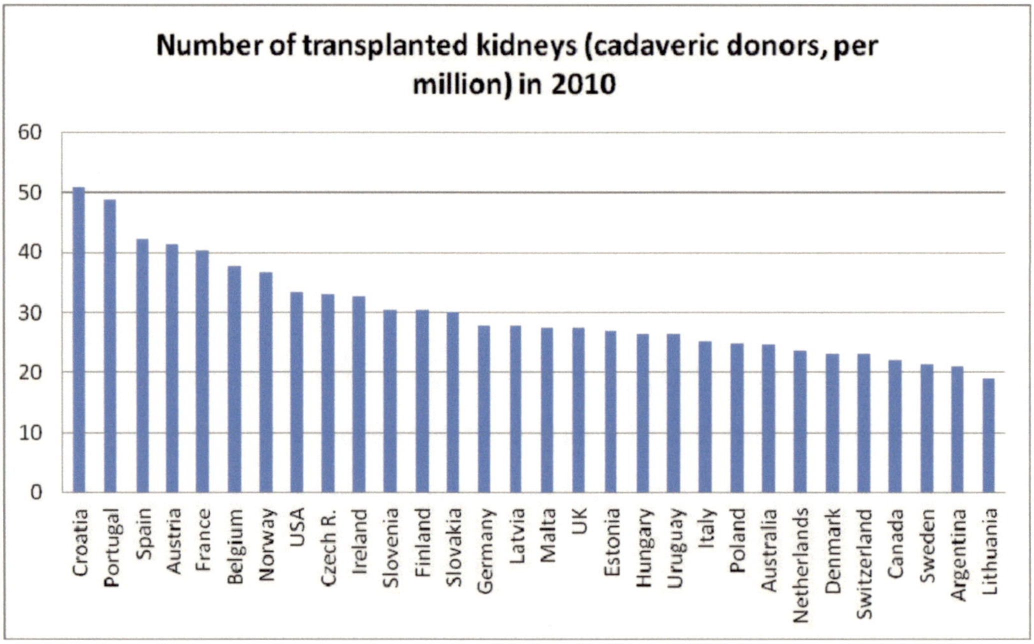

Reference: Newsletter Transplant of the Council of Europe 2011

Fig. 5. Number of transplanted kidneys (cadaveric donors) per million in 2010

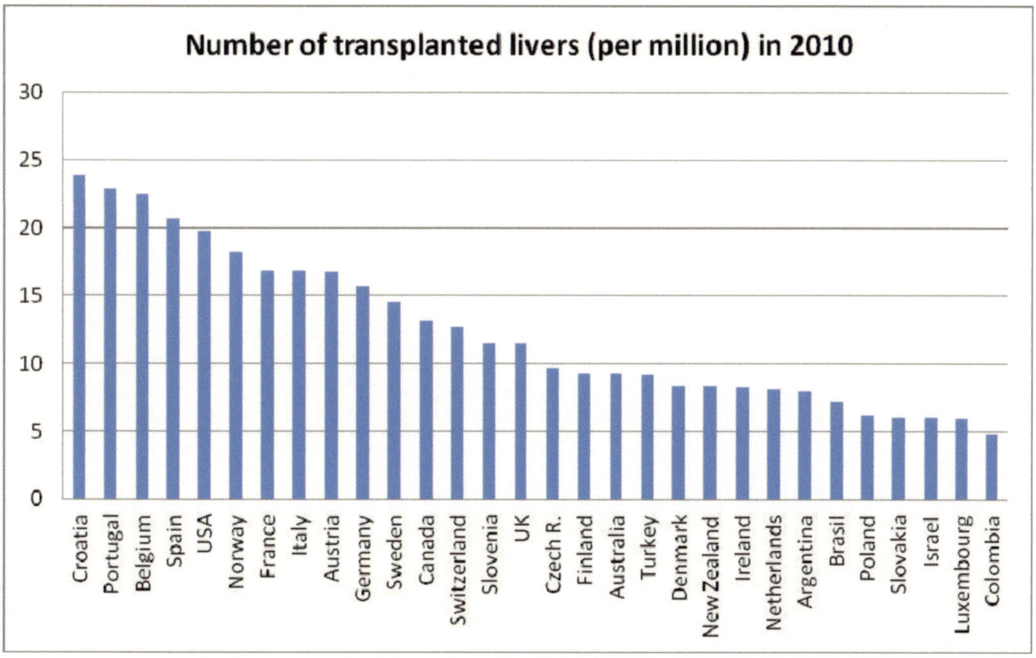

Reference: Newsletter Transplant of the Council of Europe 2011

Fig. 6. Number of transplanted livers (cadaveric and living donors), per million in 2010

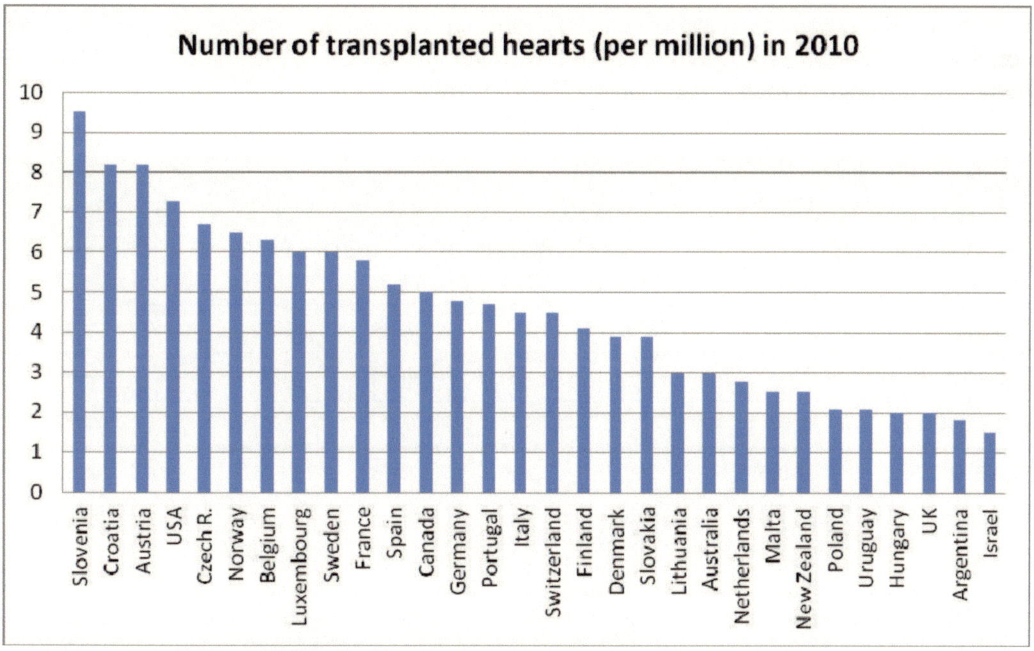

Reference: Newsletter Transplant of the Council of Europe 2011

Fig. 7. Number of transplanted hearts/per million in 2010

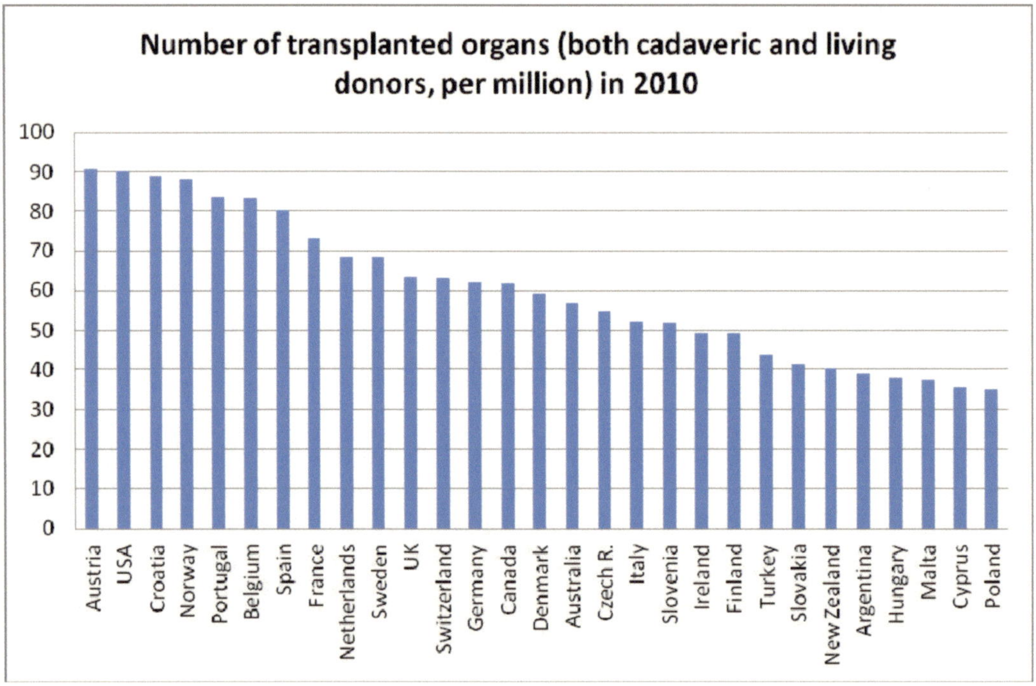

Reference: Newsletter Transplant of the Council of Europe 2011

Fig. 8. Number of total transplanted organs (cadaveric and living donors) per million in 2010

Even being the newest Eurotransplant (ET) member, in comparison with other ET member countries, Croatia ranked first in the total transplant and donation rates in 2010, and had the highest percantage of multiorgan donors (85.5%) (Table 1.).

EUROTRANSPLANT COUNTRY	POPULATION	DONORS 2009	DONORS 2010	DONOR RATE 2009	DONOR RATE 2010	TREND	% MULTI ORGAN 2010
AUSTRIA	8,357	212	189	25.36	22.61	-10.84%	76.7%
BELGIA	10,827	276	263	25.49	24.29	-4.70%	74.9%
CROATIA	4,443	77	127	17.15	28.67	+67.17%	85.5%
LUXEMBURG	0.502	0	3	0	5.97		100%
NETHERLANDS	16,065	215	216	13.38	13.44	+0,4%	68.5%
GERMANY	82,329	1196	1271	14.52	15.45	+8.42%	83.2%
SLOVENIA	2,054	33	40	16.06	19.47	+21.2%	80.0%
EUROTRANSPLANT	124,623	2009	2109	16.12	16.92	+4.96%	77.5%

* Source: Eurotransplant Internation Foundation Annual Report 2010

Table 1. Eurotransplant members; Donor/transplantation rate 2009/2010

Moreover, in 2011 this trend continues and there is an additional increase of 29.5% in the donor rate in Croatia, for the first 6 months of 2011 alone.

3. The history of Croatian deceased organ donation and transplantation system development

Croatian transplantation medicine has a long history of 40 years which has blossomed into a modern transplantation practice that successfully keeps pace with the development of all contemporary transplant surgery techniques and immunosuppressive therapy. The first kidney transplantation was performed in 1971, only 17 years after the first successful kidney transplantation in the world which occurred in 1954. The first heart transplantation in Croatia was performed in 1988, and only two years thereafter the first liver transplantation. Even as early as the 1980-ies, during the time of former Yugoslavia, the professional community felt the need to establish an umbrella organization for a transplant programme (Jugotransplant/later Crotransplant). Although for a long period of time the initial enthusiasm and development of transplant surgery techniques were not accompanied by appropriate organizational measures. Political and historical circumstances during the Homeland War (1991-1998) additionally prevented the progress and advancement of transplantation medicine during that period; all transplantation activities were brought to an almost complete halt due to moral and ethical implications. As a result, the liver transplant programme only became established as of 1998.

Originally conceived in the 1980-ies, the goal of such an "umbrella" organisation, was to provide logistical support to donor hospitals, procurement and transplantation teams, coordinate cooperation, maintain and monitor waiting lists, and carry out organ allocation in a transparent manner and in accordance with the defined criteria. The historical and political circumstances at the time (the disintegration of the former Yugoslavia and the Homeland War) did not favour such a development though. After the disintegration of Yugoslavia and the onset of Croatia's independence, the health policy searched for priorities in other areas of the health care system that had suffered the greatest losses during the war. Even so, immediately following the end of the Homeland War, there was an attempt at improving the donor rate by following the "Spanish Model". The first concrete step was taken by the adoption of the Minister's Instruction in 1998, in which the objective, measures, and manner of implementation of the Programme for Increasing the Number of Organ Donations in the Republic of Croatia were defined (Ministry of Health of the Republic of Croatia, 1998). The basic objective was to increase the organ donation and transplantation rate in the Republic of Croatia to that of other average developed European countries. The Instruction proposed the following measures for the realization of this objective:

- defining the structure (organisation) for the implementation and monitoring of the deceased donation and transplantation programmes
- organising procurement teams
- increasing diagnostic equipment availability in hospitals for determining brain death
- allotting funds for the transplantation programme
- planning and providing additional training for professionals (including training programmes regarding the psychological aspects of the family approach)

- initiating organ donation and transplantation promotion activities for public awareness
- legally recognized brain death criteria.

The gradual implementation of these measures enabled a sustained and continuous increase in cadaveric organ donations over the last 10 years. It has been followed in tandem, by an increase in the overall number of solid organ transplantations and development of new surgical techniques; in 2003 multi-organ kidney- pancreas, liver- kidney, and the transplantation of the small intestine. Additionally in 2007 Croatia became a full member of Eurotransplant and Croatian transplantation medicine has since been successfully representing a part of the integrated health care system reflective of the overall EU health system.

3.1 The condition of the organ donation and transplant program ten years ago

Only ten years ago, the professional community, political establishments, health institutions and public perceptions hit a wall. After almost 30 years of practice the transplant programme was almost completely shut down due to organ shortage. The long waiting list discouraged patients and the public. The media then reported the crushing status of Croatia's transplantation programme which when compared to similar European countries, was at the tail end of Europe, especially concerning donor rates (Fig. 2.).The future of the entire programme was at stake and the outlook was very bleak.

The lack of appropriate structure (e.g. organisation) and health administration support, coupled with faulty legislation and vague organ allocation criteria presented only some of the problems which further jeopardized the programme.

From an ethical perspective, and probably the most sensitive process of organ distribution was additionally burdened by the organ shortage, resulting in the "desperate " behaviour demonstrated by transplant centres aggressively determined to fight for the lives of "their own" patients, without taking an objective stance towards the clinical status and urgency of a possible recipient from other centres. On the other hand, the long and outdated waiting list led to frequent rejection of potential candidate patients for transplantation as being clinically unsuitable, due to their outdated or incomplete pre-transplant evaluation results. In 2000, there were approximately 900 patients on the national kidney waiting list and the average waiting time for a kidney transplant ranged between 7 and 15 years. In addition to long-term and overwhelming organ shortage, the principle frustration and weakest point moving forward at that time was the lack of appropriate central organization to comprehensively and competently manage the overall implementation and supervision of the programme.

3.2 Action taken to increase donor rate between 2000 to 2010

Since 2000, different actions have been taken on three levels which have been successfully and gradually implemented and have subsequently led to the continual increase in the donor rate in Croatia. The "key" to Croatia's success, similar as in Spain, is an integrated approach and set of initiatives designed and facilitated by the National Transplant Coordinator, to strengthen all components of the organ donation and transplantation processes; a strategy that clearly articulates jurisdiction, responsibilities and accountabilities at three levels: national, hospitals and public/individuals (Table 2.).

National level (at the Ministry of Health)
• National Transplant Coordinator appointed at the Ministry, year 2000, responsible for the National Transplant Programme planning, monitoring and implementation
• National 24 hour "duty coordination office" established at the Ministry with part-time employed Transplant Coordinators-medical students, doctors) and the following tasks:
• Keeping a National Non-donor Registry
• Keeping a National Waiting list (later assigned to Eurotransplant in 2007)
• Coordinating the donation process and providing logistical support to procurement teams and donor hospitals
• Supporting and auditing the organ allocation process (partially assigned to Eurotransplant beginning in 2007) and exchange of organs
• Keeping the Registers of Donors and Transplanted Patients (follow up)
• Processing and keeping overall data on donation and transplantation
• 2003 National Training programs for intensive care unit (ICU) doctors and hospital coordinators were launched
• 2003/04 International cooperation (exchange of livers for high urgent patients) established with Italy (Nord Italia transplant/Centro National Trapinati)
• 2004 New transplant legislation adopted
• 2006 New Financial model implemented (Reimbursement to donor hospitals)
• 2006/7 International cooperation established- Eurotransplant membership
• 2002-2010 External "audit"/inspection (Quality assurance programmes in the deceased donation process), started
• As of 2004-Procurement of hospital equipment for the purpose of diagnosing brain death / funds from the Ministry
Hospital level
• In-house transplant coordinators appointed in each hospital with ICU, and supported by the Ministry, started in year 1998
• Training Programme for Coordinators and ICU doctors, provided by the Ministry of Health (national Training Course or international Transplant Procurement Managment)
• Donor Quality Programme (donor action implemented in some hospitals as pilot project)
• Donor family psychological support /reimbursement of funeral/transport costs
Public level
• National public awareness campaign 'New Life as a Gift' launched 2005
• Since 2006, Croatia has inaugurated an official National Donor Day

• Celebration of European Donor Day (EDD);
  • Various activities aimed to increase public awareness/ every year
  • 2010 as associated partner in EU funded EDD project

• Close cooperation with patient support groups and Non-government organisation (NGO):
  • Croatian Donor Network (Donor Card)
  • Association of Transplanted Patients
  • Association of Dialysed Patients and Transplanted Patients

• Media cooperation ongoing

Table 2. Actions taken on three levels to improve donor rate

At the same time, its implementation had been strongly supported by the National Transplant Coordinator (NTC) representing the Ministry of health (i.e. health administration). Health professionals had been provided with a different kind of support in order to obtain the strategic goals - the first being primarily to increase the deceased organ donor rate. The following text describes in detail only some of the measures which have played a key role in the "phenomenon" which has occurred in the Croatian transplant programme.

4. The introduction of a key role - National Transplant Coordinator (NTC)

The introduction of the position of National Transplant Coordinator at the Ministry of Health and Social Welfare in 2000, i.e. a medical doctor full-time employed at the Ministry for the purpose of improving the transplantation system, represented a milestone and turning point in the programme. The introduction of the position of NTC precisely within the Ministry of Health and Social Welfare resulted in a solution of crucial importance for the increased number of donations and transplantations in Croatia.

The Minister at the time (as well as all Ministers thereafter, together with State Secretaries) had offered their unconditional support to the NTC, giving her "free" hands in planning and implementing measures to improve the program. Having that support, the NTC started work using all available legal instruments and the political strength of the Ministry to achieve the programme goals set forth and to introduce necessary, often "painful" changes within the health system. It is also important to point out that the existing condition of the programme was devastating and, at best described, chaotic. At that time the donor rate in major university hospitals was at an all time low, while general (county) hospitals were completely inactive. The NTC's enthusiasm, persistence, dedication and autonomy in work, and constant availability outside regular working hours had proven to be crucial in linking individuals, teams and institutions into a cooperative and harmonious whole during the initial stages of work. Such an approach encouraged the formation of a positive environment and long-term collaborative trust between professionals and the health administrations, which in the eyes of the professional community was a synonym for the "unpopular" political, rigid, slow and inefficient bureaucratic system. The wide authoritative power granted to the NTC in addition to great enthusiam and commitment of many coordinators, procurement teams, health (co)workers and individuals enabled the beginning of implementing measures following the example set forth and recommended in a European consensus document: Organ shortage: current status and strategies for improvement of organ donation (Council of Europe, 1999). By initiating close cooperation and direct communication with hospital transplant coordinators, the NTC's commitment and engagement, in tandem with the authority of the Ministry encouraged swift and efficient solutions for problems coordinators were facing, (particularly at the beginning stages of establishing the donor programme in hospitals). Simultaneously, in a dialogue with hospital managers, the NTC continued strengthening the role and authority of hospital transplant coordinators. The entire system during that period was changed by the newfound enthusiasm of many health workers as well as that of national and hospital transplant coordinator and their co-workers who worked without any financial compensation or totally inadequate financial compensation.

In close collaboration with Referral Centre for Neurovascular Disorders of The University Hospital Centre «Sestre milosrdnice», the NTC began promoting the widespread use of hospital applications (e.g. TCD and EEG) as methods used for confirming brain death. In conjunction with systematic training for the neurologists provided by the Referral Centre, the National Transplant Coordinator carried out a plan beginning in the year 2004 to acquire (TCD and EEG) hospital equipment for qualified hospital personnel. Each year selected hospitals were outfitted (by the Ministry) with the technical diagnostic equipment necessary for use in confirmation of brain death, and overall support for multi-organ and tissues explantation. Continuous improvement in education and hospital technical equipment for diagnosing brain death has been one of the measures that has enabled a 100% increase in the number of explantation centres (e.g. donor hospitals) over the last 10 years. Nowadays almost 70% of hospitals with acute beds are donor hospitals e.g. hospitals which are able to independently complete all steps of the donation process, from donor identification to its conversion into an actual/effective donor.

In 2002/2003 external audits, based on classic health inspection supervision, were performed at the five major hospitals with the aim of detecting patients' actual brain death rate occurrence and reasons for loss of donors. Inspection supervisions later grew into a form of expert-motivational supervision, which proved to be a more efficient and better accepted method of cooperation with hospitals. Upon completion of supervision followed an evaluation of rationale, corrective measures and the proposed deadline for their implementation. Such concept of supervision was based on retrospective analysis of "lost" donors, modelled after the Spanish Donor Quality Assurance Programme, the methodology of which was later described in detail in an EU project funded by the European Commission under the title DOPKI (Improving the Knowledge and Practices in Organ Donation, 2007).

It was evident that most of the hospitals were missing protocols, guidelines and criteria for each of the steps of the donation process. Very few professionals were additionally trained and skilled in communication, the family approach, or donor management at the time. Therefore, in 2002/2003 the NTC initiated preparation of new legislation along with a set of protocols and algorithms, e.g. of significant importance being donor detection and reporting the death of persons eligible as donors, that had been identified in the "Ordinance on the Reporting Procedure of the Death of Persons Eligible as Donors of Parts of the Human Body for Therapeutically Oriented Transplantation" (Ministry of Health of the Republic of Croatia, 2005).

Different training modules and programmes have been designed and launched in close collaboration with the Croatian Donor Network, panel of national experts, internationally recognised transplant managers and Non-government organisation (NGOs). Specific training modules were designed according to donor hospital objectives and combined with motivational one-day visits to the hospital. In recent years training programs were successfully extended with licensed or EU funded training modules (such as TPM, ETPOD etc.) Direct contact and visits to hospitals with training programmes adapted towards the specific problems of the hospital have remained to this day to be one of the most efficient and preferred forms of cooperation between the NTC and hospital institutions. Along with the set of protocols/ordinances and guidelines set up in regard to the donation process, the NTC had initiated the standardization of work-up protocols and criteria for admittance of patients to waiting lists; in 2005/6 , in cooperation with a panel of experts, national guidelines (Ministry of Health and Social Welfare, 2006) for kidney transplantation were prepared and a complete re-evaluation of patients on the waiting list carried out, in line with the defined standard set of tests (Ministry of Health and Social Welfare 2006). Furthermore, criteria for the organ allocation and National Waiting List management were regulated by the "Ordinance on the Criteria for the Allocation of Parts of the Human Body and the Method of Keeping the National Waiting List" (Ministry of Health, 2005).

Up until 2007, the NTC most often single-handedly organized the "round-the –clock" duty office for coordination of donor referrals, organ sharing, and procurement and transplant activities, in addition to numerous other tasks during regular working hours. Due to an employment freeze in the work force, the NTC single-handedly (with occasional short-term help from colleagues and co-workers) performed all tasks which, pursuant to the Recommendation of the Council of Europe on National Transplant Organisation (NTO), should have been under the jurisdiction of the National Transplant Organisation, i.e. an entire team of people. In 2007, the Transplantation Department was established at the Ministry as a surrogate for a National Transplant Organisation, although unfortunately, with limited scope of authority and insufficient technical capacities. Today, however, the Department has three full-time employees (a psychologist and 2 physicians) and six additional contracted transplant coordinators, mostly fifth and sixth year medical students to fulfill the required needs of maintaining a 24-hour office for referrals of potential donors, coordination and monitoring of all donation activities, and exchange of organs with Eurotransplant member countries.

The model of employment and organization of a 24-hour coordination system at the Ministry presented a big challenge for the civil service which was already stigmatized by the employment ban, non-stimulating salaries, slow administrative procedures and inability to reward its employees. Nonetheless, a successful temporary solution was found in "flexible" models of employment utilizing medical students and interns (part time contracted). The organization of the national coordination Department within the Ministry represented an economically rational substitute to contemporary NTO/agency models. At the same time, however, the work and operability of such a model (organisational unit of the Ministry) were and have been to a large extent limited by slow administrative procedures of the state administration, whose office operations, operational and technical equipment have not been suited to meet the need of a modern transplantation system (24-hour on-call duty, operational and financial interconnectivity of the entire healthcare system, swift and standardized communication, highly specific procedures, flexibility in emergencies, operative independency, appropriate authority in adopting decisions on an international level). The manner of operation of state administration and the principles of good administrative practise are in essence contrary to the principles of good "coordination" practise and consequently affect the manner of operation of national transplant organisations.

5. Network of Hospital Transplant Coordinators (HTC)

The second key element and important backbone of Croatia's organisational model is a network of in-house hospital transplant coordinators, consisting of physicians, mostly anaesthesiologists, employed full time in intensive care units in hospitals, who perform coordination in addition to their other job duties. Each acute hospital has an in-house coordinator (hospital transplant coordinator - HTC), i.e. a key donation person responsible for donor identification, management and realization of organ and tissue donation. The role of HTC has proven crucial in the early detection of each potential donor and its conversion into effective donor. Due to the complexity of the donation process in and of itself, the HTC's additional engagement was necessary outside the "routine" job duties and working hours. This included motivation, enthusiasm, training, communication and organisational skills and the creation of a positive attitude within the working community, i.e. hospitals and ICUs. The hospital in-house transplant coordinators network in Croatia consists almost exclusively of intensive care specialists (not necessarily the heads of intensive care units), whom, by the proposal of the hospital director, are appointed to the position by the Minister from the existing human resources of the hospital. Such profile of highly trained, skilled and motivated coordinators, mostly ICU doctors had proven to be another key factor for success of the donation programme in Croatia as well as in Spain (Salim et al., 2007).

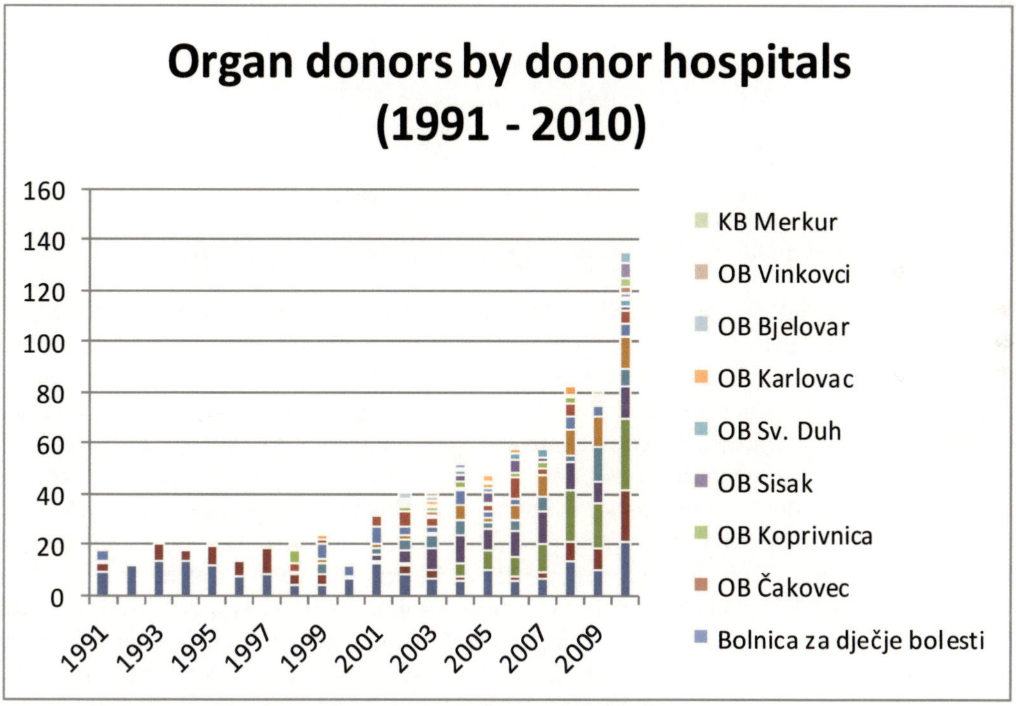

Reference: **eNTM** - http://transplantacija.mzss.hr/eNTMV2/

Fig. 9. Number of organ donors by donor hospitals (1991 – 2010)

Proof of this is particularly evident in many Croatian hospitals (Fig. 9.) (University Hospital Centre "Sestre Milosrdnice", University Hospital Centre Rijeka, Varaždin General Hospital, Sisak General Hospital, University Hospital Dubrava), which only, after appointing highly trained coordinators with professional authority, have witnessed multiple growth in donor rates.

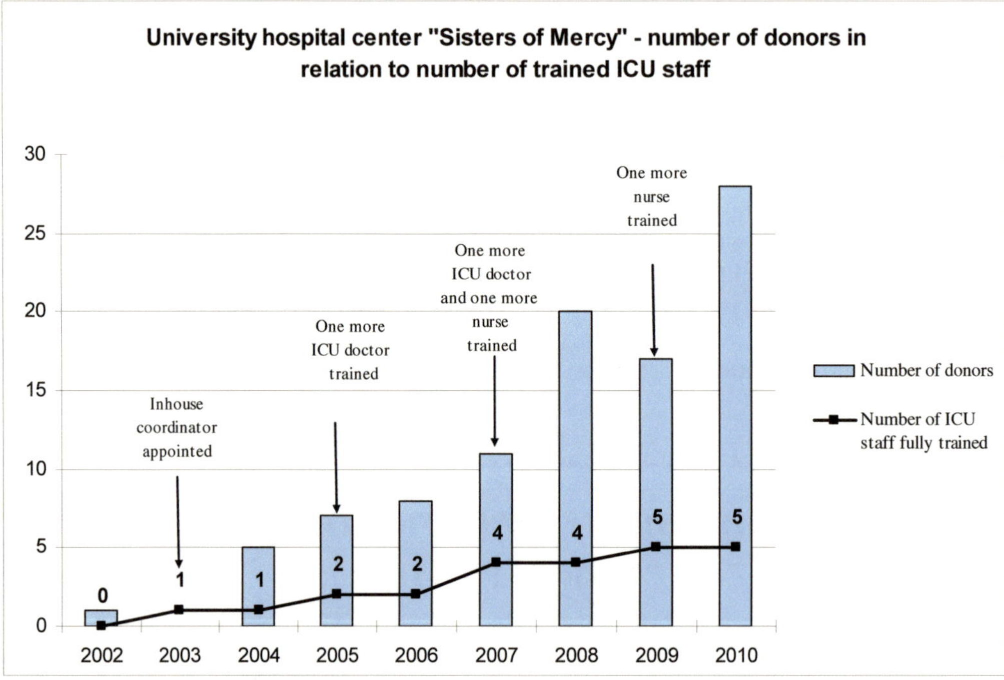

Fig. 10. Numbers of donors in University hospital centre Sestre Milosrdnice

Those highly trained hospital coordinators played a crucial role in creating a positive attitude among health care workers in intensive care units, and the implementation of good intensive care practice, i.e. care for the donor as continuation of care for the dying patient (Fig. 10.). Namely, the intensive care units staff in Croatia, like in most of countries, had and still are traditionally trained in patient care and dying patient care, but not necessarily in organ donor care. Consequently, brain death is frequently seen as a situation in which any further therapy e.g. donor maintenance is not needed. This represents the moment when the decision to continue invasive "monitoring" and therapeutic maintenance for the purpose of potential donorship, is crucial, but unfortunately in practice very often not made. (Van Gelder et al., 2008). Retrospective analysis carried out in Belgium shows that precisely such denial of therapeutic support of the dying patient is the most frequent reason for donor under detection (Van Gelder et al., 2007). The Spanish Model uses an opposite approach, which Croatia has followed and is highly successful mostly because organ donation (organ donor care) has been integrated into intensive care therapy, rather than being superimposed into it. In that way, the decision to continue of care for the dying patient (care for the purpose of organ donation), must be always made no matter what circumstances are presented by the shortage of funds or human resources. All of this reinforces the extraordinary importance of in house transplant coordinators as the key donation person responsible for the implementation of a pro-active approach, i.e. a timely detection of potential donors, clearly defined algorithms for their optimum care and unique donor treatment methodology within all intensive care units and emergency departments.

6. Financial incentives

The therapeutic promise of transplanting organs from cadaveric donors, as envisioned by the pioneers of transplantation, (Starzl, 1992) has never been realized because the demand for cadaveric organs has far exceeded the supply. In the year 2000 several possible financial incentives for deceased organ donation (such as payments, tax benefits, funeral reimbursement, and charitable contribution) were considered in the United States to determine whether any of these approaches could be used as an ethically acceptable model for a pilot trial to increase donation. The ethical methods outlined in the Table 3. (Delmonico, 2004) were developed so that they could be applied to any proposal to elucidate its propriety.

• It should preserve the concept of the organ as a donated gift • It should convey gratitude for the gift • It should not subvert or diminish the current standard of altruism • It should not be an excessive inducement that would undermine personal values and alter decision-making solely to receive the compensation • It should preserve voluntariness (e.g. so that a family member is not coerced to donate by the will of another family member solely to receive the compensation) • It should not lead to a slippery slope that fosters the sale of live human organs • It should honour the deceased (i.e. it should not dishonour the merit of an individual's life by assigning a monetary value for the individual's organs) • It should respect the sacred nature of the human body by not intruding or tampering without specific permission • It should serve the public good by maintaining the current public perception of organ donation as good • It should maintain public trust by the following: not altering patient care by premature life support withdrawal from the person who might donate and not placing transplant recipients at increased health risk by jeopardizing the integrity of the organ pool.

Table 3. Recommended characteristics of a proposal to provide financial incentives for deceased donation

Finally, a panel of experts concluded that reimbursement for funeral expenses fits within the guidelines and maintains the standards established by the ethical methods (Delmonico, L.F 2004). The importance of allotting funds for a transplant programme had already been recognized in Croatia in the late 1990-ies when the obligation to secure additional funds for the payment of the following was adopted by the Instruction of the Minister (Ministry of Health of the Republic of Croatia, 1998):

coordinator preparedness, procurement teams preparedness, preparedness of employees in centres for tissue typing, reimbursement of donor management and transplantation services costs, reimbursement of transport cost of the body of the deceased after organ donation.

Similar to the United States, reimbursement of transport cost of the body of the deceased organ donor has been implemented as the only ethically acceptable incentives on the donor side. Although there is no evidence that this kind of approach helps families to make their decision towards donation, it has been reported from HTCs that sometimes it might positively influence the family's decision. Even though such an incentive measure is definitely welcome, it does not play a crucial role in increasing donor rates. Reimbursement of donor preparation cost above the hospital budget limit, is considered to be by far the most important economic incentives (Matesanz et al, 2009). This is understandable, keeping in mind the fact that most hospitals are chronically underfunded and that financial disincentives are given at the costs of donor management and organ retrieving procedures. Furthermore, as most hospitals are neither dedicated transplant nor dialysis centres, there is no infrastructural support or financial incentive (such as removing patients off dialysis) to identify donors and procure organs.

Yet in the years preceding 2006, most donation activities in Croatia had been based on the enthusiasm and initiative of a few individuals who preformed job duties outside regular working hours and without appropriate compensation or any compensation at all. A period of eight years was required to fully implement the set of financial incentives as adopted in 1998. Nowadays transplantation procedures and donor preparation are regularly contracted and reimbursed under a special state budget item, independent of the hospital budget limits. The cost of transplantation procedures and donor preparation are reimbursed by the HZZO (Croatian Health Insurance Institute) according to the DRG (Diagnosis Related Groups) system. The amount of HRK 70,000-350,000 is reimbursed to the transplant centre depending on the complexity and type of transplantation procedure. At the same time, donor hospital receives HRK 40,000-55,000 for donor preparation and realization, depending on donor category (multiorgan, organ or tissue donor). This amount is allocated for the coordinators' extra work salary, cost of brain death diagnostics and donor evaluation tests.

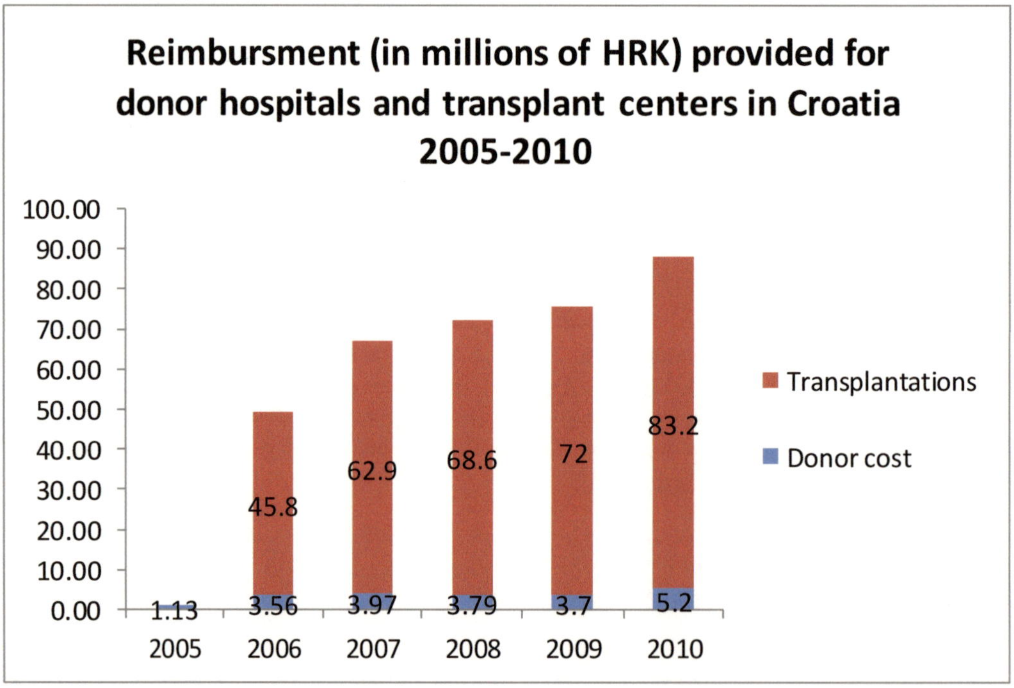

Source: HZZO report

Fig. 11. Reimbursement costs for donor hospitals and transplantation centres

7. International cooperation - Eurotransplant membership

International cooperation is recommended by the European Commission as being desirable for increasing the donor rate and harmonising the level of transplant availability among countries (European Commission June 27, 2006). Soon after 2000, due to organ shortage and the implementation of new transplant techniques it has become more evident that Croatia must find a solution for a specific group of patients (highly urgent, highly sensitised and children) and increase the chances for a timely procurement of organs for highly urgent patients and of finding a compatible organ for highly sensitized patients.

From the very beginning, Italy was considered as a good potential partner for several reasons: a neighbouring country, with developed transplantation medicine, high donor rate and the necessary organisational infrastructure, short distance, and historically based long-term cooperation and exchange of experts in the field of transplant medicine (Veneto Region and Istria and Rijeka). Underscoring the beginning of cooperation was the political significance that such regional cooperation represents, as well as unconditional support from the Italian National Transplant Organization. Following a short negotiation, a cooperation model was agreed upon which met the needs of the Croatian most endangered patient group (high urgent liver recipients). In 2004, a bilateral Agreement between the Italian National Transplant Centre and the Ministry of Health and Social Welfare of the Republic of Croatia was signed. The agreement defined the exchange of livers for high urgent patients, based on reciprocity, i.e. on "zero" balance of received and exported organs between Italy and Croatia. The cooperation resulted in a reciprocal benefit for 6 urgent patients (3 in Croatia and 3 in Italy) who received liver transplant in time to save their lives. In 2005, the extension of bilateral cooperation was discussed between an Italian and Croatian group of experts, with the aim of improving the chances for transplantation for a larger group of patients; paediatric recipients, sensitised kidney recipients, and combined transplants. Simultaneously, in light of the increasing donor rate (which presented one of the prerequisites for Eurotransplant membership), an idea arose at the Ministry for potential membership in Eurotransplant as one of the strategic goals of Croatian health policy. The feeling of historical affiliation with the West and the world view of developed counties, as well as current foreign policy efforts in Croatia's EU accession had made membership in Eurotransplant (international organization coordinating organ allocation among Austria, Germany, Slovenia, the Netherlands, Luxemburg and Belgium) one of the strategic goals of the Croatian health policy at that time. This goal, unlike many others, had from the very beginning been wholeheartedly supported by the professional community and the general public. The reason could be explained by the fact that Eurotransplant has a reputation of being one of the most prestigious international organizations with a long running tradition and expertise in organ allocation based mostly on the HLA match (of kidney allocation) and other well defined criteria. Namely, ethical dilemmas and a primary concern of the public had always focused on how to provide equal access and secure fair distribution of organs. Croatia, at that time, with its existing allocation system could hardly guarantee such high autonomy and consistency as a politically independent, international organisation, whose core business centered around an IT program for organ allocation. In 2006 Croatia became a Eurotransplant candidate member, and one year later a full Eurotransplant member. It was one of the recent accomplishments that positively influenced Croatia's National Transplant System resulting in quality improvements on several different levels; first of all the lack of a "traditional" central organization (in regards to sharing offices) was successfully overcome –

Eurotransplant membership gave Croatia a more transparent, objective, efficient and firmly structured system of organ distribution. Today, precisely this segment, which is the most sensitive towards the public, represents the most important reference and anti-corruption measure which guarantees transparency and focuses on maintaining long-term trust of the public and donor families in the health system.

Besides improving the allocation system, Eurotransplant membership had an indirect "motivational" effect on the professional community, and HTCs in particular. Namely, the loss, i.e. rejection of "marginal" organs as unacceptable or even rejection of good quality organs, used to be a "privilege" of our transplant centres, which often resulted in revolt and dissatisfaction of hospital transplant coordinators. In what was no doubt an attempt to find "ideal" organs for their recipients, transplant teams often rejected marginal organs, as unacceptable, even in times of organ shortage. Upon joining Eurotransplant, this practice as a result from a "monopolistic" position and lack of competition (in cases where only one TX centre existed) and a lack of any kind of supervision over ethical justification of such decisions, almost completely disappeared. Today, the acceptance and utilization of organs by Croatian donors fits into the Eurotransplant average (Table 4.) providing additional enthusiasm and representing an indirect incentive measure to all those caring for the donor.

KIDNEYS (2010)				
	ET	ET (%)	Croatia	Croatia (%)
Reported	4261	100 %	268	100 %
Offered	4182	98.1 %	263	98.1 %
Accepted	3925	92.1 %	246	91.8 %
Transplanted	3737	87.7 %	232	86.6 %
HEARTS (2010)				
	ET	ET (%)	Croatia	Croatia (%)
Reported	946	100 %	41	100 %
Offered	938	99.2 %	40	97.6 %
Accepted	750	79.3 %	35	85.4 %
Transplanted	631	66.7 %	33	80.5 %
LIVERS (2010)				
	ET	ET (%)	Croatia	Croatia (%)
Reported	1998	100 %	126	100 %
Offered	1996	99.9 %	126	100 %
Accepted	1955	97.8 %	125	99.2 %
Transplanted	1670	83.6 %	107	84.9 %
PANCREAS (2010)				
	ET	ET (%)	Croatia	Croatia (%)
Reported	944	100 %	38	100 %
Offered	920	97.5 %	38	100 %
Accepted	573	60.7 %	17	44.7 %
Transplanted	273	28.9 %	8	21.1 %

(ET Annual report 2010)

Table 4. Organ loss in 2010 – Eurotransplant avarage (ET) versus Croatia

Furthermore, in the field of immunogenetics, Croatia has made huge strides and significant progress in quality improvement, since this was an extremely important Eurotransplant requirement relating to the allocation criteria based on HLA matching.

Specifically, accreditation issued by the European Federation of Immunogenetics (EFI) for at least one laboratory for tissue typing was one of several prerequisites for ET full membership. The Tissue Typing Institute of the University Hospital Centre Zagreb, as the reference tissue typing centre met the requirement in May 2007, thus becoming the first Croatian medical laboratory with European accreditation. The tissue typing lab in Rijeka, although founded back in 1969, did not meet accreditation standards due to a lack of space, staff and methodological work standards. However, over the course of the next two years, and with financial and administrative support from the Ministry, the laboratory was successfully adapted, and finally met the accreditation criteria in September 2008. Currently it is the only EFI accredited centre for tissue typing in Croatia other than Zagreb.

High standards of immunogenetic testing are also required by specific Eurotransplant programmes, such as the "acceptable mismatch (AM) programme" intended for highly sensitized patients (PRA <85%). The programme offers a unique approach to the problem of highly immunized patients and significantly increases their otherwise slim chances of finding an appropriate kidney. It requires an extensive immunogenetic work-up which defines all HLA alleles for which HLA antibodies have not been created. In the case of an offered organ with precisely these antigens, the organ has to be primarily allocated to a patient from the AM programme.

There are numerous other benefits derived from Eurotransplant membership, such as a group of "high urgent" patients whose chances of a timely receipt of organs have been dramatically increased by ET membership.

8. Legislation

There are several legislative options for regulating organ donation and transplantation. Presumed consent represents one of the strategies aimed towards increasing cadaveric organ donation. In countries with presumed consent, citizens' organs are procured after their death, unless a person has specifically requested to be a non-donor. Advocates of the presumed consent approach might say that it is every person's civic duty to donate their organs once they no longer need them (i.e. after death) to those who do. People against presumed consent would argue that to implement this policy, the general public would have to be educated and well informed about organ donation, which would be difficult to adequately achieve (Hill DJ, Palmer TC, Evans DW 1999). Such presumed consent, also known as the opt-out system, is applied in over 20 European countries (Horvat, 2010). Croatia, alongside Spain, Belgium, Austria and Portugal, belongs to the group of European countries with presumed consent and the highest rate of cadaveric donors. In Croatia presumed consent has been implemented since 1988, based on the presumption of high social responsibility, transplant awareness and solidarity of our citizens and through today has remained a constant and basic value of our transplantation legislation. The new “Act on Explantation and Transplantation of Human Body Parts for Medical Treatment Purposes” (Official Gazette 177/204), adopted in 2004 together with a series of implementing by-laws, defined in detail the ethical, professional and organisational standards for organ explantation and transplantation in accordance with the most recent European Guidelines /Recommendations and Convention (*Guide to safety and quality assurance for organs, tissues and cells/ Biomedicine Convention*). The modern legal framework was one of the prerequisites for accession to Eurotransplant and the European Union. With the amendments to the Act in 2009, the Croatian legislative framework was successfully harmonised with the EU tissues and cells directives (Directive 2004/23/EU, Directive 2006/86/EU, Directive 2006/17/EU) and the benchmarks from the negotiation Chapter 28 (Consumer Health and Protection) have been successfully fulfilled (*Government of the Republic of Croatia, January 2011*). In July 2010, the EU adopted the Directive 2010/53/EU on standards of quality and safety of human organs intended for transplantation, binding all member states, and Croatia, to harmonise their national legislation with the Directive by July 2012 at the latest. Currently, the only major shortcoming of our legislation is the lack of provisions on organ donation after cardiac death. For this reason, harvesting organs from non-heart beating donors is not possible. Donation after cardiac death (DCD) constitutes a large share of the donor pool in countries such as the Netherlands (over 40% of cadaveric donors) (Moers et al, 2010), and in the United Kingdom (about 35% of the donors), whereas in Spain DCD accounts for only 5% of the share of cadaveric donors, mostly based on Maastricht type I and II. (Matesanz et al, 2009).

9. Regional cooperation and leadership in South Eastern Europe

Transplantation medicine in most South East European countries is still nonetheless presently very underdeveloped. Little data are available and few transplants are being performed when compared to other European Union countries. Meanwhile, Croatia has made a huge step forward in the last decade while other countries in the region lack the organisation and internal infrastructure necessary to support such high level programmes. Dissemination of successful Croatian strategies and acquired experience could be essential in supporting other South Eastern European (SEE) countries in the development of a deceased organ donation and transplantation program as one of the prerequisites for furthering health and socioeconomic progress in the region. SEE Health Network (SEEHN) (institutional forum set up in 2001 under the patronage of the WHO Regional office for Europe), supplied a political and legislative framework for the designation of several regional health centres, each of them specifically focusing on some public health field. In February 2011, the Republic of Croatia was officially inaugurated as the SEEHN Regional Health Development Centre on Organ Donation and Transplant Medicine, aiming to support the development of an efficient system of organ donation and transplantation in South Eastern European countries through long-term cooperation. At the 1st RHDC meeting held in Zagreb, the role, objectives, functions and collaborative partners of the newly designated RHDC were presented. National focal points (NFPs) were introduced as the RHDC liaison persons representing national health authorities of SEE Health Network region countries (Albania, Bosnia and Herzegovina, Bulgaria, the Republic of Croatia, the Republic of Moldova, the Republic of Montenegro, Romania, the Republic of Serbia, and the FYR (Former Yugoslav Republic of Macedonia). NFP's committed to start regional cooperation in the field of organ donation and transplantation medicine.

10. Conclusions

Croatia is one of the few world countries which, with relatively modest funds, has managed to reach the top ranks of the world with its transplant programme. The Croatian Model as authored by Dr. Mirela Busic incorporates successful integration of different elements of the

„best" European practices (the Spanish coordination model, the Eurotransplant allocation system, etc.) in the context of political and socio-economic circumstances of the Croatian health system (which had been severely burdened by war devastation and a post-socialist heritage). Sustainable increase in the donor rate can be attributed to the integrated and methodological approach in conjunction with a set of incentive measures, whose implementation was led by the NTC, always acting in support of the donation process as a whole and with the health professionals involved in organ donation and transplantation. Simultaneously, with the sustained development of the well structured and transparent system, enthusiasm, trust, and team work grew, while the ever present resistance, mistrust and prejudice gradually disappeared. The donation and transplantation programme in Croatia successfully linked institutions, individuals and health workers. Numerous benefits of the transplantation programme's success are reflected daily throughout the health system, in the eyes of the public, within politics, but most especially in the satisfaction of patients whose hopes and chances for a new life grow by the each day.

11. Acknowledgment

I would like to acknowledge and thank collegues and co-workers Dr. Martina Anušić-Juričić, Branka Malnar-Grubišić, Ivan Svaguša, Ivona Biškup, Ante Vulić and Lydia Raley for the techical support in the preparation of the text and data. I would also like to thank all other collegues, coworkers and collaborators involved in organ donation and transplantation activities including medical students, hospital coordinators, ICU staff, transplant teams, tissue typing staff, neurologists, radiologists, NGO's and all those who have made this possible.

12. References

Council of Europe (1999). Consensus document; Organ Shortage: Current Status and Strategies for Improvement of Organ Donation - A European Consensus, «Meeting The Organ Shortage» Editorial NEFROLOGÍA. Vol. XIX. Supl. 4. 1999. In: *Council of Europe website*, Accessed: December 20, 2010, Available from: <http://www.coe.int/t/e/social_cohesion/health/Activities/Organ_transplantation>

Council of Europe (2010). International Figures on Organ Donation and Transplantation 2010, *Newsletter Transplant,* Vol. 15, No. 1, In: *Organización Nacional de Trasplantes website,* Accessed: January 22, 2010, Available from: http://www.ont.es/publicaciones/Documents/Newsletter2010.pdf

Delmonico, LF. (2004) Financial Incentives for Organ Donation. Available from Medscape Transplantation > Overcoming Barriers to the Organ Donation Crisis Expert Column Series Posted: 01/07/2004

European Parliament, Council. Directive 2010/53/EU of the European Parliament and of the Council of 7 July 2010 on standards of quality and safety of human organs intended for transplantation. Official Journal of the European Union L 207, *Vol. 53, (August 6, 2008), pp.(14-29), ISSN 1725-2555, In:* Eur-lex website, Accessed: January 12, 2011, Available from: http://eur lex.europa.eu/LexUriServ/LexUriServ.do?uri=CELEX:32010L0053:EN:NOT

Eurotransplant International Foundation, Preliminary monthly statistics, In: *Eurotransplant website,* Accessed: February 1, 2010, Available from: <http://www.eurotransplant.org/files/statistics/2010_january1_december31.pdf>

Government of the Republic of Croatia (January 2011). Report on the Progress of Croatia's EU Accession Negotiations under the Swedish EU Council Presidency (1 July to 31 December 2009), In: *Croatian Parliament website,* Accessed: January 22, 2011, Available from: < http://www.sabor.hr/fgs.axd?id=15551>

Hill, D.J., Palmer, T.C. &Evans, D.W. (1999). Presumed Consent. If this is Introduced, People will have to have all Relevant Information. *British Medical Journal,* Vol. 318, No. 7196, pp. 1490-1490, ISSN: 0959-8138

Horvat, LD, Cuerden, MS, Kim, SJ, Koval, JJ, Young, A & Garg, AX. (2010). Informing the Debate: Rates of Kidney Transplantation in Nations with Presumed Conset. *Annals of Internal Medicine,* Vol. 153, No. 10, pp. 641-650, ISSN: 0003-4819

Hou, S. (2000). Expanding the Donor Pool: Ethical and Medical Considerations. *Kidney Int.* Vol. 58, No. 4., pp. 1820-36, ISSN: 0085-2538

Matesanz, R. & Dominguez-Gil, B. (2007). Strategies to Optimize Deceased Organ Donation. *Transplantation Reviews,* Vol. 21, No. 4, pp. 177-188, ISSN 0955-470x

Matesanz, R. & Miranda, B. (2002). A Decade of Continuous Improvement in Cadaveric Organ Donation: the Spanish Model. *J Nephrol,* Vol. 15, No. 1, pp. 22-28, ISSN 1121-8428

Matesanz, R., Marazuela, R., Dominguez-Gil, B., Coll, E., Mahillo, B. & de la Rosa, G. (2009). The 40 Donors per Million Population Plan: an Action Plan for Improvement of Organ Donation and Transplantation in Spain. *Transplantation Proceedings,* Vol. 41, No. 8, pp. 3453-3456, ISSN 0041-1345

Meeting the Organ Shortage: Current Status and Strategies for Improvement of Organ Donation. A European Consensus Document Council of Europe Website: http://www.coe.int/t/e/social_cohesion/health/Activities/Organ_transplantation Accessed:20.12.2010.

Ministry of Health of the Republic of Croatia. (1998). Instruction on the Implementation of the Organ Explantation Programme (Naputak o provođenju Programa za eksplantaciju organa). *Official Gazette (Narodne novine),* No. 75/98

Ministry of Health of the Republic of Croatia. (2005). Ordinance on the Reporting Procedure of the Death of Persons Eligible as Donors of Parts of the Human Body for Therapeutically Oriented Transplantation (*Official Gazette (Narodne novine),* No. 152/2005

Ministry of Health of the Republic of Croatia. (2005). Ordinance on the Criteria for the Allocation of Parts of the Human Body and the Method of Keeping the National Waiting List (*Official Gazette (Narodne novine),* No. 152/2005,84/07)

Moers, C., Leuevnik, H.G.D. & Ploeg, R.J., (2010). Donation after Cardiac Death: Evaluation of Revisiting an Important Donor Source, *Nephrology Dialysis Transplantation,* Vol. 25, No. 3, pp. 666-673., ISSN: 0931-0509

Salim, A., Brown, C., Inaba, K., Mascarenhas, A., Hadjizacharia, P., Pee, P., Belzberg, H. &, Demetriades, D. (2007). Improving Consent Rates for Organ Donation : the Effect of an Inhouse Coordinator Program. *The Journal of Trauma,* Vol. 62, No. 6, pp. 1411-1415, ISSN: 0022-5282

Starzl TE. (1992) The Puzzle People: Memoirs of a Transplant Surgeon. Pittsburgh: University of Pittsburgh Press: 147. ISBN: 0-8229-3714-X

Van Gelder, F., de Roey, J., Desschans, B., Van Hees, D., Aerts, R., Monbaliu, D., De Pauw, L., Coosemans, W. & Pirenne, J. (2008) What is the Limiting Factor for Organ Procurement in Belgium: Donation or Detection? What can be Done to Improve Organ Procurement Rates? *Acta Chir Belgica.* Vol. 108, No. 1, pp. 27-30, ISSN 0001-5458

5

Doctors' Attitudes Towards Opting-Out and the Implication of This Legislation for a Small Island State

Mary Anne Lauri
Department of Psychology, University of Malta, Malta

1. Introduction

The debate on whether to introduce the opting-out system is complex and involves various ethical, philosophical, psychological and legal issues. Different answers are given to questions such as "Who owns the body of the dead person? Does the State own the body of the deceased person or does the body belong to the next of kin? Should the decision whether or not to donate the organs of a dead relative be taken by the State? How informed are people about opting-out? If persons are not aware of the system, would the organs still be taken even when relatives are against opting-out?" Because there is no consensus regarding these and other questions, some sections of society and groups may present resistance to introducing the system. On the other hand, doctors' associations as well as other lobby groups argue that organs should not go to waste and agree with State intervention to retrieve more organs through the introduction of opting-out. The question asked by those in favour of opting-out is "How fair is it for thousands of people to keep on waiting for an organ transplant, when it is possible to reduce these numbers drastically by legislation?" This is the problem facing policy makers. Should the state try to encourage and facilitate a gradual change in public opinion towards opting-out or should legislation on presumed consent be introduced?

2. Legislation on organ retrieval

Different countries have different legislation on the retrieval of organs. The main two legislative frameworks are "informed consent" also known as the "opting-in system" and the other is "presumed consent", also referred to as the "opting-out system". There are variations in practice in both the opting-in as well as the opting-out system.

Opting-in, sometimes known as explicit consent requires that the individual authorises organ removal after death by for example carrying a donor card or joining a national registry (Organ Donation Taskforce, 2008). In many countries organs can be retrieved from the dead body only if permission from the family of the deceased is given. Even the presence of a donor card signed by the deceased does not give the doctors a right to remove organs from the body unless there is consent from the nearest relative. 'Nearest relative', according to the guidelines issued by the Medical Ethics Department of the British Medical Association in 2009 is defined, in order of priority, as an adult who is the deceased person's spouse or civil partner, partner living with the adult in a meaningful relationship for at least six months, child, parent, brother or sister, grandparent, grandchild, uncle or aunt, cousin, niece or nephew or friend of long-standing (British Medical Association Ethics, 2009).

In some states in the USA there is a system similar to the opting-in system with the provision that it is mandatory for medics to ask the family of the injured person whether they are willing to donate the organs before a life-support machine is switched off (Hamilton, 2003). This is known as the "required request" policy. It states that it is irresponsible as well as illegal to disconnect a ventilator from an individual who is declared dead following brain stem testing without first making proper enquiry as to the possibility of that individual's tissues and organs being used for the purposes of transplantation (Uniform Anatomical Gift Act, 1987).

The opting-out system on the other hand allows, indeed requires, doctors to take organs from the dead body if they can be used for transplantation purposes without necessarily having the permission of the family. The only restriction is that in cases where the deceased had indicated when alive his or her wish not to donate organs, doctors must respect these wishes. Countries which have introduced the opting-out system of organ retrieval include France, Italy, Belgium, Finland and Portugal. Some, like Austria have a strong/hard approach whilst others, such as Spain have a weak/soft approach. The difference between these two approaches and practices of opting-out is that the latter is more sensitive to the needs of the victim and his or her family (Organ Donation Taskforce, 2008).

Both the opting-in and the opting-out systems have their advantages and shortcomings. There is no unanimous agreement about the best legislation and code of practice. Table 1 summarises the main advantages and disadvantages of both systems.

	Opting-out system	Opting-in system
Advantages	Reduces waiting list for cadaveric organs	Altruism is encouraged
	Relieves relatives of making the difficult decision themselves	Relatives are not coerced into donating if they are unwilling to do so
	Organs do not go to waste	Relatives feel that they are doing a good deed voluntarily
Disadvantages	Could be traumatic for family members of the cadaver when they are in disagreement	Difficult for doctors to approach family when their loved one is dying or has just died
	The sense of altruism of voluntary donation is lost	Traumatised families might refuse to donate
	Doctors and other medical professionals could be perceived as insensitive fostering a lack of trust in them	Many organs go to waste and transplant opportunities are missed
	Not everyone might know when alive that there is presumed consent and might not make it known to the relevant authorities if they are against giving their organs	The family may not know the views on organ donation of their dead relative and so might find it difficult to say yes for fear of being disrespectful

Table 1. Advantages and Disadvantages of the opting-in and the opting-out

3. Is opting-out the solution?

There are various studies which indicate that introducing the opting-out system increases the number of donations (Gnant et al., 1991; Low, 2006; Rithalia et al., 2009; Roels et al., 1991; Soh & Lim, 1992). Table 2 gives the top ten countries in Europe with the highest donations and transplants per 1 million population and indicates whether they practice opting-in or opting-out in their country. Ireland is the only country out of the top ten who have the opting-in system (Europe for Patients, 2010). When this data was collected, Malta was not included in the study. The number of organs retrieved in Malta varies depending on the year and the number of accidents that take place during that year. Being a small country, the number of organs donated fluctuates between 47 pmp to 137 pmp. This is clearly above the EU average of 17.8 per million population.

Country	Donation rates per million population (1 pmp)	Opting-in or opting-out policies
Spain	33.8	Opting-out
Belgium	27.1	Opting-out
France	23.2	Opting-out
Ireland	**22.7**	**Opting-in**
Italy	21.3	Opting-out
Finland	21.0	Opting-out
Portugal	20.1	Opting-out
Austria	18.8	Opting-out
Czech Republic	18.8	Opting-out
Latvia	18.7	Opting-out

Source: Council of Europe (2007). Deceased organ donors in the European Union.

Table 2. Donation rates in the top ten countries in Europe per million population (pmp)

Several factors besides legislation may influence the number of donors per capita. Some of these factors include mortality from road traffic accidents (Coppen et al., 2005), advancement in medical technology, neurosurgical practice and paramedical care (The Parliamentary Office of Science and Technology, 2004), lack of 'transplant culture' (The Parliamentary Office of Science and Technology, 2004), family involvement (Transplant Committee of the Council of Europe, 2007), the legislative framework (English, 2007; Wright, 2007), religion and religious beliefs (Gimbel et al., 2003; Rumsey et al., 2003), the efficiency of a country's transplant co-ordination (Johnson & Goldstein, 2004); GPD and health expenditure per capita (Healy, 2005), awareness of organ donation (Oz et al., 2003), blood donation rate (Abadie & Gay, 2006), knowledge of someone who had donated an organ after death and awareness of any one who received a donated organ (Rumsey et al., 2003), education (Gimbel et al., 2003), and attitudes towards organ donation and presumed consent (Roels et al., 1997).

The impact of presumed consent legislation on cadaveric donation was studied for a 10 year period in 22 countries by Abadie and Gay (2006). The researchers found that while differences in other determinants of organ donation explain much of the variation in donation rates, after controlling for those determinants, presumed consent legislation has a positive and sizeable effect on organ donation rates. Similar conclusions were obtained by other studies. Rithalia et al. (2009) surveyed results of various studies carried out on the impact or presumed consent on donation rates in various countries with and without presumed consent and concluded that presumed consent alone is unlikely to explain the variation in organ donation rates between countries and that there must be other factors which may play a part even though their relative importance is unclear. There were a few studies which did not find a statistically significant relationship between presumed consent legislation and increase in the number of donors pmp in countries who had introduced presumed consent (eg. Coppen et al., 2005; Healy, 2005).

4. Attitudes towards opting-out

There are many studies investigating attitudes of people towards organ donation and towards opting-out. Surveys carried out in the UK before 2000 report low levels of support ranging from 28% to 57%. However a more recent survey carried out by YouGov in 2007 reported 64% of respondents supported opting-out. Another survey carried out in Scotland in 2004 showed that 53% of the participants did not agree with opting-out and 74% of the respondents agreed that the wishes of relatives should be considered before doctors are automatically allowed to take organs for transplantation (Haddow, 2006). In Malta the level of support for opting-out is even lower and only 22% agreed with this way of procuring organs in 2006. A further 20% said that they were unsure but tended towards being in favour (Lauri, 2006). In another study carried out in Spain in the 2003, only 24% of the participants agreed with the law of presumed consent. Indeed 53% considered that taking the organs without the family's permission was an abuse of authority (Conesa et al., 2003). This study was carried out after the law of opting-out had been introduced. Similarly in Belgium, a survey was carried out ten years after the introduction of presumed consent. In this country, the majority of the respondents were in favour of presumed consent however 44 % of the respondents still believed that the decision about the removal of their own organs after death should be taken by themselves only (Roels et al., 1997). In America, yet another study showed that 72% were opposed to the opting-out system (Klenow & Youngs, 1995) while in another study among actual donors, only 24% favoured a presumed consent law with an opting-out provision (Rodrigue et al., 2006). These and other studies carried out in various countries show that the level of agreement with opting-out varies. Variations in attitudes between surveys may reflect differences in methods and phrasing of questions and this has to be taken into consideration when taking policy decisions (Organ Donation Taskforce, 2008, p. 10.) However a pattern can be observed. It seems that many people are in favour of organ donation but have reservations about opting-out.

There are fewer studies which investigate the attitudes of doctors towards opting-out. Prottas and Batten (1988) found that physicians showed serious hesitation about dealing with donor families. However, in a more recent study by Schaeffner et al. (2004), researchers found that health professionals with a higher level of medical education are more likely to hold an organ donor card and also feel more comfortable in approaching relatives of potential organ donors. A study carried out by Persson et al. (1998) found that the majority of physicians in their study said that they would be willing to donate their own organs after their death but disagreed with the idea of using organs from a dead person who had a negative opinion towards organ donation. The British Medical Association which represents the majority of doctors in the UK, supports a system of soft presumed consent, with safeguards, for organ donation by deceased people over the age of 16. The association claims that in this system, relatives' views would always be taken into account (British Medical Association, 2008). They argued that having organ donation as the default position would relieve relatives from the burden of decision-making. They also point out that legislation would encourage a more positive view of the process (Organ Donation Taskforce, 2008, p. 16). This was not borne out by the studies carried out by Conesa et al. (2003) in Spain and by Roels et al. (1997) in Belgium years after the introduction of the presumed consent legislation.

The Royal College of Surgeons, the British Transplant Society and the Royal College of Pathologists have also declared their support for a system of presumed consent (British Medical Association, 2008). A survey carried out by the International Society for Heart and Lung Transplantation (ISHLT) in 2002 showed that 74% of the healthcare professionals who participated in the study and who came from 15 countries, agreed with the introduction of presumed consent however only 39% agreed that presumed consent was the single most effective way to increase organ donation. More than half of the respondents believed that donation rates could also be improved by other interventions. These included indirect compensation, better awareness and more education on organ donation among the general public, having more medical staff to talk with families and building a rapport with them and legally binding donor cards (Oz et al., 2003).

5. Reservations about opting-out

One reservation related to the introduction of opting-out is the argument of whether persons have a right over their body. Those who believe that they own their bodies and that this right is transferred to the next of kin upon one's death, argue that the State has no right to remove organs from a dead person without having the family's consent or a living will stating that the person wants to donate his or her organs (Wintor, 2008). People may have different social representations of organ donation and ownership of the body. Those who believe in an afterlife may fear that donating organs could interfere with this process (Lauri, 2009). There are others however who believe that ownership of organs rests with the State. These believe that it right and just for the State to delegate its authority to the hospital and transplant team so that these can authorize the removal of organs from dead persons and give them to patients in need of a transplant (Farrugia, 2000). Patients, they argue, should not depend on the generosity of others. Other arguments put forward by those against opting-out is the definition of brain death (Hill et al., 1999) the potential loss of choice and autonomy (Lawson, 2008) and ethical implications involved (Bell, 2006).

The difference in opinion on whether or not to introduce the opting-out system exists among the general public as well as the professionals and authorities. A quick look at the on-line comments posted on January 14 by readers of the English newspaper The Times, in answer to the article written by the then Prime Minister Gordon Brown, shows that some readers did believe that in the context of long waiting lists for organ transplants, legislation should intervene in order to save the lives of people waiting for a transplant. However, many of the readers' letters showed how talk about the opting-out system can revive the fears surrounding organ donation. Readers wrote about 'mutilated', 'violated', and 'incomplete' bodies. One reader exclaimed 'Over my dead body!', describing the system as 'corpse robbing' and used the terms 'evil', 'ungodly', and 'repugnant'. But perhaps of more concern are the objections raised by those who, in principle, are in favour of organ donation. One such person wrote that 'If people want to give the gift of life, that is their right, but it must be something that is voluntary'. Another insisted that organ donation should be an 'active choice' and another wrote that, instead of forcing the issue through legislation, the Prime Minister should be 'educating people and using a campaign to donate organs' (Webster, 2008).

This paper will contribute to the debate on opting-out by investigating the attitudes of a sample of 151 Maltese doctors towards opting-out obtained by using an on-line survey. In the second part of the paper the data collected through interviews with five doctors who are directly involved in organ donation are reported.

6. The Maltese context

Malta is a small island in the Mediterranean with a population of about 400,000 people. The National Health System is free in Malta. However many families opt to have a family doctor whom they pay for every visit. It is not rare that the family doctor often lives in the town or village of his patients and knows the families well. Neither is it uncommon for the same doctor to look after two and sometimes three generations of the same family. The family doctor is possibly the most trusted person by the family, with the parish priest being a close second. For this reason, knowing the attitudes of doctors towards the introduction of opting-out is important. Doctors are opinion leaders.

In Malta, there is one hospital which carries out organ transplants. Organs are retrieved mainly from cadaveric donors through the opting-in system. Doctors working in Intensive Care report that the rate of refusal is low. Organs transplanted in Malta are kidneys, hearts and corneas. On average, eight kidney transplants and one heart transplant are performed every year. Currently, the number of people on the waiting list for a kidney or heart transplant is 81 (P. Calleja, personal communication, August 9, 2011).

Since doctors are not requested to record the number of refusals, there is no way of knowing how many families refuse to donate. In an earlier study carried out in Malta, doctors and medical professionals concur that the number of families who refuse to donate is low (Lauri, 2008). In spite of the fact that the number of transplants has steadily increased over the years, the problem of organ shortage is still present. The question whether we should be considering the introduction of opting-out is therefore pertinent.

7. The survey

This paper investigates the attitudes of Maltese doctors towards opting-out through a questionnaire administered in June 2011. Doctors' Associations were approached and asked to send the link to an anonymous on-line questionnaire to their members. There are 1707 registered doctors in Malta (Malta Medical Council, 2010). One hundred and fifty-eight respondents answered the questionnaire six questionnaires had incomplete information. Table 3 gives the ages and gender of the respondents. The questionnaire was made up of seven questions. Question 1 asked doctors whether they agree or disagree with the introduction of opting-out in Malta. Questions 2 and 3 asked for reasons why they agreed or disagreed with the introduction of this legislation. Question 4 asked for their opinion why people sometimes refuse to give the organs of their dead relatives while question 5 was an open-ended question asking the respondents for adjectives they would use to describe 'opting-out'. Questions 6 and 7 asked for the gender and age of participants.

Age	Male	Female	Total
21-30	28	31	59
31-40	16	16	32
41-50	21	15	36
51-60	9	4	13
Over 60	11	0	11
			152

Table 3. Gender and age of respondents

8. Results

Results show that two-thirds of the respondents are in favour of opting-out. Younger doctors in the 21-31 age bracket were more in favour of introducing opting out than older doctors and female doctors were more in favour than male doctors. The association between age and being in favour or against introducing opting-out in Malta was significant (Chi-square=12.3, df=4, p=0.02). Respondents between the ages of 21 and 40 were more in favour of opting out while those over 50 were more against it.

Age	Percentage of respondents who were in favour		Percentage of respondents who were against		Total	
	Male	Female	Male	Female	Male	Female
21-30	15.9	12.6	2.6	7.9	18.5	20.5
31-40	9.3	7.3	1.3	3.3	10.6	10.6
41-50	7.9	6.6	6.0	3.3	13.9	9.9
51-60	2.0	1.3	4.0	1.3	6.0	2.6
Over 60	2.6	0.0	4.6	0.0	7.3	0.0

Table 4. Attitudes of male and female doctors on opting-out

Table 5 gives the three most common reasons given by respondents for being in favour or against opting out. Other reasons given for being in favour were that many people, even if in favour of organ donation, because of laziness or apathy never get around to applying for the card or expressing their wishes. Another reason given is that people who are actually in favour of donating their organs do not carry a donor card or register their names because they are superstitious and believe that they would be tempting faith if they do so (Lauri, 2009).

Other reasons given for being against opting-out are that such a system will hurt the family of the dead person, that Maltese culture does not favour such as system and that no one has the right to dissect a person's body without his or her explicit consent or those of the family.

		Reasons	Percentage of respondents
In Favour	1.	Organs do not go to waste	42.4 %
	2.	Family will not have to take difficult decision	39.7 %
	3.	Reduces waiting list for transplants	32.5 %
Against	1.	Cadaver does not belong to the state	19.9 %
	2.	Should encourage altruism not coercion	19.9 %
	3.	Patients may come to distrust doctors	11.9 %

Table 5. Reasons for being in favour or against opting-out

There were no significant associations between age or gender and those who gave reason 1-3 in favour of introducing opting-out. In the case of those against, there were no significant association for reason 1 however there were significant associations between age and reason 2 (chisq=16.9, df=4, p=0.002) and age and reason 3 (chisq=12.2, df=4, p=0.02), with older doctors mentioning these two reasons more frequently than the younger ones. There were no significant associations between gender and the three reasons given against opting-out.

These results support those given in the next question. Respondents were asked to describe opting-out using adjectives. A Multiple Correspondence Analysis (MCA) of the four variables (i) agreement or disagreement with opting-out, (ii) gender, (iii) age, and (iv) adjectives used to describe opting-out was carried out.

Some of the adjectives were synonyms and conveyed the same meaning. These were grouped together as shown below. Besides synonyms, some adjectives were placed in a particular group because they conveyed the same concept. For example the group of adjectives 'sensible, logical, rational, makes sense, proactive, practical, convenient' are describing opting-out from a rational, logical perspective as opposed to for example the group 'altruistic, act of generosity, benevolent, benefit for others, unselfish' which describe it from an altruistic point of view. Following are the groups of adjectives used to describe opting-out. The eleven adjectives in bold were the categories of the variable 'adjectives' which was used in the MCA.

The first five groups of adjectives used to describe opting-out in a positive light are:

- **Good**, pro-socoal, positive, fairly good idea, very good , important
- **Fair**, beneficial
- **Necessary**, essential
- **Sensible**, logical, rational, makes sense, proactive, practical, convenient
- **Altruistic**, act of generosity, benevolent, benefit for others, unselfish

Adjectives used to describe opting-out in a negative light included

- **Unethical**, immoral
- **Insensitive**, disrespectful
- **Coercive**, dictatorial, forced
- **Bad**, not the right approach
- **Arrogant**, egoistic, take advantage
- **Unnecessary**, not reasonable

In order to obtain a multivariate picture of the four variables YES/NO (agreement and disagreement with opting-out), GENDER, AGE, ADJECTIVES and their possible interactions, the MCA carried out, using SPSS Version 19, was used to extract two dimensions which between them accounted for 88% of the sample's variability on these four variables. Figure 1 shows a plot of the categories defined by the four variables against the two dimensions.

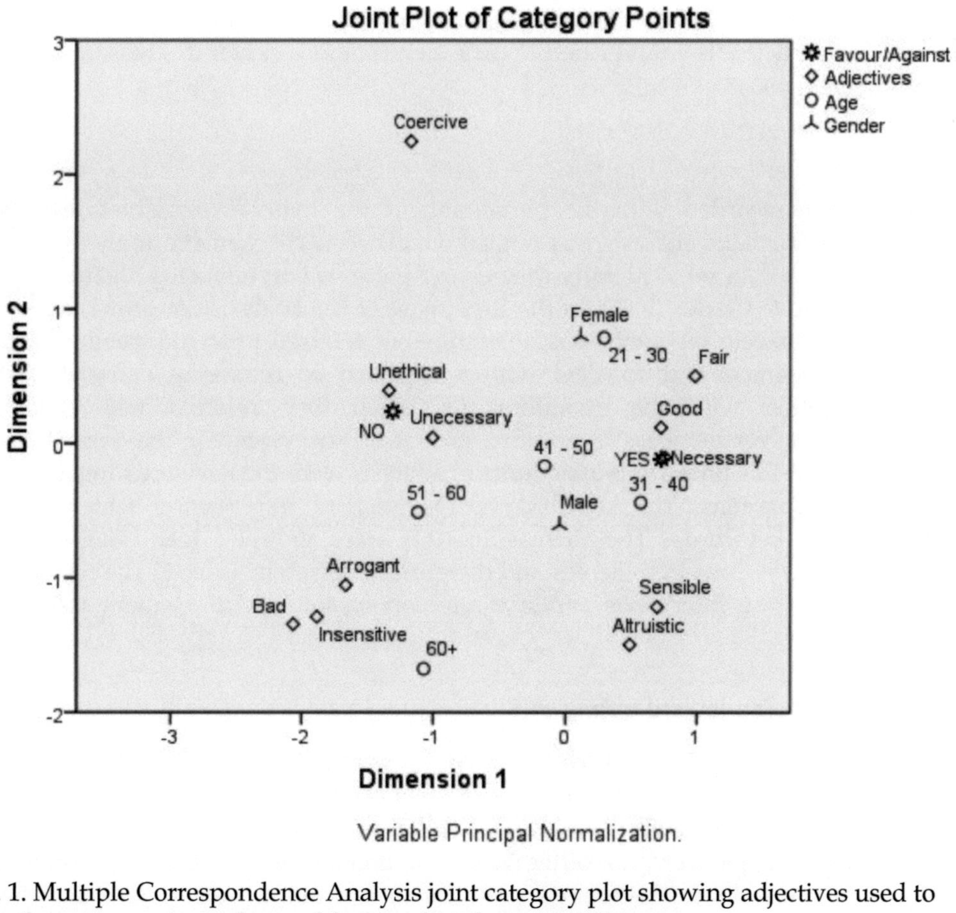

Fig. 1. Multiple Correspondence Analysis joint category plot showing adjectives used to describe opting-out, gender, and favours/not favours opting-out.

It is clear that the Dimension 1 discriminates between those in favour and those against opting-out and the corresponding adjectives describing opting-out favourably and unfavourably. Dimension 2 seems to vary along two characteristics. One of these is the age of the respondents. This dimension corresponds to moving from the highest age bracket (60+yrs) to the lowest one (21-30yrs). At the same time, this variation corresponds to a second characteristic, which reflects the nuance of the adjectives used to describe opting-out. The adjectives used by the younger age group seem to reflect the legal and ethical aspect of the issue and therefore they describe opting-out as being 'coercive', 'unethical' and 'fair'. The older age group use adjectives such as 'insensitive', 'bad', 'arrogant', 'sensible, 'altruistic' which bring out more the emotive aspect rather than the legalistic.

9. Interviews with doctors in contact with donors and recipients

The second part of the study involves the interviewing of five medical professionals who are directly involved in organ donation. These doctors meet organ donors, recipients and potential recipients waiting for an organ transplant every day and therefore are very much aware of the issues involved. Malta being such a small community, giving any information about the five participants would result in their identification and for this reason their roles will be kept anonymous.

9.1 Method

Interviews were recorded with the permission of the interviewees. Interviews were transcribed and thematic analysis was carried out. Theoretical thematic analysis involves searching across a data set to identify themes and patterns that relate to a theoretical area of interest (Braun & Clarke, 2006). In the first phase of the analysis the primary text was broken up into discrete segments which described or referred to an independent idea or concept. Each segment was labelled with a keyword or phrase. A complete list of keywords together with the quotations to which they referred was generated. This restructured version of the primary texts was the basis for the second phase of the analysis. In this phase, the basic units of analysis were the keywords together with their lists of quotations. The keywords were classified into themes which brought together related keywords. The themes in turn were grouped into categories. The classification of keywords into themes and categories is given in Table 6. The next section is an analysis of the interviews and a discussion of some of the salient issues that emerged.

9.2 Doctors' attitudes toward opting-out

In this study the five doctors interviewed were, in principal, in favour of the opting-out system but felt that the decision to introduce it could create problems and affect the respect people have towards the medical profession. They all agreed that it should be postponed to a later date when people were in a better position to understand the necessity of opting out if the need becomes acute. The reasons given for their position were various and the six main ones are discussed below.

CATEGORIES	THEMES	KEYWORDS
Refusals	Few refusals Lack of knowledge Sensitive organs	Low refusal rate Children Identifying problem areas Lack of official records Doctor-patient relationship
Families	Consulting family Permission Awareness	Must still involve relatives Family doctor Priest Imposition Difficult for doctors to ask Anonymity
Wish of the deceased	ID card Family discussion Public campaigns	Difficult decision made easier Knowing the wish of the deceased Disrespect Voluntary donation Informed consent
Altruism	Encouraging altruism Individualism	Health system Values Religion Personality traits prosocial
Anonymity	News Small country	Maltese context ITU personnel Newspapers News Television
Trust in doctors	Lack of trust Family doctor Official document	Right timing Discussion ID card Trust Respect Tarnish relationship Consult family

Table 6. Factors influencing the decision on whether to introduce opting-out

9.2.1 Low rate of refusals

Interviewees pointed out that although no statistics are kept regarding the number of refusals, they know that it is low.

> *We have to see if there is a need for it to become law. Over the past ten years, how many refusals were there? If there were refusals in England, then they need it. If we don't have that many refusals, then I don't think we need to. At the end of the day, nobody likes to have it imposed on him. It is much better to ask. (Doctor 1)*

So many people are in favour of it [donating organs], that there isn't a need in Malta. By nature, if we can help, we do so… (Doctor 5).

Here, most people do give permission for their relative's organs to be used. We rarely find people who object to it (Doctor 4)

Doctors observed some trends in families who refuse to donate. Refusals often come when the potential donor is a child. Parents find it very difficult to give permission to doctors to take organs from children. Another difficult decision is to give the eyes of the dead relative. Relatives may also refuse to donate because they are not cognizant of the procedures involved. The professionals might explain but at such a difficult moment the cognitive functions are overwhelmed and the affective element takes over.

For example, in one case, a nun who was the dead man's niece entered the room and said, "But he is still alive, look at him, feel him, he's still warm." I explained what it is. But these problems can and do arise. (Doctor 2)

9.2.2 Role of the family of the deceased

Interviewees argued that if opting-out is in place, it would be very difficult for most of the doctors to remove organs without informing the relatives and getting their cooperation. If legislation on opting-out is introduced, when relatives object to the organs being taken from the deceased, a very uncomfortable situation would arise. Although legally correct to remove the organs, going against the wishes of the relatives would increase the anguish and suffering of the family. Since family consent is still commendable, the opting-out system still presents problems similar to opting-in.

When I attended meetings with Spanish and Italian colleagues, who have the opting-out system, they claim that it is still socially necessary to inform relatives and ask for consent. (Doctor 2)

9.2.3 Altruism

Interviewees pointed out that introducing the opting-out system would remove the element of altruism from the act of donating organs. Doctors interviewed were of the opinion that altruism should be encouraged and donation should not be imposed by legislation.

If we wish to keep having high standards, then we need to accept altruism as part of our health care. We can't ignore it…. We can't reach that level. (Doctor 4)

"You have to give people the option to be altruistic." (Doctor 3)

9.2.4 Knowing the wish of the deceased

According to the research carried out by the European Commission (Europeans and Organ Donation, 2007, Special Eurobarometer 272D/Wave 66.2 - TNS Opinion and Social), more than four out of ten Europeans have already discussed with their family the question of organ donation and transplantation (p. 20). Malta stands out as the only new Member State to record a score above the European average (44% versus the average of 42% for the countries in the EU). One of the interviewees confirmed that the fact that persons would have already discussed this subject with their family has a strong influence on the willingness to donate organs of a relative.

> *Doctors find that a number of potential donors had, during their life-time, signed a consent form for donation and whilst doing this they had informed their family of their strong views in favour of donation. A signed donor card helps families reach a favourable decision. (Doctor 2)*

> *It is one of our good traits. Many times, they [the family] approach you first, before you even feel comfortable to approach them yourself… (Doctor 5).*

One of the interviewees was of the opinion that rather than introducing opting-out, Government should ask persons to decide whether they want to donate their organs or not and this is registered in their ID card. Knowing the wishes of the deceased would help both the doctor to ask and the family to decide. He also pointed out that regular campaigns should inform the public about the implications of signing this document so that there is informed consent. He pointed out that it is important to find out why people refuse and then address that particular problem.

> *Is it because people refuse on moral, religious grounds, is it they don't really care? Is it a certain apathy? Because if it is one of these, then it should be addressed rather than going to something completely different and drastic…..(Doctor 3)*

This participant claimed that in Malta this system would work out better than introducing opting-out. People would be against any form of imposition or coercion and their attitudes would ultimately undermine the aim of increasing the number of donated organs.

9.2.5 Anonymity

Another issue related to opting-out according to the participants is that in a small country, it is very difficult for donors and recipients to remain anonymous. This could create problems when all or some members of the family of the deceased person from whom the organs are taken are against the idea of donating the organs. In many countries anonymity is observed, however Malta presents a different context where, because of its size, it is very easy for persons to contact each other.

> *It depends on the local culture. Regarding cadaveric donations, in England, everything is done to make sure that the identity of the donor is not known. Now in Malta, it is useless trying to do that. Even if the entire staff is on board not to divulge information, newspapers report that there has been a fatal traffic accident and those waiting for an organ would know that there are organs available. (Doctor 1)*

If due to opting-out, people are forced to donate the organs of their relative when they do not want to, members of the family can vent their anger on the recipient and the family.

9.2.6 Trust in the medical profession

One other important argument which the participants discussed was that if opting-out is introduced, it could tarnish the trust that exists between the patient and the doctor. The medical profession has always been respected and trusted. Introducing opting-out, the respondents claimed, could tarnish this relationship.

> *If there is no trust I don't do anything….If there is lack of trust once, he will tell someone else, and it keeps happening. And once you lose it [a patient's trust], there is no way coming up. So we'd rather err on the safe side. (Doctor 5)*

Before the relatives take the decision to donate the organs of the deceased, they consult their family doctor who is always very close to the family as well as relatives. Often they also need the comfort of a priest they trust. These discussions are important. Forcing the relatives to donate when they are not in agreement is not conducive to creating a culture of trust in the medical profession.

> *Many times, you know what they are going to say before, because you build a rapport with them. It is important…If they respect you, they say 'this is the doctor who looked after my daughter, my son, parents. I trust him. I know that he did all he could to save him, now he is trying to do all he can to save someone else. (Doctor 5)*

Possibly this could be the strongest argument put forward and must be evaluated in depth. Having the citizens of a country commit themselves on an ID card about whether or not they are willing to donate, will make the relatives much more at peace with themselves when taking decisions to donate. Having one's view on the ID card implies that (i) it is easier for doctors to ask relatives (ii) knowing the views of the deceased, relatives find it easier to decide to donate (iii) more organs become available. All this would be achieved without coercion and without drastically changing the existing system.

10. Discussion

The data collected from the interviews and the survey indicate that the respondents are not in agreement as to whether opting-out should be introduced in Malta. The survey shows that 65.8% of those who answered, said that they are in favour and described donation in very positive terms. However the other 34.2% had negative attitudes towards the introduction of opting-out. Moreover the doctors who work with potential donors and recipients think that Malta, as opposed to other countries, does not need to introduce the system yet. They argue that in a small country, the relationship between the families and the family doctor, who is almost a member of the family, is still very warm and that people's respect and trust in the medical profession is also strong. This facilitates the dynamics when doctors ask for the organs of their deceased relative. When asked, the potential donor family consults with the family doctor and very often the parish priest and depending on their advice, they decide. This works well most of the time because doctors and the public are in favour of organ donation and could be one of the reasons why there are few refusals (Lauri & Zarb Adami, 2010). Introducing opting-out could create a debate which could undermine the donation process. Since in the sample we found that more than 34% of doctors are against presumed consent and since a survey carried out in 2006 showed that more than 52% of Maltese people are against presumed consent, there is a probability that the debate will backfire creating doubts in people's minds and in so doing diminishing the trust they have in hospital doctors. This may result in people becoming less positive about organ donation and less people carrying the donor card. As things are, with the opting-in system, the decision is based on trust, goodwill and altruism. If the system changes, these values may be jeopardised.

This may be a different scenario from other countries where the economies of scale are different. Maybe in other countries, because of different health schemes, the bond between the family doctor and the family is less strong and maybe the families do not consult the family doctor when they are asked to donate, resulting in many refusals. It could also be that family members and extended family are not as close-knit as Maltese families who often include two or three generations living in houses in the same square mile. Maltese families are very possessive and present a united front against anything or anybody that in any way threatens them.

Many researchers point out that most people would wish to act in an altruistic manner and help others by donating their organs after death. However what actually happens is that while the majority of people would be willing to donate organs, only a small number register their names on the Organ Donor Register or carry a donor card. This is also true for Malta. However whereas in other bigger countries, people may not have close family members who can be contacted easily, in Malta it actually takes minutes to do so, and therefore doctors can check quickly the wishes of the relatives.

The British Medical Association argue that a shift to presumed consent would prompt more discussion within families about organ donation (Organ Donation in the 21st Century, 2000). This is true, but in the case of this island, the debate will probably be a very emotional one rather than a rational one since research has already shown that the social representations which Maltese people have regarding the body and organ donation are very complex (Lauri, 2009). The majority still belief that this is a decision to be taken by the family members and nobody else. Even some doctors believe that this should be the case.

Another point made by the British Medical Association is that with a shift to presumed consent, organ donation becomes the default position and that this represents a more positive view of organ donation which is to be encouraged. This will not necessarily be the case in Malta. In fact it will probably create more negative attitudes than positive ones and would influence the metaphors people use to grapple with the issue of organ donation (Lauri, 2009). Presumed consent has not resulted in more positive views towards opting-out as can be borne out by studies carried out in other countries with presumed consent such as Spain, Brazil and Belgium.

11. Conclusion

In the case of Malta, because of its size and culture, it seems that the best way forward is to have an intensive campaign every three to five years encouraging the discussion of organ donation within the family and introducing a system whereby every citizen who applies for a formal document, in the case of our country, the ID card, are asked to register whether they want to donate their organs after their death. This document will help the family decide in the event that they are asked to donate the organs of the deceased. In a survey carried with a random sample of 400 Maltese citizens, respondents were asked whether they would donate the organs of their loved one if they knew that he or she would have wanted them to do so or would have carried a donor card. Only 9% of the respondents said they that they would not (Lauri, 2000). Having the wishes of the deceased registered on the ID card would make the family's decision very much easier.

The belief is that a shift to presumed consent is not likely to have a positive effect on donation rates in Malta at this point in time. Maybe this can be considered again in a few years' time but from the results obtained in this study, it seems that according to some doctors and the professionals working with potential donors and recipients, it is neither necessary nor judicious to introduce opting-out in Malta.

12. Acknowledgements

The author would like to thank Dr. Joseph Zarb Adami LRCP, MRCS, MDFRCA, Department of Anaesthesia, Intensive Care and Pain Therapy, Mater Dei Hospital, Malta, Mr. John Zammit DNO, PQ Health Management and Ms. Amy Zahra B.Psy (Hons.) for their kind help in writing this chapter.

13. References

Abadie, A., & Gay, S. (2006). The impact of presumed consent legislation on cadaveric organ donation: a cross-country study. *Journal of Health Economics, 25,* 599-620. doi:10.1016/j.jhealeco.2006.01.003

Bell, M. (2006). The UK Human Tissue Act and consent: Surrendering a fundamental principal to transplantation needs? *Journal of Medical Ethics, 32,* 283-286. doi:10.1136/jme.2005.012666

Braun, V., & Clarke, V. (2006). Using thematic analysis in psychology. *Qualitative Research in Psychology, 3*(2), 77-101.

British Medical Association (2008). *Organ donation – presumed consent for organ donation.* Retrieved from British Medical Association website: http://www.bma.oeg.uk/ap.nsf/Content/OrganDonationPresumedConsent

British Medical Association Ethics (2000). *Organ Donation in the 21st Century: Time for a consolidated approach.* Retrieved from British Medical Association website: http://www.bma.org.uk/images/OrganDonation_tcm41-147010.pdf

British Medical Association Ethics (2009). *Human Tissue Legislation: Guidance from The British Medical Association Medical Ethics Department.* Retrieved from British Medical Association website: http://www.bma.org.uk/images/humantissuelegislationaug2009_tcm41-190148.pdf

Conesa, C., Rios, A., Ramirez, P., Rodriguez, M. M., Rivas, P., Canteras, M., & Parrilla, P. (2003). Psychosocial profile in favor of organ donation. Transplant Proceedings, 35(4), 1276-1281. doi: 10.1016/S0041-1345(03)00468-8

Coppen, R., Friele, R. D., Marquet, R. L., Gevers, S. K. M. (2005). Opting-out systems: no guarantee for higher donation rates. *Transplant International, 18*(11), 1275-1279. doi: 10.1111/j.1432-2277.2005.00202.x

English, V. (2007). Is presumed consent the answer to organ shortages? Yes. *British Medical Journal, 334,* 1088. doi: 10.1136/bmj.39199.475301.AD

Europe for Patients, Directorate - General for Health and consumers, (2010). *Key facts and figures on EU organ donation and transplantation.* Retrieved from Europe for Patients website: http://ec.europa.eu/health/ph_threats/human_substance/oc_organs/docs/fact_figures.pdf

Farrugia E. (2000). Ethical issues of kidney transplantation. In M. N. Cauchi (Ed.), *Patients' rights, reproductive technology, transplantation* (pp. 99-105). Malta: The Bioethics Consultative Committee.

Gimbel, R. W., Strosberg, M. A., Lehrman, S. E., Gefenas, E., & Taft, F. (2003). Presumed consent and other predictors of cadaveric organ donation in Europe. *Progress in Transplantation, 13,* 17-23.

Gnant, M. F., Wamser, P., Goetzinger, P., Sautner, T., Steininger, R., & Muehlbacher, F. (1991). The impact of the presumed consent law and a decentralized organ procurement system on organ donation: quadruplication in the number of organ donors. *Transplant Proceedings, 23*(5), 2685-2686.

Haddow, G. (2006). "Because you're worth it?" The taking and selling of transplantable organs. *Journal of Medical Ethics, 32*, 324-328. doi:10.1136/jme.2005.013805

Hamilton, T. (2003, May 17). Should Organ Donation move from an opt-in system to an opt-out system? [Online forum argument]. Retrieved on 20 February, 2010 from http://www.idebate.org/debatabase/topic_details.php?topicID=216

Healy, K. (2005, April 30). The political economy of presumed consent (2005). [eScholarship article]. Theory and Research in Comparitive Social Analysis. Retrieved from http://escholarship.org/uc/item/33x4463s#page-1

Hill, D. J., Palmer, T. C., & Evans, D. W. (1999). Presumed consent. If this is introduced, people will have to have all relevant information. *British Medical Journal, 318*, 1490.

Johnson, E. J., & Goldstein, D. G. (2004). Defaults and donation decisions. *Transplantation, 78* (12), 1713-1716.

Klenow, D. J., & Youngs, G. A. (1995). An empirical exploration of selected policy options in organ donation. *Death Studies, 19*, 543-547.

Lauri, M. A. (2000). The Lay Person and Transplantation. In M. N. Cauchi (Ed.), *Patients' Rights, Reproductive Technology and Transplantation* (pp. 106-126). Malta: The Bioethics Consultative Council.

Lauri, M.A. (2006). Attitudes towards organ donation in Malta in the last decade. *Malta Medical Journal, 18(4), 25-29.*

Lauri, M.A. (2008). Changing public opinion towards organ donation. A social psychological approach to social marketing. In L. O. Pietrieff, & R. V. Miller, (Eds.), *Public Opinion Focus* (pp. 9-36). NY: Nova Science Publishers.

Lauri, M. A. (2009). Metaphors of organ donation, social representations of the body and the opt-out system. *British Journal of Health Psychology, 14*(4), 647 – 666.

Lauri, M. A., & Zarb Adami, J. (2010). The need for increasing the retrieval of organs: doctor's attitudes towards opting-out. *Malta Medical Journal, 22*(4), 14-19.

Lawson, A. (2008). Presumed consent for organ donation in the United Kingdom. *Journal of Intensive Care Society, 9*(2), 116-117.

Low, H-C., Da Costa, M., Prabhakaran, K., Kaur, M., Wee, A., Lim, S-G., & Wai, C-T. (2006). Impact of new legislation on presumed consent on organ donation on liver transplant on Singapore: a preliminary analysis. *Transplantation, 82*(9), 1234-1237.

Malta Medical Council. (2010). *Annual Report 2010.* Retrieved from https://ehealth.gov.mt/HealthPortal/others/regulatory_councils/medical_council/medical_council.aspx

Organ Donation Taskforce (2008). *Organs for Transplants: a report from the Organ Donation Taskforce.* London: Department of Health.

Oz, M. C., Kherani, A. R., Rowe, A., Roels, L., Crandall, C., Tomatis, L., & Young, J. B. (2003). How to improve organ donation: results of the ISHLT/FACT poll. *The Journal of Heart and Lung Transplantation, 22*(4), 389-410.

Persson, M.O., Dmitriev, P., Shevelev, A., Zelvys, A., Hermeren, G., & Persson, N.H. (1998). Attitudes towards organ donation and transplantation – a study involving Baltic physicians. *Transplant International, 11*(6), 419-423.

Prottas, J., & Batten, H. L. (1988). Health professional and hospital administrators in organ procurement: attitudes, reservations, and their resolutions. *American Journal of Public Health, 78*(6), 642-645.

Rithalia, A., McDiad, C., Suekarran, S., Myers, L., & Sowden, A. (2009). Impact of presumed consent for organ donation on donation rates: A systemic review. *British Medical Journal, 338*, a3162. doi: 10.1136/bmj.a3162

Rodrigue, J. R., Cornell, D. L., & Howard, R. J. (2006). Attitudes towards financial incentives, donor authorization, and presumed consent among next-of-kin who consented vs. refused organ donation. *Transplantation, 81*, 12491256. doi: 10.1097/01.tp.0000203165.49 905.4a

Roels, L., Vanrenterghem, Y., Waer, M., Christiaens, M. R., Gruwez, J., & Michielsen, P. (1991). Three years of experience with a 'presumed consent' legislation in Belgium: its impact on multi-organ donation in comparison with other European countries. Transplant Proceedings, 23, 903-904.

Roels, L., Roelants, M., Timmermans, T., Hoppenbrouwers, K., Pillen, E., & Bande-Knops, J. (1997). A survey on attitudes to organ donation among three generations in a country with 10 years of presumed consent legislation. *Transplantation Proceedings, 29*, 3224-3225.

Rumsey, S., Hurford, D.P., & Cole, A.K. (2003). Influence of knowledge and religiousness on attitudes towards organ donation. *Transplantation Proceedings, 35*(8), 2845-2850.

Schaeffner, E., Windisch, W., Friedel, K., Breitenfeld, K., and Winkelmayer, C. (2004). Knowledge and attitude regarding organ donation among medical students and physicians. *Clinical Transplantation*, 77 (11), p.1714-1718.

Soh, P., & Lim, S. M. (1992). Opting-out law: a model for Asia - the Singapore experience. *Transplant Proceedings, 24*(4), 1337-1337.

The Parliamentary Office of Science and Technology. (2004). *Postnote: Organ Transplants.* Retrieved from http://www.parliament.uk/documents/post/postpn231.pdf

Uniform Anatomical Gift Act of 1987. Retrieved from http://www.law.upenn.eduu/bll/archives/ulc/fnact99//uaga87.htm

Webster, P. (2008, January 14). Gordon Brown seeks to make everyone an organ donor - with opt-out. *The Times*. Retrieved from http://www.timesonline.co.uk/tol/news /politics/article3182388.ece?pgnum=1

Wintor, P. (2008, January 14). Brown backs opt-out system to boost organ transplants. *The Guardian*. Retrieved from http://www.guardian.co.uk/politics/2008/jan/14/uk.publicservice/print

Wright, L. (2007). Is presumed consent the answer to organ shortages? No. *British Medical Journal, 334*, 1089. doi: 10.1136/bmj.39199.492894.AD

YouGov plc. (2007). *Organ Donation fieldwork dates: 9th – 11th October 2007.* Retrieved from Britich Medical Association website: http://www.bma.org.uk/ap.nsf/Content/OrganDonationPresumedConsent

6

Organizations as Communities: Creating Worksite Campaigns to Promote Organ Donation

Susan E. Morgan
Purdue University
USA

1. Introduction

Because workplaces are communities where people spend much of their time—at least half of their waking hours—health educators have long assumed that they would be productive contexts for public education about a wide variety of health issues, including smoking cessation, health screening, and general health promotion, including physical activity, dietary improvements, and multivitamin use (Campbell, et. al, 2002; Emmons, et. al, 1999; Grosch, et. al, 1998; Sorenson, et. al, 2005). Furthermore, worksite campaigns have the potential to reach a greater percentage of a potential audience than a mass media campaign targeting the general public because the audience is "captive" in the workplace. However, using worksites to promote a health issue has often met with mixed results. Success appears to be linked to factors such as the actual reach of worksite activities, participation in activities by employees, the duration and intensity of activities, and whether campaigns target employees who are in greatest need of the intervention (Grosch, et. al, 1998; Orlandi, 1986; Pelletier, 2001).

How worksite campaign successes with other issues can translate to the education of employees about organ donation and transplantation has been largely unexplored. It is important to first consider the ways in which the promotion of organ donation differs from education about other health issues. Unlike smoking cessation, exercise, or injury prevention, becoming an organ donor does not benefit employees, at least not directly or tangibly. To become an organ donor, an employee has to die, and the contemplation of one's own death is not likely to lead to a particularly comfortable cognitive state. Many people's instinctual avoidance of the topic of organ donation itself is an obstacle that researchers and practitioners must overcome when designing an effective worksite campaign. Appeals to employees to become an organ donor must emphasize other benefits, especially the satisfaction of saving the lives of (deserving) others and perhaps even the sense that donors survive death by "living on" through their recipients.

The theoretical foundations of worksite interventions have varied considerably. Theories such as the theory of planned behavior, theory of reasoned action, and the transtheoretical model (a.k.a. the "stages of change" approach) have predominated. However, theories that create a solid foundation for some types of health interventions may not be equally suited to other health issues. This appears to be the case with organ donation, where the transtheoretical model has not been used with much success in public communication campaigns to promote organ donation, while the theory of reasoned action (and related models) have proven to be far more useful (see Morgan, 2012, for a review).

A review of the social scientific literature on the predictors of the willingness to donate organs reveals a general consensus that donation-related behaviors are a function of attitudes toward organ donation and toward becoming a donor, knowledge about organ donation (particularly knowledge that counters popular myths about donation), and the importance of the influence of family and friends. These, of course, are the same variables that comprise the theory of reasoned action. There are additional factors that appear to contribute to the willingness to donate, including existential variables such as the perception that organ donors "survive" death, a concern about saving the lives of "bad" people, the fear that signing a donor card will tempt fate and possibly bring on premature death, and a general sense of disgust from the idea of putting the organs from one person into the body of another person (Morgan, Harrison, et. al, 2008; Morgan, Stephenson, et. al, 2008). Morgan and colleagues have added these variables to the theory of reasoned action to create a model (the organ donation model) tailored to organ donation.

The operationalization of these variables has taken the form of specific features of worksite organ donation campaigns. Formative research with both general and minority populations provided important information about the specific points of knowledge that were most predictive of the willingness to donate. These include knowledge about the organ allocation system, the understanding that potential donor status will not affect the quality of medical care in an emergency, knowledge that an organ donor can have an open-casket funeral, and knowledge that a black market does not exist in the U.S. Rather than overwhelm employees with unnecessary general information about organ donation, these worksite campaigns focused on providing details about these specific points of knowledge. This information was printed on cafeteria table tents, appeared in brochures distributed to every employee, and was distributed through paycheck stuffers and email and voicemail blasts.

Organ donation worksite campaigns based on the theory of reasoned action also targeted perceptions of supportive social norms. These campaigns prominently featured employees of organizations who had been touched by organ donation. Donors and recipients were featured on billboards on roads leading to an organization's building as well as full-color posters hung on bulletin boards. Their stories appeared in newsletter articles, which provided greater details about the employees' stories, and abbreviated versions of these stories were used as paycheck/mailbox stuffers. By emphasizing to employees that they all "knew" someone who had been affected by donation, the campaign sought to capitalize on the sense of affiliation that people often feel with their co-workers. Interpersonal discussions about their co-workers' experiences offered the opportunity to exchange personal thoughts and feelings about donation. When this element of a worksite campaign was isolated and tested for its effectiveness, companies with employees personally touched by organ donation experienced greater increases in signed donor cards and/or donor registry forms. Also, the very fact that employees have crowded around an information table in a high-visibility, high-traffic area in the organization to sign up to become a donor becomes a form of social proof may be quite powerful.

Although superstitions about bringing on premature death by signing a donor card or a visceral-level disgust response at the idea of organ transplantation would be difficult at best to overcome through a worksite campaign, concerns about the deservingness of potential recipients is more easily addressed. By having transplant recipients help to staff information tables and by featuring a company's own employees in the campaign, most of whom were recipients, non-donors could establish a greater sense of connection with the sort of people who would be potential recipients of their own organs.

Three worksite campaigns will be summarized in chronological order: The United Parcel Service, The University Worksite Organ Donation Project, and The New Jersey Workplace Partnership for Life. Each campaign built upon the lessons learned in previous studies. Greater detail about the statistical evaluation of the outcomes of these campaigns can be found in publications in the social science and medical journals in which they were originally published. It should be noted that all aspects of these campaigns were subject to at least one Institutional Review Board review for ethics. Following the review of campaigns, principles for organizing worksite interventions to promote organ donation will be offered.

2. The United Parcel Service worksite campaign

The first example of a successful organ donation worksite campaign took place at United Parcel Service (UPS) during 1999-2000 (Morgan, et. al, 2002). Spearheaded by the Kentucky Organ Donor Affiliates, this worksite organ donation promotion project was a multi-channel, multi-message campaign designed to increase knowledge about facts related to organ donation, increase favorable attitudes toward organ donation, increase the rate of signed organ donor cards among audience members, and to increase the willingness of audience members to talk to family members about their decision regarding organ donation.

The worksite organ donation project consisted of a pretest/post-test comparison of two sites of a large, national package delivery corporation. A 10% stratified random sample was taken from the control and intervention sites, which were located in two separate media markets about a 90-minute drive apart. The intervention component of the project lasted for eight months and utilized multiple message strategies via both mass media and interpersonal channels of communication. The *mass media component* of the campaign included newspaper articles, notices on the intranet website, billboard ads, and radio PSAs. The *interpersonal component* of the campaign included educational sessions by the principal investigators, visits by OPO volunteers, and presentation of panels from the organ donor quilt. OPO volunteers staffed tables at the multiple locations at the intervention site several times throughout the campaign, distributing literature, giveaways promoting organ donation, and t-shirts. Volunteers asked employees if they had signed an organ donor card or the back of their driver's licenses, and offered to witness signatures for those who wanted to consent to becoming potential organ donors. Volunteers also shared personal information about their experiences regarding organ donation and answered questions about organ donation facts and processes.

The evaluation of the campaign demonstrated that these strategies were highly effective with a diverse population. Respondents at the intervention site were more likely to sign an organ donor card, have more favorable attitudes toward organ donation generally, and to feel more comfortable about talking to family members about their decision to donate than respondents at the control site. Among those people who had not yet signed an organ donor card, the campaign successfully raised their intention to do so in the future.

However, there were a number of limitations to the UPS study. First, there was no way of determining which facets of this multi-channel, multi-message campaign produced the strongest effects. Similarly, it was not possible to determine the most cost-efficient means of reaching people with the most powerful message. For example, there was no way to tell how many people accessed the organization's intranet site and read the facts about organ donation. Finally, it was unclear to what degree personal encounters with organ donor recipients or organ donor family members contributed to the traditional means of educating people about organ donation.

3. The University Worksite Organ Donation campaign

Because the UPS worksite campaign used only one company and could not pinpoint the campaign elements that contributed to campaign success, a subsequent campaign using six matched worksites was planned, using universities as the sites for two types of campaigns (contrasted against control sites). The University Worksite Organ Donation Campaign was conducted at the University of Arizona, University of Alabama, Rutgers University, Texas A&M University, University of North Carolina at Charlotte, and Pennsylvania State University. This project represented a more theoretically rigorous test of the campaign strategies initially tested in the UPS campaign. Instead of simply dividing sites into intervention and control, as with the UPS campaign, a third condition was added to test the advantages offered by a full intervention (which included the interpersonal component included in the UPS campaign) over a mass-media-only intervention, which is cheaper and easier to implement, but may ultimately be less effective (Morgan, et. al, 2010).

The campaign heavily utilized internal media including campus papers and faculty/staff newsletters in addition to more traditional outlets such as billboards and radio. In one of the quasi-experimental conditions, only media messages (including those that featured the stories of members of the university community) were used to promote organ donation. In mass media-plus-interpersonal condition, the media campaign was supported by ten on-site visits by OPO staff and volunteers over the course of an academic year.

As with the UPS campaign, a pretest/post-test design was used to evaluate the effects of each type of campaign. A random stratified mail survey demonstrated that compared to the control condition, there was a statistically significant advantage to adding on-site visits on whether respondents reported signing a donor card or talked to family about organ donation. However, the media-only campaign did not produce results that were statistically different from the control condition. The project organizers argue that the outreach component offers community members the opportunity to "put a human face" on the issue of organ donation because many volunteers are transplant recipients or donor family members. Additionally, the site visits provide an opportunity to ask questions about organ donation that may linger even after seeing ads or billboards promoting organ donation.

Because universities are large employers that are present in every state, offer their own set of media outlets (including newspapers and radio stations), and are effectively matched on a number of vital characteristics, they are an ideal set of organizations to test these campaign principles. However, it is difficult to generalize to worksites that are not university-based. Universities tend to employ a greater proportion of well-educated people than most employers. University worksites are also comprised of a large number of buildings housing employees, which creates difficulties in reaching employees in one (or just a few) centralized locations. In addition, a year-long campaign such as the one conducted at university worksites is probably not feasible for most OPOs and their workplace partners.

4. The New Jersey Workplace Partnership for Life

In order to test the generalizability of the findings of the University Worksite Organ Donation Campaign with a wider variety of organizations, a larger-scale series of worksite campaigns was developed in New Jersey (Harrison, in press; Morgan, Harrison, et. al, 2010). This project reached over 30,000 employees in 45 companies in industries including health care, pharmaceuticals, manufacturing, law, education, and municipalities. Companies were divided into three quasi-experimental conditions that replicated those of the University Worksite Organ Donation Project (mass media campaigns contrasted against campaigns that also included on-site visits by staff and volunteers). In addition to expanding the number and diversity in the type of companies reached, campaigns were reduced to a 10 week time period.

In addition to "myth buster" messages designed to educate employees about the most common misconceptions about organ donation, companies in the mass media condition publicized the stories of co-workers who had been touched by organ donation. About half of all companies had employees willing to share their stories; in the event that an employee story was not available, stories about people in the same industry or the same town were used instead to maximize a sense of affiliation. All media messages were disseminated through internal (not external or paid) media, including email, cafeteria table tents, newsletters, posters, paycheck stuffers, and LCD boards.

Depending on the size of the company, which ranged from 100 employees to nearly 4,000 employees, on-site visits to companies in the high-intensity campaign group were conducted 3-4 times over the course of the 10-week campaign. Tables were set up in high-traffic locations, including lobbies and cafeterias and were typically staffed by two project team members and a volunteer from the organ procurement organization, usually a transplant recipient. A panel from the state's donor family memorial quilt was on display to further promote a sense of personal connection with the issue. Small giveaways such as pens, magnets, and sticky note pads helped to attract attention to the table, where staff members then used a set script to engage employees in a discussion about any questions about donation or the state's organ donor registry.

Results from pretest/post-test surveys of a random sample of employees confirm previous findings that campaigns which include on-site visits are more successful than those that use only internal media to disseminate information about organ donation. Mass media campaigns, which utilized only internal forms of media (newsletters, posters on bulletin boards, paycheck stuffers, etc.) increased the rate of donation among non-donors by an average of 13.6%.

5. Best practices for Worksite Organ Donation campaigns

A blueprint for successful campaigns (from both a pragmatic as well as theoretical point of view) is slowly emerging. While it is ideal practice to ground interventions on a theory of behavior change, it is probably sufficient for practitioners to simply follow in the footprints of previous campaigns as closely as possible. Similarly, the effectiveness of any campaign requires evaluation of audience members' knowledge, attitudes, and beliefs before and again after the campaign and to compare these results to a matched control group (generally, an organization of similar size and composition). Again, a full evaluation may be outside of the realm of possibility for most practitioners, but a brief survey of, for example, the number of people who have definitively committed to becoming a potential organ donor before the campaign and again after the campaign would provide a reasonably good means of measuring whether the campaign succeeded in its goals.

One type of campaign practice that many practitioners appear to find difficult to resist (in part because managers of organizations generally offer access to this channel the most readily, often to the exclusion of other channels) is the „lunch and learn." In this format, campaign staff show up to an appointed conference room or other meeting space during the lunch hour and present information about organ donation to employees who are interested in learning more about organ donation. As one might expect, the people who need accurate information about organ donation the most (in other words, people who are the most likely to believe in common myths about donation) are also the least likely to voluntarily attend such a meeting. Additionally, any „improvements" noticed in donation-related outcomes (such as donor registrations) are likely to be very small and only among people who were already inclined toward such behaviors.

Fortunately, it is entirely posssible to replicate successful worksite campaigns. Worksite campaigns that include the following six elements are more likely to result in a greater number of donor registrations.

First, it is important to utilize both mass media and interpersonal communication channels. Messages distributed through each channel will have strengths and weaknesses that can be compensated for by messages delivered through the other channel. Mass-produced educational materials (such as educational brochures) should have high production values; otherwise, the credibility of the campaign can be called into question. However, no matter how well produced, messages delivered through mass media channels (including emails, posters, etc.) can seem impersonal. Moreover, they lack the ability to be tailored to each individual employee's personal misgivings about donation. This is why on-site visits by trained staff members and/or volunteers are of central importance. From experience, the ideal number of visits should be 2-3, spaced about 2-3 weeks apart over a 6-9 week period to maximize the effect of the educational intervention by offering opportunities to address concerns about donation in person while avoiding „intervention fatigue" by employees and management.

Second, having access to multiple intra-organizational communication channels will support the success of a worksite campaign for a couple of reasons. Not only are these channels free, but the use of these channels signals to employees that the campaign is being supported by top management. Intraorganizational „mass"communication channels that are frequently used include company intranet websites, newsletters, company mail, email, voicemail, and bulletin boards in hallways, stairwells, and breakrooms (for posters).

Third, whenever it is possible, solicit employees' own stories about how they (or close family members) been touched by organ donation, either because they (or a loved one) received an organ transplant or because someone close to them died and became a donor. These stories can be featured in campaign materials to great effect. Not only do they personalize the issue of organ donation and make it more „real" to employees, these stories identify a readily identifiable point-person for employees to talk to about donation. However, it is good idea to ensure that these informal „spokespeople" are reasonably knowledgeable about donation before the campaign begins.

Fourth, the ability to conduct on-site visits in high-visibility, centrally-located gathering places is of great importance to the success of worksite campaigns. Not only does a central location help to maximize the likelihood that all employees will be exposed to campaign messages and have the opportunity to interact with campaign staff, it also helps to create „buzz" about the campaign among employees. The more you can gather people around an information table to talk to staff, the more likely it is that other employees will want to listen or talk. To increase the chances that people will come over to an information booth or table, it is important that staff members do not sit (unless medically necessary) and that they distribute something that is perceived to be useful or interesting that is free. (There are many low-cost giveaways available through numerous vendors. Pens are popular for good reason. Check samples from vendors to make sure they write well. No one likes a lousy pen.)

Fifth, the use of well-trained volunteers who follow scripts on how to address the most common concerns about organ donation will ensure that myths about donation are „busted" smoothly and convincingly. Although there is a line of thought that simply sharing „personal stories" about transplant experiences will motivate members of the public to commit to donation, there is ample evidence that knowledge already exists about the need for donation as well as the life-saving potential of organ donation; sharing personal stories does not overcome the most common objections to becoming a potential organ donor. In other words, stories must be accompanied by information that is specific to each individual employee's concerns. Teaching staff and volunteers how best to quickly and succinctly disseminate information about donation in response to common inquiries is a far more effective strategy. Numerous manuals for training staff and volunteers on communication protocol are available by request from volunteer coordinators working for organ procurement organizations in the U.S.

Sixth, because worksite interventions represent a significant investment of time and energy, it is best to concentrate efforts on large organizations of 500 employees or more. Donation is a low-incidence event; the likelihood that any one individual will become a potential donor is very low. Currently, only about 1 in 100 people die in such a way that they would be eligible to become an organ donor. Without any public education intervention at all, about half of eligible donors have either already declared their wishes to donate or their family members will consent to donation in the absence of documentation of their deceased loved one's wishes. Thus, a large number of people need to be reached effectively with a campaign to increase the actual number of donors by even one person.

6. Costs associated with worksite campaigns

Although worksite campaigns can be conducted in a way that minimizes direct financial expenditures, there are other types of costs that must be considered. The largest cost for campaign organizers is time. Potential worksites to host a campaign must be selected, after which possible appropriate contacts to correspond with about the project. Next, meetings have to scheduled to do an initial presentation of the campaign and its goals. A second round of meetings with „gatekeeping" managers (and union representatives, where applicable) is inevitable, particularly with the largest organizations. Organizations with unionized employees will require the permission and involvement of unions in order to gain permission to distribute printed materials, for example, and may present a set of complications that are difficult to forsee. (Involving national leaders of unions may prove to be an investment of time that can be worthwhile if a campaign targets organizations within the same industry, such as auto manufacturing.)

Meetings are not the only expenditure of time involved with the development of a worksite campaign. The process of creating and tailoring campaign messages can involve a significant investment of time. Similarly, the process of arranging for the distribution of these messages can take many hours. Training, scheduling, and supervising volunteers and/or staff members is an ongoing commitment. Finally, creating a final report for the organization reporting on activities and outcomes (such as number of new donor registrations) is an important deliverable that is valued by many organizations.

Time is one type of intangible expense associated with worksite campaigns. Opportunity costs are another type. The energy expended on organizing and executing a worksite campaign is energy that cannot be devoted to other types of activities that could also advance donation. Thus, it is important to invest time wisely.

Additionally, there are still a few direct financial costs for a worksite campaign which can be detailed. First, educational materials for all employees should be printed. Even at pennies or centimes per print, printing charges will add up if an organization has thousands of employees. Second, incentives for employees to visit an information table staffed by volunteers (or paid staffers) will need to be purchased. Small giveaways are usually colorful and attract attention and can provide an excuse for volunteers to begin a conversation with a line like, „We're talking to people about donation today. Have you considered registering as a potential organ donor? Third, direct costs are often incurred by campaigns if they reimburse staff members for mileage or gasoline as well as meals during the time that they work. (These same costs are incurred during the training process for volunteers who are willing to work for this type of campaign.)

Finally, it can be a good practice to give a token gift to the organizational liaison who has worked with your team to coordinate campaign activities and the dissemination of educational materials. Many people readily agree to help and quickly discover that the job is bigger than they had anticipated. If you would like to build a list of references that you can provide to future potential worksite campaign locations, it may be a wise investment to make sure your liaisons think of you fondly.

Gaining (and maintaining) access to large organizations for worksite campaigns appears to be the principal challenge facing these campaigns, which nevertheless hold the promise of reaching many thousands of people with organ donation information as well as easy opportunities to become potential organ donors.

7. Conclusion

In conclusion, worksite organ donation campaigns hold considerable promise for the future. "One important finding [from worksite campaigns]...is that [they]... may be more powerful in increasing the target behavior of individuals... Such group interventions are also certainly more cost-effective than individual interventions. Worksite programs take advantage of social support, peer influence, and preexisting group loyalties, which may be important because people often find behavior change difficult on their own" (Perkins, 1990, p. 182). Professionals seeking to disseminate compelling and accurate information about organ donation would do well to conduct worksite campaigns not only because they provide a large "captive audience" for information about organ and tissue donation and the importance of talking to family members about their donation decisions, but because information can be framed in ways that matter to employees.

8. Acknowledgments

The author would like to acknowledge the excellent contributions of the many people who have helped to create and evaluate the successful worksite campaigns discussed in this chapter. They include Tyler Harrison, Jenny Miller Jones, Lisa Volk Chewning, Tara Artesi, Jessica Melore, Michael Stephenson, Walid Afifi, Shawn Long, Tom Reichert, Tom Cannon, and the many extraordinary volunteers whose lives have been touched by organ donation.

9. References

Campbell, M.K., Tessaro, I., DeVellis, B., Benedict, S., Kelsey, K., Belton, L. (2002). Effects of a tailored health promotion program for female blue-collar workers: Health works for women. *Preventive Medicine, 34,* 313-323. ISSN 0091-7435

Emmons, K.M., Linnan, L.A., Shadel, W.G., Marcus, B., & Abrams, D.B. (1999). The working healthy project: A worksite health promotion trial targeting physical activity, diet, and smoking. *Journal of Occupational and Environmental Medicine, 41,* 545-555. ISSN 1076-2752

Grosch, J.W., Alterman, , T., Petersen, M.R., & Murphy, L.R. (1998). Worksite health promotion programs in the U.S.: Factors associated with availability and participation. *American Journal of Health Promotion, 13,* 37-45. ISSN 08901171

Harrison, T. R., Morgan, S. E., Chewning, L. V., Williams, E., Barbour, J., Di Corcia, M., & Davis, L. (in press). Revisiting the worksite in worksite health campaigns: Evidence from a multi-site organ donation campaign. *Journal of Communication.* ISSN 0021-9916

Heaney, C A. Goetzel, R Z. (1997). A review of health-related outcomes of multi-component worksite health promotion programs. *American Journal of Health Promotion. 11*(4):290-307. ISSN 08901171

Morgan, S.E. (2012). Public communication campaigns to promote organ donation: Theory, design, and implementation. In R. Rice and C. Atkin (Eds.) *Public communication campaigns.* Thousand Oaks, CA: Sage Publications. ISBN 9781412987707

Morgan, S.E., Harrison, T.R., Long, S.D., Afifi, W.A., & Stephenson, M.T. (2008). In their own words: A multicultural qualitative study of the reasons why people will (not) donate organs. *Health Communication, 23,* 23-33. ISSN 1041-0236.

Morgan, S.E., Harrison, T.R., Chewning, L.V., DiCorcia, M.J., & Davis, L.A. (2010). The Workplace Partnership for Life: The effectiveness of high- and low-intensity worksite campaigns to promote organ donation. *Communication Monographs, 77,* 341-356. ISSN 0363-7751

Morgan, S.E., Miller, J., & Arasaratnam, L.A. (2002). Signing cards, saving lives: An evaluation of the Worksite Organ Donation Promotion Project. *Communication Monographs, 69,* 253-273. ISSN 0363-7751

Morgan, S. E., Stephenson, M. T., Harrison, T. R., Afifi, W.A., & Long, S.D. (2008). Facts versus "feelings": How rational is the decision to become an organ donor? *Journal of Health Psychology, 13,* 644-658. ISSN 1359-1053

Morgan S.E., Stephenson M.T., Afifi W., Harrison T.R., Long S.D., & Chewning L.V. (2010). The University Worksite Organ Donation Project: a comparison of two types of worksite campaigns on the willingness to donate. *Clinical Transplantation, 25,* 600-605. ISSN 0902-0063

Orlandi, M.A. (1986). The diffusion and adoption of worksite health promotion innovations: An analysis of barriers. *Preventive Medicine, 15,* 522-536. ISSN 0091-7435

Pelletier, K.R. (2001). A review and analysis of the clinical and cost-effectiveness studies of comprehensive health promotion and disease management programs at the worksite: 1998-2000 update. *American Journal of Health Promotion, 16,* 107-116. ISSN 08901171

Perkins, K. A. (1990). Applicability of health promotion strategies to increasing organ donation. In J. Shanteau & R. J. Harris (Eds.), *Organ donation and transplantation: Psychological and behavioral factors*. Washington, DC: American Psychological Association. ISBN 978-1557980793

Sorensen, G., Barbeau, E. Stoddard, A.M., Hunt, A.K., Kaphingst, K., & Wallace, L. (2005). Promoting behavior change among working-class multiethnic workers: Results of the health directions-small business study. *American Journal of Public Health, 95,* 1389-1395. ISSN 0090-0036

7

Increasing the Likelihood of Consent in Deceased Donations: Point-of-Decision Campaigns, Registries, and the Law of Large Numbers

Tyler R. Harrison
Purdue University
USA

1. Introduction

The need for organ donation is growing while the number of those dying in ways to be eligible to donate (i.e. head trauma and auto accidents) is decreasing (Punch et al., 2007). In the U.S. alone there are over 111,000 people waiting for an organ transplant, with that number continuing to grow on an almost daily basis (United Network for Organ Sharing (UNOS), 2011). Additionally, over 7,000 individuals in the U.S. have died each year for the past ten years while waiting for a transplant, and over 100,000 have died within the past 15 years (Organ Procurement and Transplantation Network (OPTN), 2011). While few countries have been able to consistently increase the number of donors from year-to-year (with Spain being a notable exception), there are still large numbers of individuals who are eligible to donate and do not. One key factor in that helps explain lack of consent by family members to donation in the U.S. has been lack of knowledge of a deceased's wishes. When family members know of a desire to donate, rates of consent to donate are in the 85 - 95% range compared to 25 - 55% when they do not know the deceased's wishes (e.g. Rodrigue et al., 2005; Siminoff & Lawrence, 2002). Additionally, some research has shown that knowing an individual's wishes to donate made the family 6.9 times as likely to consent to donation (Siminoff & Lawrence, 2002). Thus, increasing declarations of intent or consent through registries is one way to insure family members know of a loved one's wishes to donate.

In the U.S. there is a rapidly growing body of research focusing on campaign strategies to increase the number of individuals who have declared their intent to donate. While many of these campaigns are successful (e.g. Feeley et al., 2009; Morgan et al. 2002; Morgan, Harrison, et al., 2010), many also suffer from limited reach or impact (e.g. Quinn et al. 2006; Fahrenwald et al., 2010), and may thus be a questionable use of resources for non-profit organ procurement organizations. While new strategies such as social media (i.e. facebook) are being investigated for their ability to generate new potential donors, the results of those studies are not yet know. However, a series of recent studies (Harrison et al., 2008; Harrison et al., 2010; Harrison et al., 2011; King et al., under review) have demonstrated the ability to overcome this limited reach and provide dramatic increases in the rates of joining organ donor registries (ranging from 200% to over 500% with net increases in the tens of thousands of new registrations) by utilizing point-of-decision campaigns targeting potential donors at Division of Motor Vehicles (DMV) offices where individuals apply for driver's licenses. These campaigns have taken advantage of the large push by HRSA/DoT to establish registries in every state in the U.S., and many of these registries are operated through DMVs or their equivalents.

Utilizing estimates on family consent rates, this chapter explores differences in potential rates of donation to demonstrate how increasing the number of individuals who have declared their intent to become donors can significantly increase rates of organ donation. Additionally, this chapter explores the importance of registries and examines different approaches to increase the number of individuals who join organ donor registries at DMV branches. These strategies include: training clerks how to ask individuals to join the registry and address myths the public may express; focused volunteer trainings of people touched by donation with an emphasis on persuading the public to become donors by communicating effectively their stories of donation, addressing myths and barriers to donation, and providing mechanisms for action; point-of-decision campaign materials to establish normative influence, address barriers, and prompt action; and mass media campaigns to prime individuals to take action to be a donor when they utilize DMVs. The relative effectiveness (both in terms of creating new registrations as well as cost per registration) of these strategies is explored in this chapter.

While these campaigns have largely been conducted in the U.S., a review of barriers to donation internationally reveals similar barriers, although with culturally specific differences to those found in the U.S. (e.g. Conesa et al., 2006; Molzahn et al., 2005; Topbas et al., 2005), especially among minority populations. Many of the campaign strategies discussed in this chapter are easily modified to address different cultural and national concerns, and this chapter presents suggestions for adapting campaign strategies and materials to address these differences. Ultimately, we argue for the importance of registries (in non-presumed consent countries) and focused point-of-decision and interpersonal campaigns for use internationally.

2. The law of large numbers: DMV-based registries and potential consent and recovery rates

In 2002 The Lewin Group concluded that the "effectiveness" of donor registries could not yet be established, largely as a function of the relatively short period of time that registries have been in existence. Since that time, almost every state in the U.S. has developed either a DMV, internet, or DMV/Internet based registry. While many states have created registries, the rate of individuals joining these registries varies dramatically. For example, at the start of a recent project to increase rates of joining the registry in Michigan, only about 11% of individuals had joined the Michigan Organ Donor Registry (Harrison et. al. 2010). While this number has since increased dramatically, the percentage is still very low compared to the over 70% of the public who have joined the registry in Utah, Montana, Alsaka, Oregon, and Washington. On average, 40% of Americans have joined an organ donor registry to date. (Donate Life America, 2011). However, some OPOs are reluctant to put resources towards public education campaigns to increase registries, perhaps because of a lack of full understanding of the report, and the belief that registries are *not* effective. For many, the current definition of a successful registry appears to necessitate yielding actual organ donors; this is not appropriate given the current level of registry utilization and the number of years that registries have existed. If we accept the statistics that approximately 1% of the population will die in such a way that they could become a potential donor, states with only ten thousand registrants can be expected to yield a maximum of 100 potential donors over the registrants' *lifetime*. Comparatively, states with 1,000,000 registrants can expect to have 10,000 potential donors over the course of a lifetime. Complaining that a registry has yielded only one or two donors since a registry was established a few years ago is tragically shortsighted given the long-term potential of registering large numbers of confirmed potential donors through DMVs.

Obviously, though, some individuals would become organ donors regardless of the presence of state registries. One indication that donor registries can be a highly efficacious way to increase the number of actual donors comes from HRSA/DoT funded project conducted with Intermountain Organ Recovery System in Utah. The project began in 2002 consisted of both media and grassroots activities. The results were dramatic. The percentage of Utahans between 16 and 74 registering to become donors rose from 58.4% to 63%. While a 4.6% increase may seem modest, it represents an additional 70,224 potential donors in just less than three years bringing the total number of people registered as donors to over one million. Of all medically eligible deaths, 97% of people on the registry went on to become donors, while only 61% of non-registrants became donors. Further, the importance of using the DMV as a portal for entry to the registry was demonstrated: 99% of registrants came from the DMV, while comparatively very few signed up online (Health Resources Services Administration (HRSA), 2006).

A few examples may be useful to illustrate the full potential of how increasing the number of individuals who have declared their intent to become organ donors can actually increase the number of organ donors. Obviously, calculations of potential donors are based on many assumptions. The calculations presented below use a consent rate of 50% if the family does not know the wishes of the deceased, and 95% if they do (with over 36 states having passed first person consent laws (Donate Life America, 2011), and many OPOs moving toward enforcing first-person consent laws, this number is likely to be on the low side). Additionally, the calculations assume that 1 in 100 individuals will die in a way to make them eligible to become a donor. Further, the calculations assume an average of 3 organs are recovered from each donor. Assuming a population of 5 million, over the course of a lifetime we can expect 50,000 potential donors and 150,000 potential organs to become available for transplantation. With these assumptions in mind the table below illustrates potential consent and organ recovery rates for registries with 11% (low), 40% (current average), and 76% (current high) of the population having declared their intent to donate.

While there is certainly room to adjust the assumptions in these calculations (in either direction), these figures provide an excellent illustration of the law of large numbers in relation to organ donation registries, and the need to judge the effectiveness of registries over extended periods of time. Using these assumptions, a state with a current population of 5,000,000 and a well-filled organ donor registry could potentially save an additional 51,300 lives through transplantation compared to a state with no registry. Additionally, in the absence of in-house medical transplant procurement managers, such as in the Spanish Model (Vidal et al. 2007), well-filled registries are likely to provide consent rates at or above those found in Spain. Thus, there seems to be ample indication that donor registries have the potential to serve a very important role in increasing the rate of organ donation in the U.S. and other countries.

5,000,000 population	11% Registered Donors	40% Registered Donors	76% Registered Donors
Number of individuals on registry	550,000	2,000,000	3,800,000
Number of consents from registry	5,225	19,000	36,100
Number of consents not on registry	22,250	15,000	6,000
Total number of consents	27,475	34,000	42,100
Total % of consents per eligible donors	54%	68%	84%
Number of potential organs recovered	82,425	102,000	126,300
Number of consents if no registry	25,000	25,000	25,000
Consents as a result of registry	2,475	9,000	17,100
Potential organs recovered as a result of registry	7,425	27,000	51,300

Table 1. Examples of potential rates of consent and organ recovery by percentage of public on registry based on population estimate of 5,000,000

3. Filling organ donor registries

When looking at the numbers for an average size state in the U.S., getting 3.6 million individuals to join an organ donor registry is obviously an enormous task. The structure of the registry itself is very important, as are strategies to encourage individuals to join the registry.

DMVs that operate organ donor registries possess two key characteristics that give them substantial advantages over other venues for implementing campaigns to join donor registries. First, they reach almost all individuals over 16 years of age. Most DMVs require individuals to come in person to obtain their first driver's license or state ID card, and many require return visits every four to six years for renewals. Thus, in many states tens of thousands of individuals come through branch offices on a monthly basis. Reaching this large of a population through any other sort of intervention would be almost impossible. Second, at DMVs in states that host registries, individuals actually have to make a decision about whether to declare their intent to become organ donors. Many states require clerks in branch offices to ask members of the public if they want to join an organ donor registry. At that point and individual must decide either yes or no. Campaigns in worksites, public health fairs, flea markets, or elsewhere do not actually mandate decision-making. If an individual is unsure of their intentions toward donation they can delay their decision; this option to delay decisions may be a factor that contributes to the relatively low rates of sign-ups at many community outreach events. Targeting individuals at a place and time when a decision is required is likely to help those who are favorable but undecided to declare their intentions to become a donor.

3.1 Public education strategies to fill organ donor registries

Over the past decade, also largely as a result of funding from HRSA/Division of Transplantation, there has been tremendous growth in the U.S. in the creation and evaluation of campaigns to increase the number of individuals declaring their intent to become organ donors. Rather than reviewing the growing body of literature focused on worksite interventions, university-based campaigns, or community outreach events, the following section focuses specifically on campaigns targeting DMV branches. While campaigns in DMVs are successful at reaching large numbers, the limited amount of time spent in DMV branch offices limits the amount of information an individual is likely to process. Individuals who have substantial objections to donation may need more information or more time to be persuaded before declaring their intentions to donate. Thus, DMV campaigns may not be able to persuade those who have substantial objections to donation, suggesting the need for ongoing or more in-depth campaigns (such as those discussed in Morgan's chapter in this volume) to affect attitude and behavior change. However, getting large numbers of individuals on an organ donor registry should be a major priority given the potential increases in consent rates.

A series of recent campaigns have worked toward developing best practices to increase rates of joining organ donor registries by targeting both employees and members of the public at DMV branches. These campaigns include a pilot study in Charlotte, North Carolina focusing primarily on point-of-decision materials targeting African Americans at DMV branch offices (Morgan, unpublished manuscript); clerk trainings at DMV branches in multiple counties across Kentucky (Harrison et al., 2008) and Florida (Rogrigue et al., under review); and a series of phased interventions across Michigan targeting the general public and featuring point-of-decision materials, an interpersonal component, and a mass media intervention (Harrison et al. 2010; Harrison et al. 2011; King et al. under review).

3.1.1 African Americans and organ donor registries in North Carolina

The reasons for African Americans' reluctance to donate have been the subject of considerable speculation. In addition to lack of awareness and lack of knowledge (Morgan et al., 2003; Yancey et al., 1997), religion (Reitz & Callender, 1993; Wittig, 2001; Yancey, et al., 1997) preference for directed donation (Arnason, 1991; Hall, et al., 1991; Lange, 1992; Reitz & Callender, 1993), medical mistrust (e.g. McNamara, et al., 1999; Plawecki, et al., 1988; Reitz & Callender, 1993; Siminoff & Arnold, 1999; Siminoff & Chillag, 1999; Spigner, et al., 1999; Yancey, et al., 1997; Yuen, et al., 1998), and a desire to maintain bodily integrity (McNamara, et al. 1999; Rubens & Oleckno, 1998; Spigner, et al., 1999) are the major reasons cited by researchers for African Americans' unwillingness to donate organs.

Morgan and Cannon (2003) conducted a study of 300 African American adults in New Jersey, which demonstrated that there are key barriers that require particular attention when targeting African Americans with organ donation messages. Respondents were asked eight knowledge questions about organ donation. The level of knowledge displayed by people who had already signed organ donor cards was significantly higher (an average of 5.14 correct responses) than those who had not signed a card (an average of 3.72 correct responses). Five items in particular strongly distinguished donors from non-donors: the belief that racial discrimination plays a role in organ allocation, the belief that organ donation is associated with additional medical costs, the belief that organ allocation is more likely to favor the rich over the poor, a misunderstanding of brain death, and the belief that a black market for organs exists in the U.S. These are clearly important knowledge items to target in future organ donation promotion efforts in the African American community since they clearly (and strongly) differentiate donors from non-donors.

A campaign targeting African-Americans in Charlotte, North Carolina was one of the first projects focusing specifically on DMV branch offices targeting African Americans. For this project, brochures developed by The Coalition for Donation that targeted African Americans were further tailored to the specific concerns and needs of African Americans listed above. The rationale for using the DMV as an important site for the dissemination of organ donation information is because people are asked whether they want to be organ donors at the DMV, precisely at a time when they are unlikely to be carefully considering this issue. The campaign was successful with the targeted population. The campaign produced a 6% increase in the rate of donor registrations (from 23% to 29%) in less than one year. As a relative increase over the baseline, this represents a 26% improvement in registration rates among African Americans, and resulted in thousands of new and unique registrations. Registrations also increased among non-African Americans, who were not targeted by the campaign. However, this rate of increase was less than half of that of African Americans (Morgan, unpublished manuscript), demonstrating the importance of well-tailored and targeted messages.

3.1.2 The drive for life campaign

A second strategy for DMV based campaigns involves training DMV clerks about organ donation, and how to talk to the public about donation. While creating and managing organ donor registries through DMVs has many advantages, one of the disadvantages is that the clerks who staff DMV offices are not specialists in organ donation. Their primary job is to handle the business of the state as it relates to motor vehicles. As such, it is unrealistic to expect DMV employees to be passionate or knowledgeable about organ donation. The personal experience of two of the investigators involved with the project was that DMV clerks sometimes provided misinformation about organ donation unwittingly, and in the worst cases, actively discouraged members of the public not to designate their donor status on their license. Of course, this should not be surprising since DMV clerks cannot be expected to be better educated about organ donation than the general public. Even when OPOs provide periodic "training" (presentations) with clerks, these trainings are often sporadic, brief, and not tailored to the interactions that can be expected to occur between DMV clerks and members of the public. Thus, it appears that two barriers to the utilization of DMV-based donor registries are DMV clerk inaction (e.g. not asking people whether they would like to be a donor before laminating their licenses), and the dissemination of inaccurate information (e.g. "I won't do it myself because I know they'd let me die to get my organs").

A DMV clerk training intervention was designed to coincide with the start of a new DMV based registry that was approved by the Kentucky legislature in 2006. Just prior to the launch of the registry Harrison and colleagues (2008) conducted trainings of DMV clerks in 8 counties. Additionally, 4 counties were chosen as control counties and were matched as closely as possible on demographics. An initial survey of DMV clerks revealed attitudes and knowledge about donation that were not significantly different than that of the general population of the rest of the state. While not unexpected, this particular group of clerks had voluntarily set up a non-profit organization to promote donation and were highly supportive of the organ donation and the organ donor registry. However, even with knowledge on par with that of the general public, the clerks were tasked with talking to the public about organ donation and asking them to join the new registry.

To help overcome knowledge barriers and to increase confidence in communicating with the public about organ donation, Harrison and colleagues (2008) created a one-hour training program that covered the fundamentals of how the new registry worked (e.g. who has access to the registry, how names can be removed, etc.), basic myths and facts about organ donation based on common misperceptions that keep people from becoming donors (e.g. belief in a black market, religious beliefs about donation, brain death, medical mistrust, deservingness of recipients, problems with organ allocation, etc.). Additionally, the clerks were trained in communication techniques to enhance their persuasiveness, or at least neutrality, in asking people to join the registry (e.g. framing questions in the positive, providing short answers to questions, maintaining positive nonverbal cues, etc.). Additionally, clerks were provided with a training manual full of facts about the registry, communication strategies, and facts and myths about donation, "at-a-glance" answers to common misperceptions, and a script on the best way to ask people to join the registry. Clerks were surveyed after the trainings and there were significant increases in knowledge and attitude across all dimensions related to organ donation.

Overall, the trainings of drivers license bureau clerks proved to be highly successful, with rates of joining the organ donor registry for the first six months after the trainings 14% higher than control counties and 9% higher than the overall statewide average. This translates into thousands of new registries each month as a direct result of clerk trainings, and potentially into thousands of lives saved over time. However, over time the rates of new registries started to decrease, in spite of our best efforts to provide motivation to encourage clerks to maintain their positive communication strategies. These motivational strategies included letters from recipients and donor families, competition between branches, and on-site visits to check in with clerks, and did result in short term recovery after these motivational efforts.

In a similar study, Rogridgue and colleagues (under review) developed a series of interventions targeted at DMV staff in Florida, including training DMV staff about myths and barriers to organ donation and the importance of positive communication with members of the public. In addition to the standard brochures related to organ donation, the intervention also included periodic visits by staff and volunteers to provide information to the public about donation. During the intervention period rates of registration increased by approximately 10% (i.e. from 32.4% to 35.9%), although increases varied by region, with areas with higher minority populations seeing lower increases. As with the Kentucky DMV study, after the initial intervention period rates of joining the registry decreased slightly in intervention counties, even though presumably the same clerks who were trained were still interacting with the public. The gradual decreases found in both studies involving clerk trainings suggests an area of future research: how to keep clerks motivated to put on a positive face toward organ donation when faced with countless negative reactions.

3.1.3 The Michigan Tell Us Now DMV campaign

While some DMVs require clerks to ask the public to join the organ donor registry, other states have different requirements. Michigan's policy has been that the public must directly request the clerk in order to join the registry, rather than having clerks ask if they wish to join. As such, training clerks about organ donation was not a viable option. Additionally, this policy likely contributed to Michigan having one of the lowest percentages of the public joining the registry in the entire U.S. A series of phased interventions were constructed by Harrison and colleagues (Harrison et al. 2010; Harrison et al. 2011; King et al. under review) to help overcome this barrier to joining the registry and increase the number of people in Michigan who had declared their intent to become donors.

There were three primary elements to the Michigan interventions. First, point-of-decision (POD) materials were placed in all branch offices in intervention counties. POD materials were designed to prime the public about donation and ran for the entire six months of each intervention in each county. Messages were designed using principles from the Organ Donor Model (Morgan et al., 2002) to address knowledge and social norms about donation. The placement of materials was determined by principles of communication design (e.g. Aakhus, 2007; Harrison et al. 2010; Jackson, 1998) to encourage positive interactions about organ donation. Materials for each set of interventions modified for the target audiences of each county. Additionally, materials were designed to be encountered at every step of the process until the final interaction with the DMV clerk where they could designate themselves as donors on the registry.

Materials included posters (see figure 1) featuring local community members who had been touched by donation to encourage positive social norms about donation. Local community members were chosen over celebrities as one of the key barriers to donation in the U.S. is the belief that the rich and famous are far more likely to get transplants than a member of the general public (Morgan et al., 2005). Additional materials included footprints with organ donation messages (placed along common routes throughout the DMV offices), "clerk cards" (see figure 2) that were handed to individuals on check-in with a simple message to give the card to a clerk if they wanted to be a donor, and counter-mats (see figure 3) where customers signed paperwork at clerks' stations which again prompted them to be donors. Additionally, standard information brochures were available throughout the offices.

The second component of the intervention included a mass media campaign. The mass media campaign ran in conjunction with POD materials for the first four months of the campaign in each intervention county. Mass media components included a series of 30 or 60 second radio PSAs featuring stories of individuals touched by organ donation, and concluded with a tag line asking customers to "Tell Us Now" that they wanted to be a donor. In addition to radio PSAs there were a series of billboards (see figure 4) using the same stories and visuals that appeared in the POD materials. These billboards were placed on the approach to each DMV branch office to further prime individuals to think about becoming a donor prior to entering the branch office. In more heavily populated areas billboards were placed on the outsides of buses running through target neighborhoods. Again, materials were tailored to the primary target audience of the campaign.

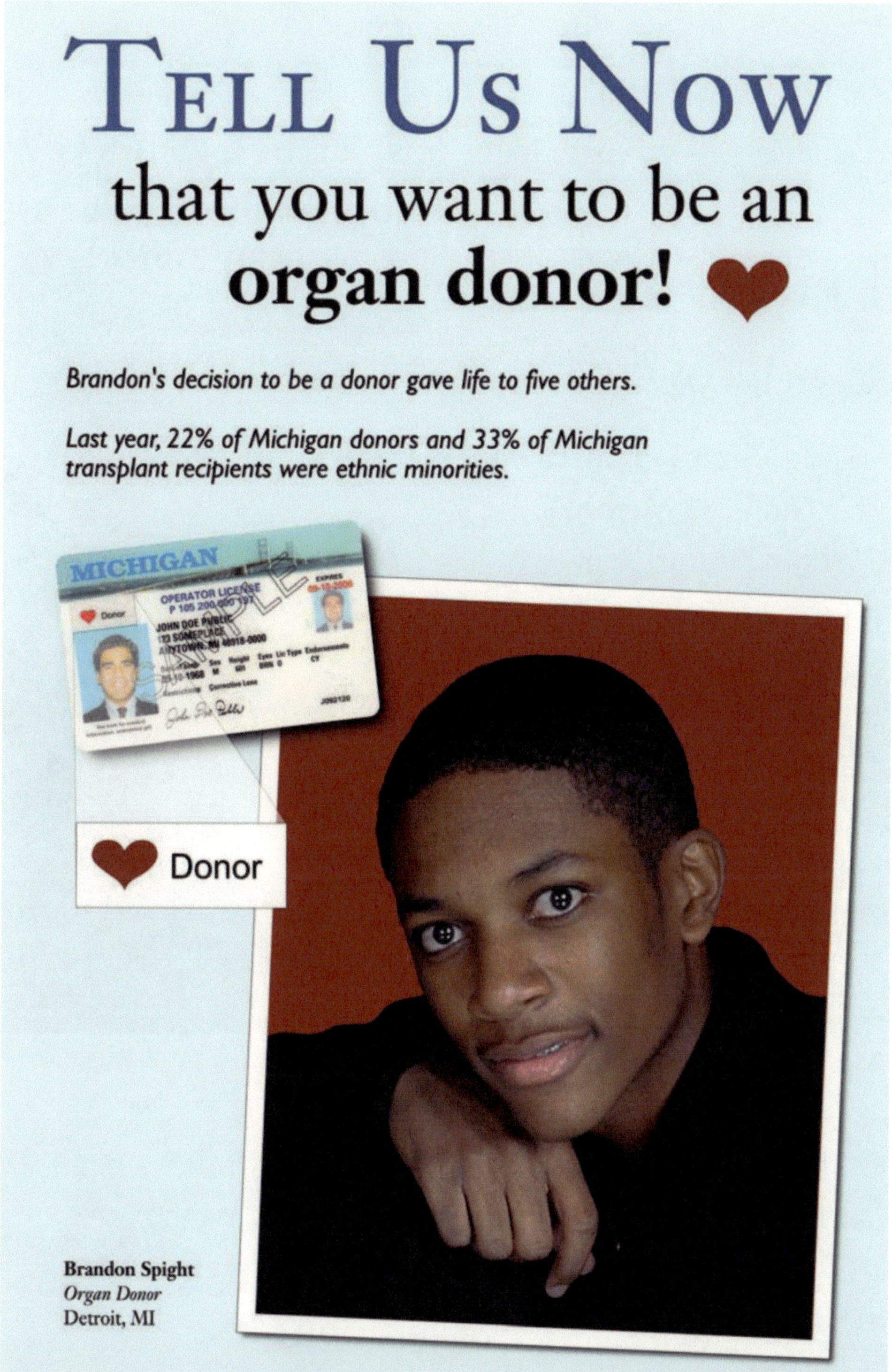

Fig. 1. Example of Poster Featuring Local Community Member Touched by Donation.

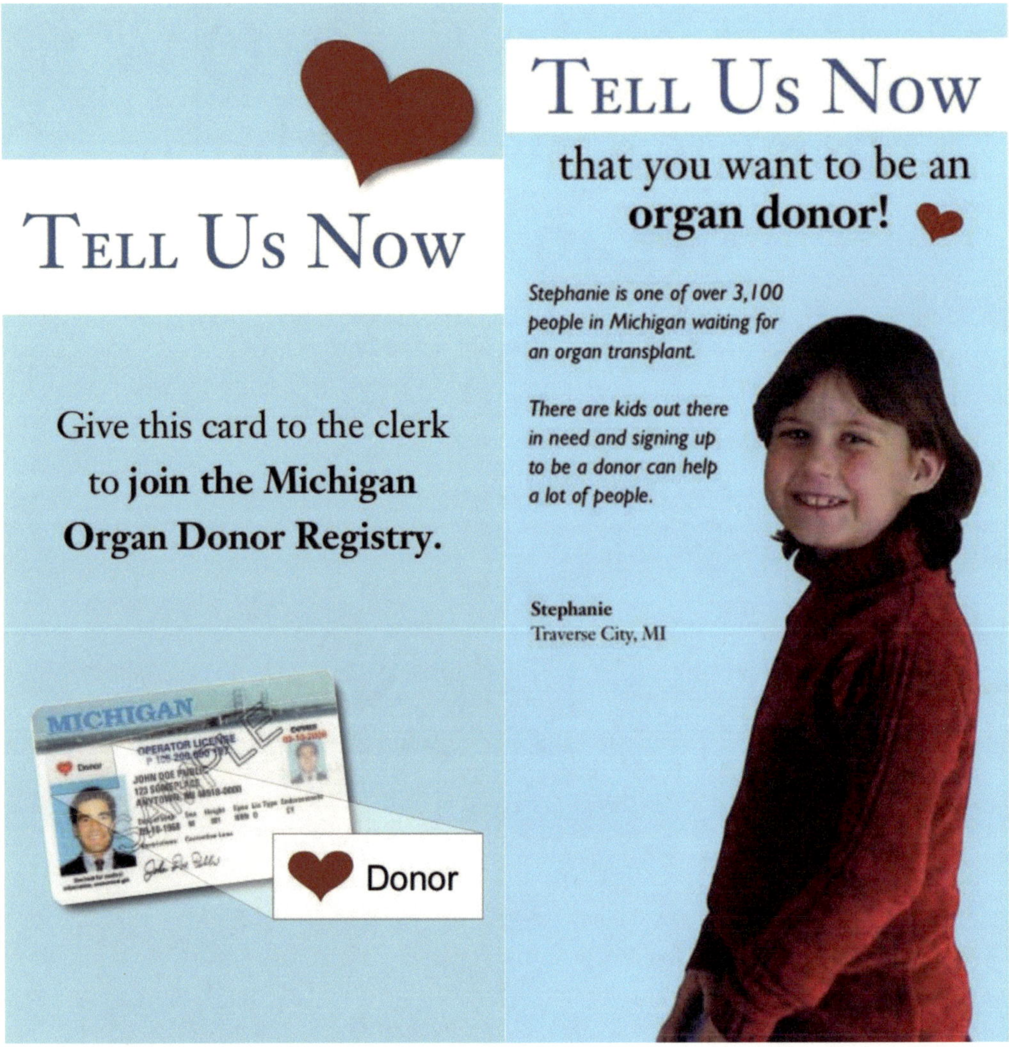

Fig. 2. Example of Clerk Card Front and Back

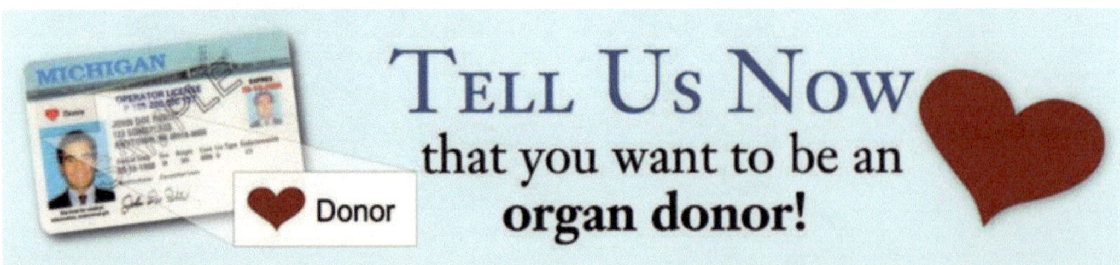

Fig. 3. Counter Mat

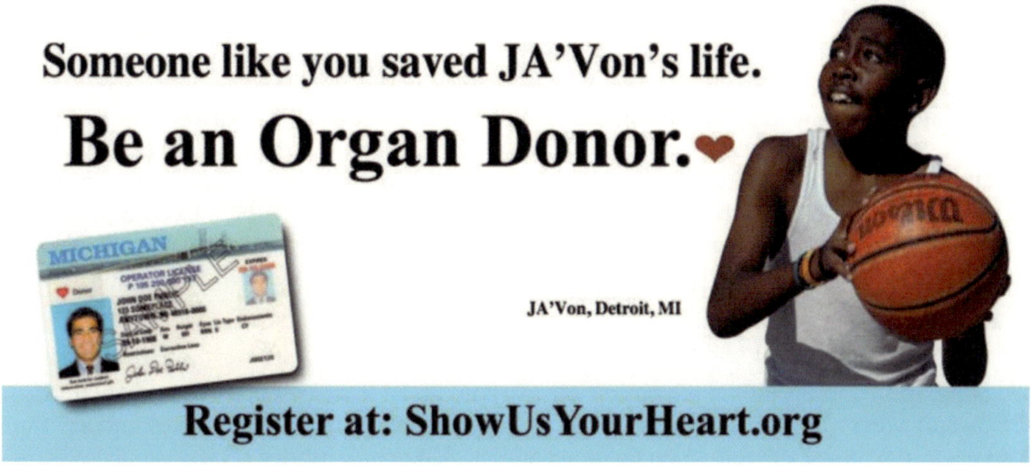

Fig. 4. Sample Billboard

A final component to the intervention consisted of an interpersonal intervention where volunteers associated with the local organ procurement organization (OPO) covered shifts in branch offices to talk to members of the public about joining the registry. Most volunteers had been touched by organ donation, either as recipients, in need of a transplant, or donor family members. The interpersonal component occurred during months 3 and 4 of the 6-month intervention. During these two months all other elements of the campaign (POD, mass media) were also included. All volunteers underwent specialized training that was modified from the Kentucky project and from two previous worksite campaigns (Morgan, Stephenson et al. 2010; Morgan, Harrison et al. 2010). The training was necessary because simply being touched by donation does not mean an individual knows all of the facts about donation or the best ways to talk to the public about donation. Volunteers wore "uniforms" with polo shirts displaying the "Tell Us Now" logo. Volunteers were placed in branch offices for four four-hour shifts per week and greeted every individual who entered DMV branch offices, handed them a "clerk card", and if any individual showed extra interest or had questions, talked to them about organ donation.

The first two phases of our interventions took place in predominately Caucasian counties (Harrison et al. 2010). Results showed that media messages plus POD materials were able to increase the number of people joining the registry by 200% and the addition of the interpersonal component raised that rate to between 300 and 380%. When mass media and interpersonal components were removed, POD materials continued to generate an approximately 200% increase compared to baseline. When we conducted our campaign in predominately African American neighborhoods using messages tailored for that population we saw even more dramatic results (Harrison et al., 2011). In zip codes with a population of 80% or more African Americans, we saw increases of 380% for media and POD materials, and over 1250% increase with the addition of the interpersonal component. POD material alone still resulted in increases of over 250% compared to baseline. Surprisingly, given many of the concerns expressed by African Americans about organ donation, we were able to increase the number of people registering to be donors to the same rate as Caucasians. Overall, in just over a year of interventions across five counties we were able to add over 60,000 unique registries above baseline data.

At the completion of the intervention in our initial 5 counties, POD materials were placed throughout DMV branch offices across the state, and an evaluation was completed on the impact of POD materials in the absence of mass media or interpersonal components (King et al., under review). When POD materials were introduced at DMV branch offices in an additional 34 (much smaller population) counties, registrations increased approximately 50% (i.e. from 9.1% to 14.6%), and over the course of 6 months generated almost 9,000 new and unique registrations over baseline. While POD materials alone do not generate as many registries as when combined with the interpersonal component, the placement of POD materials is essentially a one-time occurrence. As such, the return for very limited investment of resources is quite large.

3.2 Cost effectiveness of DMV campaign components

Creating and running public education campaigns can be a very expensive endeavor. Most OPOs and other non-profit and governmental agencies have limited resources and are thus looking to maximize the return on those resources. King et al. (under review) analyzed costs per registry for the different campaign strategies in the Michigan projects. The most cost effective way to increase registries is by using just POD materials. The cost per registry in the 34 counties that received only POD materials was $1.34 per registry. The campaigns that included the media components cost between $12 and $34 dollars per registry (the cost varied as a result of population size, the cost of the media market, and differences in registration rates of the different counties). However, given the apparently limited impact of the media, removing that cost from the estimates, and including only the POD materials and costs associated with managing volunteers, King reports costs ranging from $1.30 to $3.10. While POD materials may generate registries for the lowest cost, they don't reach as wide an audience, and many people who might be persuaded to join the registry are missed as a result. Based on the massive increases found when volunteers were on site, it appears that the use of POD materials with an interpersonal volunteer component may give not only the best value, but also reach a much broader segment of the population, resulting in higher overall numbers on organ donor registries. Regardless, if we go by earlier assumptions on rates of consent and eligible donors, adding 200 names to a registry should result in one new donor over a lifetime. Even at a cost of $34 per registry, the cost is only $6,800 to secure one donor (with an average of three organs). On the low end of $1.30 per registered donor, the cost per actual donor is closer to the $250 range. It is hard to imagine anyone objecting to spending $250 - $6,800 to save three lives. These figures suggest that OPOs should take a long-range view of public education, registries, and the donation process and commit the resources necessary to fill organ donor registries. While there are not direct cost comparisons available for clerk trainings, trainings in the Kentucky project cost approximately $35 per clerk (food during the training and a $25 gift card to a local store to compensate for their time) plus the cost of someone to do the trainings and follow up. This is a very low cost investment considering the ongoing benefits of clerk interactions.

Unfortunately, at this stage no research has been done to examine how many individuals who sign up on the registry actually become donors. However, given the arguments made earlier in the chapter, this is not an appropriate evaluation. Registries are designed for long-term benefits, with the number of donors considered over an average lifetime. What we do know is that if a potential donor is listed on a registry, they are significantly more likely to become actual donors than if they were not on the registry. The estimates provided earlier demonstrate how significant organ donor registries can be.

3.3 Structural issues for organ donor registries

We concur with The Lewin Group report (2002) that a successful registry is one which registers as many willing citizens as possible as potential donors. Registries that make it inconvenient for people to join will clearly miss many thousands of opportunities for people to join, thus reducing the potential pool of declared donors for whom "first person consent" can be secured, or in the cases of "registries of intent", providing evidence to family members of the wishes of the deceased. DMV-based registries are convenient and are squarely in the path of the majority of Americans. Any barriers to registering at DMVs (including the lack of information to make an on-the-spot decision) should be removed to further maximize utilization of the registry (The Lewin Group, 2002). Based on experiences from the previous campaigns, I suggest the following as guidelines in thinking about the development of the most effective registries.

- Registries should be housed with an agency that requires all (or at least the vast majority) of its citizens to actually come in person on a semi-regular basis and complete some form of mandatory transaction.
- Clerks should be trained in how to (persuasively) ask if an individual would like to join the registry, and to provide brief, accurate answers to questions about organ donation.
- The process should be as simple as swiping an ID card through a machine or hitting a single key to indicate desired status.
- Well-designed POD materials should be placed strategically to enhance their effectiveness as individuals engage in their normal transactions.
- Space should be provided for volunteers to set up information booths and to greet and talk with customers about organ donation.
- There should be an online version of the registry. Online registries should be easy to complete, not require a witness or the mailing in of a secondary card to verify signatures, and should have the full force of joining in person. One possible way for verification is through asking for a national identity number, social security number, or state ID number.
- Registries should have an easy mechanism in place so individuals can remove their names if they change their minds.
- While registries of consent seem to be working well in the U.S., cultural or national considerations should be taken into account and registries of intent may suffice in some contexts.
- Data should be updated in real-time and registry information should be easily accessible to those who are authorized for access.

DMV-based registries have an additional potential advantage for OPOs: They provide the opportunity to measure, in real time, actual behavior change occurring in each part of the OPO's territory. This means that concentrated bursts of public education outreach efforts with a particular population in a particular city can be evaluated on the basis of whether an increase in donor registrations has occurred. These numbers can be compared to baseline measures (the previous six months, or the number of registrations during a particular month the previous year). Of course, not all people who have been swayed by a particular outreach effort will find themselves at the DMV within weeks or months of an intervention; however, an increase in registrations will nonetheless provide a measure of the impact of a relatively large-scale intervention (e.g. a special effort to organize many churches to observe a Donor Sabbath, or the success of a media-based campaign during Donor Awareness month).

4. International perspectives and adaptation

One of the most important factors involved in consent to donation of a loved one's organs appears to be knowledge by the family of the wishes of the deceased. While registries are an excellent way to document these wishes and to provide compelling proof to the family of those wishes, registries may not be feasible in all countries or systems of organ donation. For example, in countries that have an "opt-out" system, whereby everyone is presumed to be a donor unless they have made notification of their desire not to be a donor, a registry of those wishing to be organ donors seems counterproductive. However, many of the countries that have an "opt-out" system still rely on family consent before recovering and transplanting organs (see Gevers, et al. 2004 for discussion of policy versus practice). While countries like Spain have tremendous success at achieving family consent, other countries have much lower rates of success. Campaigns that work toward some degree of documentation or family notification can serve much the same purpose as a full-fledged registry. As with registry-based campaigns, though, the focus should be on reaching large segments of the population and providing some sort of clear documentation of the wishes of the individual.

Countries who are developing systems of organ donation or who follow an "opt-in" model should consider the creation of regional or national registries. If countries are in the early stages of such a process, developing a unified data set and using common programs and programming languages will make for a system that is more easily accessed, expanded, and shared. Additionally, the more types of data that an be included on the registry, the more useful of a tool it becomes for evaluating trends and developing campaigns to target specific populations that register at lower rates to become potential donors. Examples of data that are useful from a campaign/evaluation perspective include zip code data, gender, race/ethnicity, and age. While many other types of data are useful, this type of information is often collected during DMV or identity card processes.

While many of the messages used in the campaigns are targeted toward specific U.S. population groups, many of the barriers to donation are very similar across different cultural and ethnic groups (e.g. lack of knowledge about brain death, fears of a black market, medical mistrust, perceived religious beliefs) and messages can be easily adapted to meet the needs of specific target audiences. To create effective persuasive informative campaigns, researchers and practitioners should attend to both the type and quantity of information sources (Ganikos, et al., 1994) as well as the type of message. Previous studies have shown that some types of knowledge can be low and yet not affect the willingness to donate, while other types of misconceptions can be critical to the decision to donate (Morgan & Miller, 2002; Morgan et al., 2003). Therefore, focusing on specific knowledge barriers rather than on general awareness is more likely to yield positive campaign effects. Additionally, while communication norms are different based on country, culture, and ethnicity, training key gatekeepers, volunteers, or staff members about best communication practices is key. This includes developing scripts about how to get individuals to declare intent to donate, addressing common myths and barriers to donation, telling personal stories about donation, and talking to family members about consenting to donation. Finally any campaign should be constructed on solid theoretical foundations. Variations of the Theory of Reasoned Action or the Theory of Planned Behavior that target knowledge, attitude, and social norms have seemed to work well for campaigns about deceased donation. More recently there has also been a focus on non-cognitive barriers to donation (see Morgan, 2012 for an excellent review of theoretical approaches to organ donation campaigns).

5. Conclusion

When families are aware of the wishes of a deceased loved one, rates of consent to donation are much higher than when they are not aware of those wishes. One mechanism to insure families have knowledge of a loved one's wishes is through an individual's enrollment on an organ donor registry. Organ donor registries run through DMV offices (or some similar type of agency or structure) take advantage of the law of large numbers and have the ability to quickly add large numbers of individuals to organ donor registries, thus increasing rates of consent and ultimately saving lives. Additionally, campaigns that focus on training clerks about how registries work, common facts and myths related to organ donation, and how to communicate about organ donation is one strategy that has proven effective in increasing the number of individuals who join organ donor registries. Additionally, providing theoretically driven, well-designed and well-placed POD material, and having volunteers or OPO staff members engage in interpersonal communication about organ donation increase the rates at which individuals join registries. These strategies have proven successful across multicultural populations, and campaign messages can be easily tailored to the concerns of different countries or cultures.

6. Acknowledgements

The author would like to acknowledge the many individuals whose intellectual contributions, boundless energy, support, and creativity were invaluable toward the success of several of the projects discussed in this chapter. They include Susan Morgan, Mark Di Corcia, Andy King, Elizabeth Williams, Paula Hopeck, Tammie Havermahl, Monica Johnson, Jenny Miller Jones, Rebecca Ivic, Mary Ganikos, and the many remarkable volunteers and staff members whose dedication to organ donation continues to make work like this possible.

7. References

Aakhus, M. (2007). Communication as design. *Communication Monographs*, Vol. 74, pp. 112–117, ISSN 0363-7751

Arnason, W. B. (1991). Directed donation: The relevance of race. *Hastings Center Report*, Vol. 21 No. 6, pp. 13-19, ISSN 0093-0034

Conesa, C., Rios, A., Ramirez, P., Canteras, M., Rodriguez, M. M. & Parrilla, P. (2006). Attitudes toward organ donation in rural areas of Southeastern Spain. *Transplantation Proceedings*, Vol. 38, pp. 866 - 868, ISSN 0041-1345

Donate Life America, (2011). Number of organ, eye, and tissue donors continues to rise. Retrieved August 15, 2011 from http://donatelife.net/number-of-registered-organ-eye-tissue-donors-continues-to-rise

Fahrenwald, N. L., Belitz, C., & Keckler, A. (2010). Outcome evaluation of 'Sharing the Gift of Life': An organ and tissue donation educational program for American Indians. *American Journal of Transplantation*, Vol. 10, pp. 1453 - 1459, ISSN 1600-6143

Feeley, T. H., Anker, A. E., Watkins, B., Rivera, J., Tag, N., Volpe, L. (2009). A peer-to-peer campaign to promote organ donation among racially diverse college students in New York City. *Journal of the National Medical Association*, Vol. 101, pp. 1154 - 1162, ISSN 0027-9684

Ganikos, M. L., McNeil, C., Braslow, J. B., Arkin, E. B., Klaus, D., Oberley, E. E., & White, M. F. (1994). A case study in planning for public health education: The organ and tissue donation experience. *Public Health Reports,* Vol. 109, No.5, pp. 626-631, ISSN 0033-3549

Gevers, S., Janssen, A., Friele, R. (2004). Consent systems for post mortem organ donation in Europe. *European Journal of Health Law*: Vol. 11, No. 2, pp. 175-186. ISSN 0929-0273.

Harrison, T. R., Morgan, S. E., & Di Corcia, M. J. (2008). The impact of organ donation education and communication training for gatekeepers: DMV clerks and organ donor registries. *Progress in Transplantation,* Vol. 18, pp. 301 - 309, ISSN 1526-9248

Harrison, T. R., Morgan, S. E., King A. J., Di Corcia, M. J., Williams, E. A., Ivic, R. K., & Hopeck, P. (2010). Promoting the Michigan Organ Donor Registry: Evaluating the impact of a multifaceted intervention utilizing media priming and communication design. *Health Communication,* Vol. 25, pp. 700 - 708, ISSN 1523-0236

Harrison, T. R., Morgan, S. E., King A. J., & Williams, E. A. (2011). Saving lives branch by branch: The effectiveness of driver licensing bureau campaigns to promote organ donor registry sign-ups to African Americans in Michigan. *Journal of Health Communication,* Vol. 16, No. 8, pp. 805 - 819, ISSN 1081-0730

Health Resources Services Administration, (2006). Retrieved August 10, 2006 from http://newsroom.hrsa.gov/newssummary/march2006.

Jackson, S. (1998). Disputation by design. *Argumentation,* 12, pp. 183–198, ISSN 0920-0427

King, A. J., Williams, A. E., Harrison, T. R., & Morgan, S. E. (under review) The 'Tell Us Now' Campaign for Organ Donation: Impact of Point-of-Decision Messages Promoting a DMV-Based Registry.

Lewin Group, The (2002). Guidelines for donor registry development conference: Final report. Contract HHS-GS-23F-9840H. Accessible from www.hrsa.gov.

Molzahn, A. E., Starzomski, R., McDonalk, M., & O'Loughlin, C. (2005). Chinese Canadian beliefs toward organ donation. *Qualitative Health Research,* Vol. 15, pp. 82 - 98, ISSN 1049-7323

McNamara, P., Guadagnoli, E., Evanisko, M. J., Beasley, C., Santiago-Delpin, E. A., Callender, C. O., Christiansen, E. (1999). Correlates of support for organ donation among three ethnic groups. *Clinical Transplantation,* Vol. 13, pp. 45-50, ISSN 0902-0063

Morgan, S. E. (unpublished manuscript). Final report of the Grassroots and media campaign to promote organ donation among African Americans in North Carolina.

Morgan, S. E. (in press). Public communication campaigns to promote organ donation: Theory, design, and implementation. In R. Rice & C. Atkin (Eds.) *Public Communication Campaigns.* Thousand Oaks, CA: Sage Publications. ISBN

Morgan, S.E. and Cannon, T. (2003) African Americans' knowledge about organ donation: Closing the gap with more effective persuasive message strategies. *Journal of the National Medical Association,* Vol. 95, No. 11, pp. 1066-1071, ISSN 0027-9684

Morgan, S. E., Harrison, T. R., Long, S., Afifi, W., Stephenson, M., and Reichert, T. (2005). Family discussions about organ donation: How the media influences opinions about donation decisions. *Clinical Transplantation,* Vol. 19, pp. 674 - 682, ISSN 0902-0063

Morgan, S. E. and Miller, J. (2002). Beyond the organ donor card: The effect of knowledge, attitudes, and values on willingness to communicate about organ donation to family members. *Health Communication*, Vol. 14, No. 1, pp. 121-134, ISSN 1523-0236

Morgan, S. E., Miller, J., and Arasaratnam, L. A. (2002). Signing cards, saving lives: An evaluation of the Worksite Organ Donation Promotion Project. *Communication Monographs*, Vol. 69, No. 3, pp. 253-273, ISSN 0363-7751

Morgan, S. E., Miller, J., and Arasaratnam, L. A. (2003). Similarities and differences between African Americans' and European Americans' attitudes, knowledge, and willingness to communicate about organ donation. *Journal of Applied Social Psychology*, Vol. 33, No. 4, pp. 693 – 715, ISSN 0021-9029

Morgan, S. E., Harrison, T. R., Chewning, L. V., Di Corcia, M., & Davis, L. (2010) The effectiveness of high- and low-intensity worksite campaigns to promote organ donation: The Workplace Partnership for Life. *Communication Monographs*, Vol. 77, pp. 341 - 356. ISSN 0363-7751

Morgan, S. E., Miller, J., & Arasaratnam, L. A. (2002). Signing cards, saving lives: An evaluation of the Worksite Organ Donation Promotion Project. *Communication Monographs*, Vol. 69, pp. 253 – 273, ISSN 0363-7751

Morgan S.E., Stephenson M.T., Afifi W., Harrison T.R., Long S.D., & Chewning L.V. (2010). The University Worksite Organ Donation Project: a comparison of two types of worksite campaigns on the willingness to donate. *Clinical Transplantation*, DOI: 10.1111/j.1399-0012.2010.01315.x ISSN 0902-0063

Organ Procurement and Transplantation Network, (2011). Retrieved August 15, 2011 from http://optn.transplant.hrsa.gov/latestData/rptData.asp

Punch, J.D., Hayes, D. H., LaPorte, F. B., McBride, V., & Seely, M. S. (2007). Organ Donation and Utilization in the United States, 1996 – 2005. *American Journal of Transplantation*, Vol. 7 (part 2), pp. 1327 – 1338, ISSN 1600-6143

Quinn, M. T., Alexander, G. C., Holingsworth, D., O'Connor, K.G., & Meltzer, D. (2006). Design and evaluation of a workplace intervention to promote organ donation. *Progress in Transplantation*, Vol. 16, pp. 253 – 259, ISSN 1526-9248.

Reitz, N. N. & Callender, C. O. (1993). Organ donation in the African American population: A fresh perspective with a simple solution. *Journal of the National Medical Association*, Vol. 85, pp. 353-358, ISSN 0027-9684

Rodrigue, J. R., Cornell, D. L. & Howard, R. J. (2005). *The American Journal of Transplantation*, Vol. 6, pp. 190 – 198, ISSN 1600-6143

Rodrigue, J. R., Krouse, J., Carroll, C., McMillen, L., Giery, K. Fraga, Y., Frost, T., & Edwards, E. (under review). A Department of Motor Vehicles intervention yields moderate increases in donor designation rates.

Rubens, A.J., & Oleckno, W. A. (1998). Knowledge, attitudes, and behaviors of college students regarding organ and tissue donation and implications for increasing organ/tissue donors. *College Student Journal*, Vol. 32, pp. 167-178, ISSN 0146-3934

Siminoff, L. A., & Lawrence, R. H. (2002). Knowing patients' preferences about organ donation: Does it make a difference? *The Journal of Trauma: Injury, Infection, and Critical Care*, Vol. 53, pp. 754 – 760, ISSN 0022-282

Siminoff, L. A., & Arnold, R. M. (1999). Increasing organ donation in the African American community: Altruism in the face of an untrustworthy system. *Annals of Internal Medicine*, Vol. 130, pp. 607-609, 0003-4819

Siminoff, L. A. & Chillag, K. (1999). The fallacy of the "gift of life." *Hastings Center Report,* Vol. 29, pp. 34-41, ISSN 0093-0334

Spigner, C., Weaver, M., Pineda, M., Rabun, K., French, L., Taylor, L., & Allen, M. D. (1999). Race/ethnic-based opinions on organ donation and transplantation among teens: Preliminary results. *Transplantion Proceedings,* Vol. 31, pp. 1347-1348, ISSN 0041-1345

Topbas, M., Can, G., Can, M. A., & Ozgun, S. (2005). Outmoded attitudes toward organ donation among Turkish health care professionals. *Transplantation Proceedings,* Vol. 37, pp. 1998 - 2000, ISSN 0041-1345

United Network for Organ Sharing (UNOS), 2011. www.unos.org, retrieved August 15, 2011.

Vidal, M. M., Castell, R. C., Zapata, D. P., & Duarte, G. P. (2007). Transplant procurement management: Transplant coordination organization model for the generation of donors. In R. Valero (Ed.) *Transplant Coordination Manual,* pp. 9-26. Limpergraf, S.L.: Barbera del Valles, Spain, ISBN 978-84-612-0565-3

Wittig, D. R. (2001). Organ donation beliefs of African Americans residing in a small Southern community. *Journal of Transcultural Nursing,* Vol. 12, No. 3, pp. 203-210, ISSN 1043-6596

Yancey, A. K., Coppo, P., & Kawanishi, Y. (1997). Progress in availability of donors of color: the national marrow donor program. *Transplantation Proceedings,* Vol. 29, pp. 3760-3765, ISSN 0041-1345

Yuen, C. C. Burton, W., Chiraseveenuprapund, P., Elmore, E., Wong, S., Ozuah, P., & Mulvihill, M. (1998). Attitudes and beliefs about organ donation among different racial groups. *Journal of the National Medical Association,* Vol. 90, pp. 13-18, ISSN 0027-9684

8

Social Capital and Deceased Organ Donation

Chloe Sharp and Gurch Randhawa
University of Bedfordshire
UK

1. Introduction

At present, the UK has one of the lowest numbers of deceased donors when compared to other European countries at 12.8 per million people (pmp) to the EU average of 17.8 pmp (Council of Europe, 2007). To tackle this, the NHS Blood and Transplant's (NHSBT) strategic plan 2011-2014 aims 'to increase organ donation by 60% in 2013-14 and sustain and improve thereafter', by seeking 'opportunities to achieve self-sufficiency in donation and transplantation across the UK, taking into account the changing donor pool' (p.11).

Deceased organ donation policy to address this has been argued across a wide range of fields, such as medicine, philosophy and social sciences to try to seek a way to increase Organ Donor Register numbers. The current system is an opt-in system, whereby an individual expresses their wishes to become a donor and what organs to donate through the Organ Donor Register. The aim to increase organ donation so significantly by the NHSBT, may be an indicator that the current system is not working. To try to remedy this, 'nudges' have been implemented, where individuals have to compulsory declare their wishes on their driving license as suggested by behavioural economists (Cabinet Office, 2010). When an individual applies for their driving license, they have three options; 'yes, I would like to register, I do not wish to answer this question now and I am already registered on the NHS Organ Donor Register' (Directgov online, 2011). Other more overarching policies have been considered in the literature such as paid donation (Radcliffe et al., 1998; Erin and Harris, 2003) and presumed consent (Lawson, 2008) to try to increase numbers as they have been viewed to gain a higher number of donors pmp in other countries.

This chapter will provide a way of viewing current and potential policies through applying a social capital viewpoint. The first part of this chapter will provide a brief overview of social capital and its most prolific writers. Gift exchange theory and aspects of social capital will be analysed in the second part in relation to deceased organ donation, for example, trust, reciprocity and social networks. This section will also consider prosocial behaviour, civic engagement and active citizenship from the social capital perspective. The third and final part will focus on the limitations, challenges and opportunities that face the application of social capital to deceased organ donation and organ donation policy.

2. Development of social capital theory

One of the main challenges to the use of social capital is the plethora of definitions, interpretations and forms of measurements (Claridge, 2011). Social capital has, however, become popular in recent years and has become significant in politics and governance, in particular the 'Big Society', in Mr Cameron's attempt to promote 'socially integrated behaviour' (Guardian online, 2010). Attention will now turn to brief outlines of the approaches of the main theorists; Bourdieu, Coleman and Putnam.

Levels of analysis	Bourdieu	Coleman	Putnam
Individual / class faction	➢ Titles / names ➢ Friendships / associations ➢ Memberships ➢ Citizenship		
Family / community		1.0 Family size 2.0 Parents' presence in the home 3.0 Mother's expectation of child's education 4.0 Family mobility 5.0 Church affiliation	
Community / region			➢ Memberships in voluntary organizations ➢ Voting participation ➢ Newspaper readership

Source: Claridge (2011) web page (with permission from author)

Table 1. Social Capital theorists and different levels of analysis

2.1 Bourdieu

Social capital is viewed as 'the sum of the resources, actual or virtual, that accrue to an individual or group by virtue of possessing a durable network of more or less institutionalised relationships of mutual acquaintance and recognition' (Bourdieu and Wacquant, 1992, p.119). The underpinnings of social capital were viewed as social networks and relationships according to Bourdieu, built on class and social hierarchy. His ideas were influenced by the work of Marx as he believed that social capital highlights conflict and power (Field, 2003). Social capital was something that individuals had to work at and the value of individual ties depended on the amount of connections they had and the capital gained from each connection (Bourdieu, 1980). Field (2003) argues that Bourdieu's views of social capital neglected any exploration into the 'dark side' of the concept and is orientated towards being individualistic.

2.2 Coleman

Coleman's work differed from Bourdieu's, as Bourdieu's focused on the outcome of the individual rather than the group or societies (Claridge, 2011). Coleman (1988; 1990) defined social capital as 'the set of resources that inhere in family relations and in community social organisations and that are useful for the cognitive or social development of a child or young person. These resources differ for different persons and can contribute an important advantage for children and adolescents in the development of their human capital' (Coleman, 1994, p.300).

Coleman was a functionalist sociologist believing that every section of society has a function. Functionalists view society on a macro scale, making their theories generalised about wider society, and norms and moral values are based on consensus that are maintained through socialisation. Social capital for Coleman was a function, it was seen to be in the shape of 'obligation and expectation, trust, information, norms and penalties that discourage their transgression, relational authority and social organisation and social network' (Poder, 2011, no page number). Attributes of social structures can encourage or inhibit social capital, such as altruism. These are utilised by individuals within society and for Coleman, social capital was an 'unintended result', it was something that individuals could have if they invested in social structures. Social capital may be viewed as a resource because it is created by the norm of reciprocity, reciprocity through networks, rather than on an individuals, where relationships are influenced by trust and shared norms (Field, 2003).

Coleman argued that sociological and economic concepts can be married together to create links between micro and macro levels within society. He was influenced by the work of Becker, an economist who applied economic principles to education, family and health through the perspective of rational choice theory. Rational choice theory purports that individuals act in their own interest and interactions are viewed as exchanges. Coleman argues that individuals and society are interdependent and individuals are motivated by egoism, relationships are created and sustained to become social structures and resources for individuals. Rational choice theorists believed that individuals were agents who wanted to satisfy their own self-interest. However, Coleman suggested that it is social relations that help 'establish obligations and expectations between actors, building the trustworthiness of the social environment, opening channels for information, and setting norms that endorse particular forms of behaviour while imposing sanctions on would-be free-riders' (Coleman, 1988, p.102).

Social capital for Coleman was a way of explaining how people are able to cooperate with each other against the tide of the assumptions made by rational choice theory. Coleman viewed social capital as a way of contributing to human capital, which links with education and health. He believed that social capital contributes towards collective action, Coleman argued that social capital was a public good that is created by and benefits from all of those who are part of the structure (Field, 2003), therefore co-operation is required as it is in the individual's self-interest.

2.3 Putnam

According to Putnam, a political scientist, social capital is characterised as 'features of social organisation, such as trust, norms, and networks, that can improve the efficiency of society by facilitating coordinated actions and cooperation for mutual benefit' (1993, p.169). Putnam's notion of social capital are 'moral obligations and norms, social values (especially trust) and social networks (especially voluntary associations)' (Siisäinen, 2000, p.1). Social capital increases the likelihood of collective action by 'increasing the potential costs to defectors; fostering robust norms of reciprocity; facilitating flows of information, including information on actors' reputations; embodying the successes of past attempts of collaboration; and acting as a template for future cooperation' (Putnam, 1993, p.173).

Putnam's notion of social capital was influenced more by Coleman than Bourdieu's ideas of social networks. Putnam viewed civic culture as a way of determining the success of democratic performance, being made up of a society that has high levels of trust, solidarity and a public who were interested in public affairs. Civic culture is founded on generalised reciprocity, this is where a person may help someone and expect the favour to be returned in the future by someone else when it is needed. This brings together the individual and the collective as the consequences for both are positive. Generalised reciprocity is a notion that has been previously explored by social exchange theorists such as Sahlins (1978).

Putnam et al. (1983, 1993) suggested that generalised reciprocity is unequal within society due to differing socio-economic statuses (Almond and Verba, 1963). The difference between civic and uncivil society is heavily influenced by Colemans' (1988) view of social capital, in particular networks, trust and norms of reciprocity. Putnam suggests that the demise of social capital in the United States of America has contributed towards an increase in crime and violence and an ineffective health care system as 'For a variety of reasons, life is easier in a community blessed with a substantial stock of social capital' (1995, p.67). In societies where there is generalised reciprocity, collective action is taken based on networks and civic culture and sustained more through reciprocal social relationships than voluntary associations. The decrease in social capital in the USA may be traced back to de Tocqueville according to Field (2003), who also felt that a high level of civic engagement improved democratic societies. The decline of social capital may be due to four reasons; individual's being time poor due to long working hours for both parents in families, increased travel times, television and age as younger generations are less likely to belong to clubs, vote and read newspapers (Putnam, 2000).

Putnam is well-known for his ideas of 'bridging' and 'bonding'; bonding social capital is good for 'undergirding specific reciprocity and mobilizing solidarity' (Putnam, 2000, p.22-23), between people with similar backgrounds such as a similar age or religion, or are family and friends (Woolcock, 2001). It serves as 'a kind of sociological superglue' in maintaining strong in-group loyalty and reinforcing specific identities, however, it reinforces homogeneity (Field, 2003). Bridging is 'better for linkage to external assets and information diffusion', and provides a 'sociological WD-40' that can 'generate broader identities and reciprocity' (Putnam 2000: 22-3). Connections are across a number of networks, such as work friends or acquaintances (Woolcock, 2001) bringing people together from diverse social divisions where, ties are weak according to Granovetter (1973) and structural gaps exist (Burt, 1995).

Bonding creates a sense of belonging but bridging creates positive societies. Putnam (1995) views bonding and bridging as being 'reinforced reciprocally' (Poder, 2011, page unknown). Both are appropriate for meeting different needs of individuals, bonding is beneficial for maintaining and reinforcing in-group relations and identities, whereas bridging is beneficial for linking external assets and disseminating information that generates reciprocity (Putnam, 2000). In addition, Woolcock (2001) has added linking social capital where connections are made with individuals far outside of one's community, reaching a wide range of resources.

Siisiäinen (2000) explains that trust in society is 'generalised trust' and links with generalised reciprocity. Trust links with the notion that individual agents help the common good because they trust that their action is 'rewarded' through the development of collective social relations (Newton, 1999). Generalised trust is the basis for 'brace reciprocity' and networks, 'trust creates reciprocity and voluntary associations, reciprocity and associations strengthen and produce trust' (Siisiäinen, 2000, p.3-4). In turn, this creates civic culture, breaking this cycle through actions such as disorder or not trusting society, creates non-civic culture. Putnam did have difficulty explaining where social trust began, it is complex and within post-industrial societies can come from two sources; reciprocity and civic engagement Putnam et al. (1993). He has been criticised for his lack of clarity of where social capital begins and how it can be maintained (Misztal, 2000) and assumes there are links between trust and social networks (Sztompka, 1999).

Field (2003) argues that Putnam's theory resonates with Durkheim's ideas of solidarity, his theory differs from Coleman and he is clear in not basing his ideas on rational choice theory. Putnam disagreed with Tönnie's notion of *Gemeinschaft* (organic community) and *Gesellschaft* (social organisation). He believed that family was less important than the coming together of different and distinct groups (Putnam et al., 1993) and collective action could be achieved through these 'horizontal' ties. Putnam and Coleman highlight the significance of social relationships where high levels of social capital may make up for lack of economic resources (Ryan et al. 2010).

3. The bigger picture

Up to this point, the main theorists' views have been briefly explained, now attention will turn to gift exchange theory and the finer details of social capital in relation to deceased organ donation, such as trust, reciprocity, social networks and civic behaviour. It may be noted that a definition of social capital that applies to deceased organ donation has not been specified as a result of the brief descriptions of the three theorists' approaches. Each of the approaches will be drawn upon as they all contribute towards the analysis of deceased organ donation, however Putnam's theory may be the most relevant, as it draws upon community level approaches.

3.1 Gift exchange theory as a starting point

Social capital may be considered a modern manifestation of gift exchange theory, devised by Mauss (1923). After observing archaic, money-less societies, Mauss postulated three obligations within gift relationships; the obligation to give, the obligation to receive and the obligation to reciprocate. Gift exchange theory carries some similarities to social capital, in that exchanges have wider implications for social relations and the creation of social cohesion and the key aspect of Mauss's theory, reciprocity. Gift exchange theory has been widely applied to deceased organ donation and transplantation (Sque and Payne, 1994) as it has been described as the 'gift of life' in previous health campaigns. It is believed to apply because the notion of the gift encompasses the ethos of giving, however, it has been criticised for being a simplistic and misleading metaphor (Siminoff and Chillag, 1999) and coercive (Scheper-Hughes, 2007).

Social capital has been analysed in relation to gift exchange theory by Dolfsma et al. (2008). They suggested that social capital results from 'concrete interaction (gift exchange) between concrete individuals' (p.322). A gift exchange creates a relationship that can be revisited at a future point in time and could be referred to as social capital (Bourdieu, 1986; Nahapiet and Ghosal, 1998). Gift exchange plays a significant role in the creation of social relations and networks (Cheal, 1988; Gouldner, 1960). Social capital itself may be the byproduct of the obligation to repay, featured in Mauss's theory where the recipient repays back society rather than the individual through generalised reciprocity (Dolfsma et al. 2008), this may not be immediately. Giving gifts creates social indebtedness which perpetuates the exchange process (Belk and Coon, 1993). Social capital is the reciprocal aspect of the gift exchange process, according to Coleman (1994) the repayment can be used when they require it, however trust and the context will influence this. Dolfsma et al. (2008) outlines that social capital as an outcome of the gift exchange system enables an understanding of the creation, maintenance and demise of social capital. The obligation to repay is the key to the creation of social capital.

Lessons that can be learned from the gift exchange theory analysis in relation to deceased organ donation are the 'tyranny of the gift' (Fox and Swazey, 2004) and the 'spirit of the gift' (Mauss, 1923). The 'tyranny of the gift' explains the burden that the recipient feels when reciprocating the gift as they may want to repay the donor, however they are no longer alive and it is not possible to repay them in equal terms as Mauss's theory prescribes. With regards to social capital, recipients may consider 'paying it forward', either becoming a donor or creating voluntary associations to help others. This notion links with Putnam's generalised reciprocity.

With regards to the 'spirit of the gift', this provides a mystical sense to the gift as this concept in relation to organ donation suggests that the identity of the giver is carried in the gift. This is one of the challenges that come with giving organs to anonymous strangers. In terms of social capital, this may make the connection between the donor and recipient stronger than other forms of formalised prosocial behaviour and perpetuate the need to reciprocate.

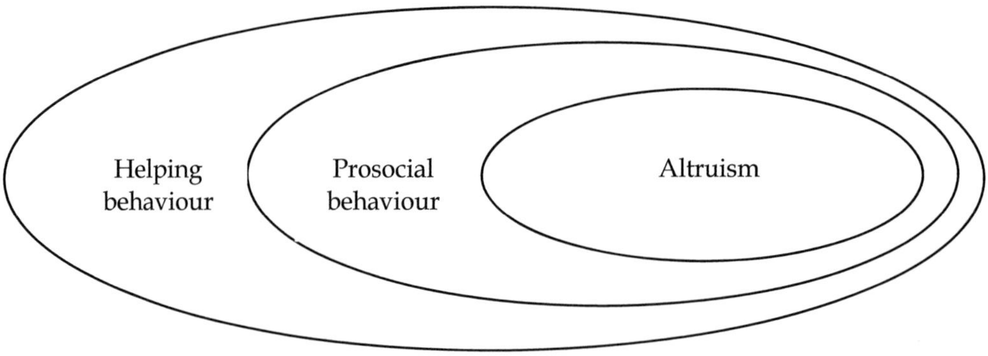

Source: Bierhoff (2001) 'Relationships between the concepts of helping, prosocial behaviour and altruism' p.286

Diagram 1. Helping and prosocial behaviour and altruism

At this point, it may be said that helping behaviour, prosocial behaviour and altruism may be defined differently (Bierhoff, 2001). Helping is where individuals support one another, prosocial behaviour is where the action is intended to benefit the welfare of the recipient, not driven by professional obligations and the recipient is a person, not an organisation. Altruism is a type of prosocial behaviour is constrained by the motivation of the individual's empathy. These definitions according to Bierhoff (2001) may be useful in defining further the type of behaviour that is being displayed by donors and donor families. Donors give organs to help others and this may be motivated by altruism, this is one of the challenges that Titmuss found in his work on blood donation and will be discussed later.

3.2 Social capital and deceased organ donation: Giving the 'gift of life'

From an extensive literature review, it is suggested that social capital can provide a useful way of viewing deceased organ donation and its policies, using lessons from gift exchange theory as a springboard. Social capital considers the multi-layered links within society such as micro-, meso- and macro (Schuller et al., 2000)(Table 2). For example, the micro level considers the individual and psychological theories, such as self-efficacy, and influences on decision making on health behaviours (Campbell, 2002). The micro-level may also account for the socio-demographics and socio-economic status of the individual such as their level of income and education. These may in turn have an impact on the kind of community that the individual resides in, whether they feel safe and they belong to this community and also their access to health services and specialist service information, such as organ donation and transplantation. The meso level is community, this may be in the form of neighbourhood groups, taking urbanisation into account, the social environments within these communities and the perceived norms. Existing communities could hold potential for health promotion in accessing groups of people and tailoring messages. Communities may be in the form of neighbourhood groups or business acquaintances (Narayan and Cassidy, 2001). The macro level takes into account wider society such as social, economic and political aspects and in relation to deceased organ donation may be influenced by the imagined 'other' who may be the organ recipient, a stranger in society. It could take into account the social norms of organ donation and laws, policies and governing bodies around organ retrieval.

Micro	Individual
Meso	Group/Community
Macro	Society

Table 2. Different levels of social capital

From table 3, it is possible to see from the items highlighted in green, that deceased organ donation spans across different levels of society and social capital theory at different points in time. There is the point when the individual signs the register, the family consenting to donation, the donation process and the repercussions of the donation in a social sense. Heffron (2000) explains the different types of ties, these are strong (repeated) or weak (temporary); vertical (through hierarchical structure) or horizontal (decentralised authority); open (civic engagement) and closed (protected membership); geographically wide or close; instrumental (membership for individual needs) or principled (membership as solidarity). Reasons for donating are complex as it may involve many factors on different levels as illustrated by Table 3.

	Bonding	Bridging	Linking	
Macro- level	Honours and law	Diplomacy, war	International Law	**Sanctions**
	Patriotism and trust *(Trusting strangers/Social norms towards donation)*	Treaties	Human rights, aid *(Right to live/ Helping others)*	**Norms**
	Nation or race *(Perceived recipient/ Imagined 'other')*	Trading links etc	UN etc *(NHS/Perceived distribution and allocation of organs i.e. locally, nationally or internationally)*	**Networks**
Meso-level	Exclusion *(Myths and concerns such as transplantation occurring when alive and death anxiety)*	Group conflict	Enforcement	**Sanctions**
	Community customs *(Death rituals)*	Out-group understanding	Mutual respect *(Between donor family and recipient/ Community views towards donation)*	**Norms**
	Neighbourhood or workspace *(Building trust/ discussion about donation)*	Links between communities *(Organ donor family and recipient)*	Links between strata	**Networks**
Micro-level	Withdrawal of affection	Shame and reputation	Shaming and formal sanction	**Sanctions**
	Love and care *(wanting to help others)*	Reciprocity etc	Generosity *(The organ as a selfless gift rhetoric)*	**Norms**
	Parents and siblings *(Make final decision/discussion/ trust)*	Acquaintances, friends, etc *(Building trust/ discussion about donation)*	Links to powerful	**Networks**

Source: Halpern (2005) p. 27

Table 3. Amended conceptual map of social capital

Moseley and Stoker (2010) suggested the social norms at present is for people to agree with organ donation in principle, but not to sign up to become organ donors, there is no social sanction in shaming for those who are not donors. Also, there may be perceived sanctions for becoming donors, which may link with the disapproval of family members whose beliefs may be based on myths of organ donation, illustrating the need for education and family discussion.

To some degree, the organ transplantation process is a type of bridging social capital as it is bringing together people across different networks, the ties are weak as the connection occurs once but at the same time is strong as characterised by the 'spirit of the gift'. They are vertical as the process occurs through the NHS hierarchical structure, and is instrumental as it fulfils the needs of the recipient. After the transplantation event, individuals would have experienced organ donation, either donor families or recipients may create organisations to help and support one another.

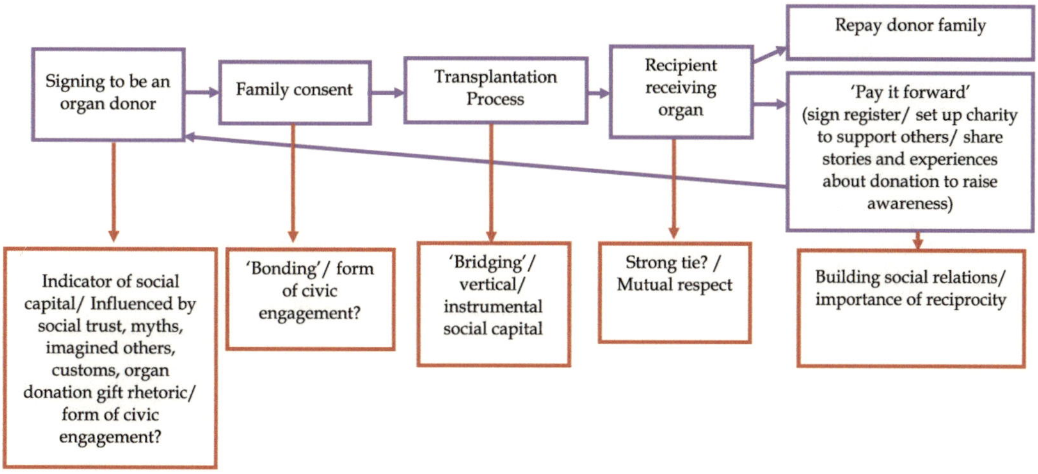

Diagram 2. Social Capital in Deceased Organ Donation

Morgan et al. (2006) commented on social capital in relation to the cohesiveness of local communities and 'bonding' social capital within these, leads to the unwillingness to donate outside of them. This may be due to low levels of bridging, where ties are loose with other social groups and cultural differences may the way that imagined others in society are perceived. Another explanation may be due to kinship and group belonging, this limits exchange with outsiders. Their view of social capital would link in the diagram to signing to be a donor in that there may be a perception that organs only should be given to kin or those within the same group, this may be religious or ethnic for example. Their research was based on White, Black Caribbean, Black African, South Asian and mixed race, the majority of respondents being White. This may also link with national identity, multiculturalism, racism and prejudice.

This connection where there is a preference of organs going to kin or others that individuals are familiar with could link with Lam and McCullough (2000) work where 'social distance' described this phenomenon. Social distance was illustrated by participants who stated that they would be 'willing to donate organs to people similar to themselves before they will donate to strangers at large. This is an issue of similarity to and distance from the individual based on family ties and kinship, rather than a matter of racial prejudice' (Lam and McCullough, 2000, p.455-456).

3.3 Structural and cognitive social capital and organ donation

Organ donation may be considered to fit Uphoff's framework as it views social capital as being structural and cognitive. According to Uphoff (2000), structural social capital are rules, roles, procedures and networks that contribute towards mutually beneficial collective action (MBCA) and cognitive social capital are mental processes that are reinforced through culture and are in the form of norms, beliefs and values contributing to MBCA.

The structural element of social capital may relate to the procedures around becoming an organ donor, the organ removal and transplantation process and networks within this process between the donor family, health care team and recipient. The cognitive aspect of social capital may relate to the norms and beliefs towards organ donation. Uphoff explains that these two forms of social capital are interdependent, the structural aspects can be observed but the cognitive aspects cannot.

	Structural	Cognitive
Sources and manifestations	Rules and roles, networks and procedures. Organ donation and transplantation process/ Healthcare team training/ Stories in the media about donation	Norms, values, attitudes and beliefs Towards organ donation (myths/concerns, helping behaviour and morals) influenced by religion, culture, and society
Domains	Social organisation NHS Blood and Transplant/Government/Local hospitals/Transplant Team	Civic culture Society
Dynamic factors	Horizontal and vertical linkages Networks within the organ donation and transplantation process	Trust, solidarity, cooperation and generosity (Sense of belongingness) Possible reasons for donating organs
Common elements	Expectations that lead to cooperative behaviour	

Source: Uphoff (2000) p.221

Table 4. Structural and cognitive levels of social capital

It may be argued that individuals are not fully informed as they are not being told in detail about organ donation through the adverts and when signing up to register. At this point, it is emphasised that organ donation is a personal decision that should be fully informed, the term 'cooperative behaviour' is part of this model and it is not advocated that organ donation is this as it would suggest coercion. This model illustrates the interaction between the structural aspects and cognitive aspects. Cognitive aspects of social capital in relation to deceased organ donation.

The structural and cognitive forms of social capital are evident in Bourdieu, Coleman and Putnam's work at a descriptive level, however, not at an analytical level (Uphoff, 2000). Uphoff believed that roles and rules, as well as norms, values and attitudes produce expectations about the way in which people act. According to Healy (2006), these expectations of how the donation process should be experienced may be facilitated by 'cultural account of organ donation', where there are 'feeling rules' (p.117). In other words, literature provided by the hospital is intended to guide individuals in how they should be feeling about donating organs and the expectations that other actors, such as other family members, health care teams, have of them.

Networks are viewed by Uphoff as patterns of social exchange that exist over time and are perceived to be important for social capital. In relation to organ donation, exchange of information may be viewed as a form of social capital. In the study by Darr and Randhawa (1999) social networks were viewed to be key in disseminating information about organ donation. This may be linked to social capital because according to Coleman (1994), information provides a basis for action. Thus, if information is being circulated based on falsities or myths, such as the need for body totality, this may influence the action that individuals take.

The property of social capital raises interesting questions, some forms of social capital are "collective goods", they are not owned property of those who are benefitting from them (Coleman, 1988). This is an interesting notion because it begins to question the property of organs. This is usually debated within the literature about the commercialisation of organs. However, if organs are viewed as "collective goods" because they are given to strangers who are part of the wider collective, would it be the individual who owns it or the donor family?

In relation to welfare policy, Le Grand (1997) suggests that human motivation and behaviour impacts on policy. Those who 'finance, operate and use the welfare state are no longer assumed to be either public spirited altruists (knights) or passive recipients of state largesse (pawns); instead they are all conserved to be in one way or another self-interested (knaves)' (p.149). This may suggest that individuals are motivated by their self-interest and this may have implications for organ donation policy. These type of self-interest based arguments link with the beginning of the chapter for payment or reward based donation policies.

3.4 Social capital and blood donation

By taking these aspects into consideration, when looking at organ donation's current and alternative policies through a social capital lens, it may explain the issues of altruistic donation and potential issues in the use of alternative policies. Social capital has not yet been applied directly to deceased organ donation in this sense, however it has been applied to health in terms of quality of life and wellbeing (Campbell, 2002). The closest comparison that can be made is to the account of applying social capital to blood donation. Alessanderini and Carr (2007) found that social trust is currently low in Australia due to increased alienation but through participatory policy-making, this has had positive implications for blood donation as individuals feel involved. Alessandrini et al. (2007) suggests that social capital should be considered in blood donation but recognises the demographic factors which will impact on it.

Blood donation is viewed as the benchmark of the measurement of levels of social capital alongside voting behaviour according to Mohan et al. (2004). Blood donation and voting have similarities because individuals visit a centre to perform the action, but for deceased organ donation it is in two private forms. The individual filling in a form to illustrate their willingness and the families making a decision about their recently deceased loved one. Both decisions are made in an isolated environment, where it may not be further spoken of, making it difficult to sow the seeds for social capital to flourish. The individual's decision may be made impulsively when given the chance, when 'nudged' on the DVLA form or presented with opportunities on the GP registration form or Boots Advantage card form. Aside from these opportunities, individuals may not consider organ donation deeply if they were undecided when asked on the forms. But for others, deep consideration may be needed before signing the forms and they may forget about signing up altogether. The decision for the family is made at a time of great difficulty and at some stage of the bereavement process.

Putnam (2000) prosocial behaviour which is formal such as blood donation, benefits strangers, and can be viewed as an indicator of social capital. Social capital has been linked with blood donation and organ donation by Mohan et al. (2004) who view donation as a measure of social capital and was compared with electoral behaviour. They illustrate the limitations of the studies that showed links between blood donation and social capital. It may be that blood donation has been linked with electoral behaviour as forms of measuring social capital, perhaps because they are both public acts in that for both one goes to the polling station or the bloodmobile collection point to perform the act. Organ donation, however, is private and may not be viewed as a measure for social capital because it is performed by donor families and not the individual. However, signing the organ donor register may be a measure of social capital because it is the individual's confirmation of their wish logged on the ODR where the statistics about UK donor numbers are available. This comparison may be limited though as, blood donation and voting is something that can be done a number of times in one's lifetime, organ donation may help someone at some point in the future, if their family allow it. Blood donation and voting are personal decisions, but donation is a family decision. Blood donation and voting have tangible outcomes that the individual can experience, but organ donation is something that happens after one dies.

3.5 Analysis of individual aspects of social capital in relation to organ donation

3.5.1 Norms

Moseley and Stoker (2010) in their research, they challenge the social norm and civic behaviour based on information circulated within networks. In their study, there was an information exchange within existing virtual social groups such as blogs and Twitter where one's decision to become an organ donor was told to others. Education has been a source for sparking family discussion in a recent Maastricht programme in The Netherlands (Reusbaet et al., 2011), whereby adolescents were educated in organ donation and they spoke to their families about it, rather than leaving it to older generations and parents to raise the topic with their children. Raising awareness and educating people about donation had a direct impact on engagement with organ donation. For example Vinokur et al. (2006) showed that pupils shown educational materials about organ donation were more likely to contact the organ donor registry. Through a social capital lens, the key is not just about educating people, but the ongoing information exchanges that occur within social networks.

3.5.2 Generalised reciprocity

Adler and Kwon (2002) suggested that generalised reciprocity 'resolves problems of collective action and binds communities. It transforms individuals from self-seeking and egocentric agents with little sense of obligation to others into members of a community with shared interests, a common identity and a commitment to the common good' (p.25). From this perspective, low organ donation may be viewed as a social problem that can be solved through collective action, knowing that this act will help others and will build up a sense of community and contribute towards the 'common good'. Rather than an individual issue, where past research has focussed on attitudes and behaviours in decision making, perhaps organ donation could be looked at from a wider perspective that helping a stranger will not only help one person, but many others.

Portes (1998) argued that it was obvious why the "recipients" of social capital wanted the benefits of it, but what about the "donors", what motivates them? He argued that a tie did not constitute returned benefits, he supported Putnam's et al. (1993) notion of trust and norms in motivating "donors". This has been dismissed by critics who believe that individuals are egoistic (Adler and Kwon, 2002). But Portes (1998) suggest that individuals are motivated by 'consummatory' motives which are 'deeply internalised norms, engendered through socialisation in childhood or through experience later in life by the experience of a shared destiny with others' (Adler and Kwon, 2002, p.25). Another motive may be 'instrumental' which are norm based, influenced by rational choices and obligations created through gift exchange or what Portes calls 'enforced trust' by the broader community.

Coleman referred to social capital contributing to the sanction of free-riding; this is a phenomena that Sýgora (2009) has expanded upon in his chapter *'Altruism Reconsidered'*. This links with Trivers (1971), an evolutionary psychologists work and social exchange theory where individuals would receive the benefits of others without providing any input. For altruistic systems to be successful, such as organ donation, free-riders should be sanctioned (Sýgora, 2009, p.31) and may be problematic for social capital because it would stagnate the reciprocal element. But, it may spur on social capital and reciprocation as the individual may feel guilty taking something that they were not willing to give.

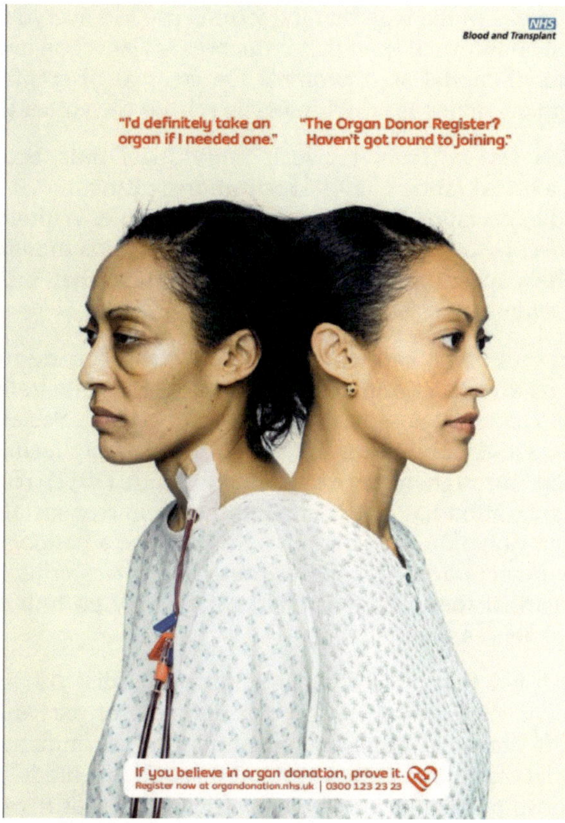
NHS
Blood and Transplant
"I'd definitely take an organ if I needed one."
"The Organ Donor Register? Haven't got round to joining."
If you believe in organ donation, prove it.
Register now at organdonation.nhs.uk | 0300 123 23 23

Source: Organ Donation online (2011a)

Diagram 3. Advert as part of current campaign

In this poster, one can see that if one is willing to take an organ they should be willing to donate. The emphasis has moved away from the notion of the gift and towards obligations and reciprocity. This the byproduct of social capital and later stage of the giving process rather than focusing on the creation of the 'gift relationship'. However, this image may be seen as a way of making individuals feel guilty and emotionally blackmailed into donating and focuses on the recipient rather than the donor and reasons to donate such as altruism. It does not currently promote reciprocity in the form that will promote social cohesion and contribute towards society. In Alessandrini's (2007) research, 1.7% donated blood as they felt guilty, most people donated blood as they felt they were socially responsible (24.6%), received personal satisfaction (28.3%), wanted to give back to the community (31.3%) and wanted to do good (13.8%). These notions relate to civic engagement and helping the common good which will be explored later in the chapter.

3.5.3 Trust

Within social capital, trust is a perception that the individual has towards known others in their immediate and wider communities, but also towards strangers and wider society. The definition of trust is problematic as it varies across disciplines Tonkiss and Passey (1999) illustrate that social capital theorists view trust as instrumental in economic terms, but imply moral and normative values in the way that the term is used in everyday language. They felt that trust is a feeling on an informal level that influences social action and interaction. Trust is a recurring issue in social capital as it prompts the creation of social networks which are sustained through common values as individuals can rely on each other (Furbey et al., 2006).

However, Beem (1999) states 'Trust between individuals thus becomes trust between strangers and trust of a broad fabric of social institutions; ultimately, it becomes a shared set of values, virtues, and expectations within society as a whole. Without this interaction, on the other hand, trust decays; at a certain point, this decay begins to manifest itself in serious social problems… The concept of social capital contends that building or rebuilding community and trust requires face-to-face encounters'. (p. 20)

Gilchrist (2004) found that social capital is a 'collective asset made up of social networks based on shared norms and trust and mutuality' (p.4). This illustrates the importance of social networks in the creation and sustaining of social capital. Social capital accounts for perceptions of trust in society and strangers which may impact feelings of belonging and wanting to help others through organ donation. Putnam (2011) recently theorised that multiculturalism and migration has contributed to the decline of social capital in the UK. In a sense deceased organ donation decisions may link to one's national sense of belonging, trust in society and strangers and perhaps wanting to express criteria for preferences for recipients of one's organs if they fear that their organs may go to a community that they have had negative experiences with.

Homans's (1950) suggested that gift exchange generated social cohesion and people may invest in relationships. Social capital may be an outcome of exchange relations through social interactions. Gift exchange literature purports that the initiation, maintenance and possible decline of social capital can be understood through this model (Dolfsma et al. 2008). Within the gift relationship, there is an element of 'trust' in that the gift will be put to its appropriate use and also the gift will be reciprocated.

3.5.4 Social solidarity

Solidarity is a notion that has been given attention in bioethical issues according to Nuffield Bioethics online (2011) and is being examined further. The term is viewed to be ambivalent, but may 'inform questions on bioethics where philosophical and policy issues do not turn only on individualised ethics' (webpage). However, social solidarity can be defined as 'the integrative bonds that develop between persons and the social units to which they belong. Solidarity is potentially composed of both behavioural and affective components, but as research on social networks has shown, the two are frequently unrelated - structural or situational factors may encourage or constrain behavioural interaction independent of the strength or closeness of the relationship' (Molm et al., 2007, 207).

Through analysing Mauss's gift exchange theory, Douglas (1990) suggested that it is in the interests of the members of the collective to participate and exchange gifts and services with others (Komter, 2005). This links with social capital and the notion that deceased organ donation is in the interest of individuals. More organs will be available, meaning that individuals will benefit from this 'resource' if they require an organ if they are ill. By collectively dealing with the issue, the byproduct of this may be the strengthening of social relations and the building of social solidarity. Mauss (1923) concurs that gifts create social bonds and in an analysis of Titmuss's work, Rose (1981) suggested that the NHS assisted the social solidarity of Britain. Titmuss (1971) in his study compared paid and unpaid blood donation in the USA and UK respectively and found that the UK blood quality was better. It is debated whether Titmuss suggests that altruism was a motivating factor behind donating blood, or whether it was other, more selfish factors such as increasing individual's self-esteem. However, his work heavily influenced policy on blood and organ donation policy.

The main criticism of Titmuss's work is the notion that donation is based on pure altruism, similar to that of charitable giving, without obligation to reciprocate. Sýgora (2009) added that giving to charity benefits the altruistic and egoistic motives, Komter illustrates 'feelings of being morally obliged to return a gift and not purely altruistic motives are the main psychological impetus to reciprocal giving' (2006, 46-48). She found the motives behind giving, the role of gratitude helped maintain social relations and refers to Simmel's work, 'By mutual giving, people become tied to each other by a web of feelings of gratitude. Gratitude is the motive that moves us to give in return and thus creates the reciprocity of service and counterservice' (Komter, 2006, p.67). Reciprocity is a key factor in the creation of the 'cement of society' (ibid, p.203).

Putnam (2011) recently argued that the lack of homogeneity, in the shape of multiculturalism in Western societies is leading to atomised societies, not cohesive ones. Diversity was considered to strengthen social capital, but Putnam challenges this. At this point, it may be theorised that social and national identity and to some extent, for migrants or second generation migrants, ethnic identity may play a role. Perhaps linked with multiculturalism is the fragmentation of what 'Britishness' or 'Englishness' is, this is another area entirely and is outside the scope of this chapter, but is worth acknowledging at this point.

3.5.5 Altruism

Altruism is 'to act on concerns for others' welfare as well as their own' according to the social psychologist Farsides (2007). Altruism has been defined earlier in this chapter and, but this definition highlights self-interest behind altruistic acts. Durlauf and Fafchamps (2004) did view a link between altruism and social capital 'One... claim often made in the literature is the idea that social capital favors altruism and raises concerns for the common good - the 'touchy-feely' side of social capital... Even a minor increase in altruism can raise social efficiency, [as shown] in a standard Prisoner's Dilemma game...Altruism provides an efficient solution to free-riding - a principle that most religions seem to have discovered centuries ago.' (Durlauf and Fafchamps, 20-21). Free-riding is a weakness in altruism (Sýgora, 2009) and in social capital (Adler and Kwon, 2002). Smith (2007) believes that the link between altruism and social capital may be a two-way relationship, social capital may encourage altruism, facilitate reciprocity and perpetuate further interaction, creating further social capital.

Sýgora (2009) suggested that deceased organ donation is a form of charity, similar to that of alms-giving found in religion. However, charity is perhaps a uni-lateral form of giving, whereas lessons from gift-exchange theory when applied to deceased organ donation would suggest that some level of reciprocation exists from recipients. Individuals may not be able to fully repay the donor family, however, they would be able to help others in the future, through 'paying it forward', as mentioned earlier when discussing generalised reciprocity.

Whether altruism exists is debatable, from a socio-biological perspective such as Dawkins or an economic viewpoint, such as Adam Smith, both fields converge their views that individuals act for their own self-interest. But altruistic acts may be strategic according to List (2007) in that individual's help people only if they are to be benefited in some way. Komter (2006) found that the individual's expressed altruistic motives, such as love and solidarity but it is gifts may have a 'strategic aim'. Gifts benefit a person in need but simultaneously appease the donor's conscience.

However, if altruism does exist, Alessandrini (2007) highlights that it is socially constructed (Bishop and Rees, 2007; Healy, 2006) and Rushton (1980) argues that it is something that is taught and practiced. Titmuss (1970) found that none of the donor's answers were completely altruistic, there was 'some sense of obligation, approval and interest, some feeling of "inclusion" in society; some awareness of need and the purpose of the gift' (p.238). More recently, Healy (2006) argued institutional and individual aspects of altruism and suggests that it was the NHS which collected the blood that created the bond to wider society and enabled donors to give their blood for personal reasons and to help the general demand. He states 'the ways in which society organises and structures its social institutions...can encourage or discourage that altruistic in man' (p.225). Etzioni (2003) suggests that 'It cannot be stressed enough that the reference here is not to altruism, which critics correctly point out often is an insufficient motive for action... .Rather reference is making organ donation a part of one's sense of moral obligation, something one cannot look in the mirror or face friends without having lived up to' (p.1).

The Behavioural Insights Team, part of the Cabinet Office, influenced by behavioural economics suggest that people make choices in their own interest, especially when unaware of the facts Thaler and Sunstein (2008). In relation to organ donation, they suggest a libertarian paternalistic approach, libertarian where there is no government coercion and paternal as the government are able to nudge. The government is trying to create prosocial behaviour and have created the behavioural insight team, aka the 'nudge unit'. Halpern (2005) suggests that social networks aspects could be combined with behavioural economics.

Smith, a medical scholar, suggested there are four attributes of altruism; 'a sense of personal responsibility for another's well-being...a sense of compassion for another...a sense of empathy...an uncalculated selfless commitment to the needs of others' (1995, p.787). The consequences of altruistic acts are 'a vicarious pleasure in the welfare or happiness of others; a sense of relief when another's needs appear to be met; good equated with caring for others' (cf. Rapport and Maggs, p.498). Smith's arguments concur with debates around communitarianism and individualism and Dworkin (1992) 'civic republican' and 'altruistic citizen' (p.209). Dworkin stated that the altruistic citizen is driven by the well-being of others and the civic republican is driven by acting as a member of a community. To encourage the altruistic citizen to behave altruistically towards the community, he suggests integration as a mechanism that has been highlighted as being challenging by Putnam.

3.5.6 Civic engagement and civil society

Civil society is the connection between welfare and citizenship and active citizenship is the crux of civil society because it addresses the obligation towards the common good and builds a 'good society' of trust, compassion and participation. Civil society includes the 'market, and "kinship, family and community systems" ... and "the education system, the union movement, local government, the media, voluntary organisations and ... the church"'(cf. Sibeon, 1997, p.81). However, in the 1990s there was a debate around civil society, whether it is based on civic trust and goes back to collectivism as it purports a new form of communitarianism (Etzioni, 1994; Fukuyama, 1995). Communitarianism '...seeks to make organ donation an act people engage in because they consider it their social responsibility, something a good person does, akin to volunteering' (Etzioni, 2003, p.1).

The Borrie Report (1994) states that social capital is made up of institutional relationships of civil society which is built upon solidary individualism and active citizenship and includes extended families, community groups and religious organisations (p.307-308). Beveridge suggested New Labour's focus on active citizenship is a response to globalisation pressures. The sense of social citizenship should be based on agreed principles on rights, duties and responsibilities of the state and individuals to maintain state welfare in the future (Pratt, 2006). To some degree this is still the current political agenda as Cameron's Big Society advocates community and empowerment through social action (Cabinet Office, 2011).

If civic engagement is part of social capital, then who owns it? Putnam was reluctant to ascertain whether it was a private or public good, 'Social capital has both an individual and a collective aspect—a private face and a public face. First, individuals form connections that benefit their own interests. One pervasive stratagem of ambitious job seekers is "networking," for most of us get our jobs because of whom we know, not what we know—our social capital, not our human capital… If individual clout and companionship were all that there were to social capital, we'd expect foresighted, self-interested individuals to invest the right amount of time and energy in creating or acquiring it. However, social capital also can have "externalities" that affect the wider community, so that not all the costs and benefits of social connections accrue to the person making the contact… Social capital can thus be simultaneously a "private good" and a "public good." (Putnam, 2000, p.20).

3.6 Grass-roots approach to health promotion

As social capital does emphasise the importance of communities, this would naturally lead onto the recommendation of a grass-roots approach where messages are tailored to established communities. Schuller et al. (2000) explains that social capital may be used in this functionalist way but social capital itself does not encourage this. Health care professionals, local community leaders and organ recipients from the local community to attend events to increase awareness of organ donation and promote discussion. Social networks are emphasised in social capital, networks can be created and established through making contact with communities, such as neighbourhood or religious. Overall, the sum will be greater than all parts.

Taking a grass-roots method to promoting organ donation is not new, by taking a social capital stance, its importance as an approach is emphasised. Darr and Randhawa (1999) in the UK and American scholars such as Callender (1989) and Hall et al. (1991) advocate a grass-roots approach. Recently Whitelaw (2011) in the Guardian argued that face to face events help, as taking a grassroots approach has helped elsewhere. They illustrate that in July 2009, Kidney Research UK had a Peer Educator programme which was tailored to their audience, it was either religious in nature or for Joe Bloggs on the street, and started people talking about it through social networks. Social networks are a key element of information dissemination, people share experiences and information but for organ donation it may be wrong information which may be perpetuating the current situation as there is lack of knowledge. In addition, Channel 4's 'Battlefront' is taking a 'grass-roots' approach to increasing awareness amongst teens at the UK's Underage Festival, backed by Alexandra Burke, a pop singer.

Organ donation online (2011b) showed that in their campaigns aimed at Black African, Black Caribbean and South Asian groups, they were hosting events at shopping centres, faith sessions, facebook social media, thus linking in with social capital. These sources pull upon ethnic minority groups, further research may be required as to how indigenous population feel, as resources may be seen to be focusing away from them. Hosting events are not just a method of raising awareness, but may have wider implications such as increasing trust (Beem, 1999), particularly in organ donation, helping to dispel myths which may circulate social networks and act as a source of social capital in an information sense.

Through the grass-roots approach, social capital is formed through a bottom-up approach to promotion and engagement, as opposed to a one-size-fits-all top-down approach. NHSBT would be sending the message that the NHS will come to the community to speak to people about donation rather than people having to come to them or briefly consider it as part of a form filling exercise. For some people, it may be a big decision as it encapsulates many factors such as religious, cultural and social concerns. Individuals may have many unfounded issues about donation that they have nobody to speak to about when filling in the forms. People are time poor, as Putnam pointed out and are bombarded with adverts on a regular basis, organ donation adverts may be being lost and may not be relevant. However, it may be expensive and time-consuming to put events like this together. Information would have to be tailored to each group and staff would have to make time to be available, when they are already extremely busy. Also, which groups that are targeted to be given information would have to be justified and the impact of the event may be difficult to measure.

In addition to a grass-roots approach, education should be increased and information held on the organ donor register could be analysed. Children could become more involved in organ donation education, recently reported Adams (2011) as they are viewed to be more altruistic at this age. As argued before, altruism is in itself a contested issue, but through educating children, it may spark discussions about death and organ donation with parents. Through education, social norms may be challenged as myths are dispelled. Geographic information from the Organ Donor Register may enable the mapping of where the donation 'hot spots' are and how these correlate with social capital in these areas, strong and weak.

4. Opportunities and limitations

4.1 Opportunities

Through the social capital lens, it may be possible to consider the current and potential policies in a different way. The Organ Donation Taskforce (2008) illustrated that presumed consent was considered due to erosion of trust between patients and health care professionals. When the aspect of trust is considered through a social capital lens, its importance is magnified. Presumed consent removes the altruistic and reciprocal element, which could potentially, if capitalised upon, contribute towards a civic society. This may be similar if organ donation was to be commercialised, it would remove reciprocity.

4.2 Limitations

Social capital takes into consideration a wide variety of factors that were not considered through gift-exchange theory. As it may exist on a number of different levels in different forms, there are a number of challenges and questions to face when applying social capital to deceased organ donation:

Limitation	Explanation
Encouraging preference-based donation?	Does social capital highlight the limitations of 'gifting' organs, in that people do not feel comfortable donating to people who may be different from them? Portes (1998) explained that people are willing to give up something for another person in the same social structure and Randhawa (1998) highlighted preferences to donate organs to other individuals that they have biological or sociocultural connections with. These issues link with Putnam's bonding social capital, therefore, preference-based donation, whereby individuals can choose who their organs go to in a multi-faith, multi-cultural society. It is something that is being considered in living donation (Dor et al., 2011) however, it may exacerbate in-group identities, fragmentation and alienation within the UK.
How much social capital?	As a relatively small number of transplants are occurring, how much social capital could be built from it? There are low levels of organs available and more transplants would be possible if more organs were available and in the long run could be a source of social capital.
Low levels of societal trust	There may be low levels of trust in strangers and society (World Values Survey, 2006) and may link with issues of social distance, as people would want to help those they know before strangers. It may be naïve to think that people will contribute so readily to people they do not know to help the common good, does it link with rational choice theory and strategic decisions in that there is no perceived benefit from helping strangers?

Limitation	Explanation
Reciprocity	The reciprocal element can only come from those who have received organs. Is the current number of people on the organ donor register a measurement of social capital? How accurate is this data? Family refusal rate may decrease this. Further analysis is required, such as who make up the demographics of these individuals that have signed up.
Community	How do individuals define community, is it possible to make ties across borders, local communities and neighbourhoods through grassroots events? The ties would be 'weak' as they would not be repeated over time, but it would increase education.
Social and health inequality	Is social capital reproducing class through limited access to health information about organ donation through DVLA and Boots advantage card? Those who are at the lower spectrum may not drive or afford to shop at Boots.
Social media	Is Twitter, facebook and blogging over-used for networking or an untapped source for raising awareness about donation? According to a social capital blog, America is changing the way that social capital is being measured and now includes 'frequency of using the internet to express opinions about political and community issues' (webpage).
Human capital	Do individuals feel that they can donate, if people are ill or old they feel they cannot according to Bekkers (2006). People should be made aware that people can donate into old age and with certain illnesses in a way that would discourage them from viewing donation in a negative way.
'Dark side' of social capital	Does organ donation highlight power struggles? Is there too much focus certain groups of the population such as BME and can this make indigenous population feel excluded?
Unsuccessful transplants or transplants that last for a short time	Would these potentially erode trust or the reciprocal aspect of organ donation as social capital is temporal?
Role of the media	TV, news and film may be the source of information about organ donation rather than community leaders at present. There may be inconsistency in messages about donation, there should be more positive stories and it should be less sensationalised, like that in Spain. The media could highlight that donors are good citizens, making this the social norm, rather than organs being gift or hero due to the implications of these terms.
Future of transplantation	Transplantation is ever expanding into unexplored areas, people may not feel comfortable about the future of donation. Perhaps if it was in the public domain and individuals participated in it policy making, people may feel comfortable about its progression.

Limitation	Explanation
Can it fit in with the Big Society?	The Big Society may be viewed as an ethos of creating a community-led and empowered nation. Organ donation may be seen is a concrete example of how to help many other people in society and be socially responsible and contribute to the common good.
Current economic Milieu	In hard times, budget cuts may be seen to be eroding society, such as decrease in social housing and cuts in benefits, perhaps leading to more social instability and movement, decreasing the likelihood of the maintenance of established communities. However at the same time, lack of economic resources may increase levels of social capital.
Unclear as to building and maintaining it	There are deeper issues that underlie social capital such as roles of families, which are becoming broken.
Social norm	This is to accept organ donation in principle but not to donate, there is no sanction for not donating, if donation was the norm, would people feel coerced into giving?
A romantic or Marxist idea?	Putnam argued that social capital has demised due to being time poor, lack of membership to clubs and not reading the newspaper. Does that mean that coming together as a country to help tackle the issue is a romantic idea or a Marxist idea in that people will unite in what they believe in? Would people believe in it enough, even after being educated about it?
Lack of national identity	There may be a feeling that there is a lack of national identity in Britain which manifests itself in difficulty to help strangers and may challenge the notion of pulling together to tackle the problem of donation. However, this may not be the case, as helping those in need may be viewed as helping the human race or 'brothers' and 'sisters' and national identity is not part of it.
Individualistic Society	Social capital may be lower in individualistic societies such as the UK **(Hofstede, 2011)**, which may challenge the creation and maintenance of it through donation.

Table 5. Limitations of links between social capital and organ donation

5. Conclusion

Social capital offers a unique and useful way of examining deceased organ donation and to simultaneously consider many aspects that may be inhibiting the success of altruistic approaches to donation. This is a theoretical position on the connection between social capital and deceased organ donation and does not claim for these to be empirically founded in any way. Social capital is a cohesive and holistic way of viewing deceased organ donation as it marries together micro, meso and macro levels of analysis and illustrates the importance of building up an individual's trust in society and in organ donation. It is not denied that there are many flaws to this theory, it is a malleable concept, making it flexible to facilitate the notion of deceased organ donation but its elasticity can lead to it being difficult to fully apply to all areas. The purpose of this chapter is to highlight organ donation as a form of civic engagement and illustrate why gifting and altruistic donation may be difficult to facilitate in a society that may have low levels of cohesion, trust, sense of national identity and community. The author hopes to evoke discussion through viewing deceased organ donation through a social capital lens to consider many other factors that are not considered through gift exchange and altruism, that they perhaps are cogs of a bigger machine.

6. References

Adams, S. (2011) *Let children decide to be donors, says GOSH doctor*, http://www.telegraph.co.uk/health/8752867/Let-children-decide-to-be-organ-donors-says-GOSH-doctor.html [last accessed 16/09/2011]

Add http://www.nhsbt.nhs.uk/strategicplan/ at the end of the reference [last accessed 15 September 2011]

Adler, P. & Kwon, S. (2002) Social capital: Prospects for a new concept, *Academy of Management Review*, 27 (1), 17-40

Alessandrini, M., Carr, A. & Coghlan, P. (2007) Building social capital through blood donation: the social futures project, *ISBT Science Series*, 2, 46-52

Alessandrini, M.J. & Carr, A. (2007) The Politics of organ donation: chasing a rainbow? *The International Journal of Humanities*, 5 (3), 153-166

Alessandrini, M.J. (2007) Community volunteerism and blood donation: Altruism as a lifestyle choice, *Transfusion Medicine Review*, 21 (4) 307-16

Almond, G.A. & Verba, S. (1963) *The civic culture*. Princeton: Princeton University Press

Battlefront (2011) http://www.battlefront.co.uk/ [last accessed 20 September 2011]

Beem, C. (1999). *The Necessity of Politics. Reclaiming American public life*, Chicago: University of Chicago Press.

Bekkers, R. (2006) Traditional and health-related philanthropy: The role of resources and personality, *Social Psychology Quarterly*, 68, 349-366

Belk, R.W. & Coon, G.S. (1993) Gift giving as agapic love: an alternative to the exchange paradigm based on dating experiences, *Journal of Consumer Research*, 20 (4), 393-417

Bierhoff, H. W. (2001). Prosocial behaviour. In M. Hewstone & W. Stroebe (Eds.), *Introduction to social psychology*, Third Edition, Oxford: Blackwell

Bishop, J. P. & Rees, C.E. (2007) Hero or has-been: Is there a future for altruism in medical education? Advances in Health Sciences Education, 12 (3), 391-399

Borrie Report, The (1994) *Commission on Social Justice*, Viking Press, London.

Bourdieu, P. (1980) Le capital social: notes provisiores, *Actes de la Recherce en Sciences Sociales*, 31, 2-3

Bourdieu, P. & Wacquant, L.J.D. (1992) *An Invitation to Reflexive Sociology*. Chicago and London: University of Chicago Press

Bourdieu, P. (1986) The forms of capital. In J.G. Richardson (ed) *Handbook of Theory and Research*, New York: Greenwood

Burt, R. (1995) Le capital social, les trous structuraux et l'entrepreneur, *Revue Française de Sociologie*, 36 (4), 599-628

Cabinet Office (2010) *Applying Behavioural Insights to Health*, London: Cabinet Office

Cabinet Office (2011) *Big Society – Overview*, http://www.cabinetoffice.gov.uk/content/big-society-overview [last accessed 15 September 2011]

Callendar, C.O. (1989) The results of transplantation in Blacks: just the tip of the iceberg, *Transplantation Proceedings*, 21, 3407-3410

Campbell, C. (2000) Social capital and health: contextualising health promotion within local community networks. In: Baron, Stephen and Field, John and Schuller, Tom, (eds.) Social capital: critical perspectives. Oxford University Press, Oxford

Cheal, D. (1988) *The Gift Economy*, London and New York: Routledge

Claridge, T. (2011) *Social Capital Research*, http://www.socialcapitalresearch.com/definition.html [last accessed 15/09/2011]

Coleman, J.S. (1988) Social capital in the creation of human capital, *The American Journal of Sociology*, 94 (Supplement), 95-120

Coleman, J.S. (1990, 1994) *Foundations of social theory*, Cambridge: The Belknap Press of Harvard University Press

Council of Europe http://www.coe.int/t/dg3/health/themes_en.asp [last accessed 15 September 2011]

Council of Europe, (2007) http://ec.europa.eu/health/ph_threats/human_substance/oc_organs/docs/fact_figures.pdf+organ+donation+statistics+europe [last accessed 15/09/2011]

Darr, A. & Randhawa, G. (1999) Public opinion and perception of organ donation and transplantation among Asian communities: An exploratory study in Luton, *International Journal of Health Promotion Education*, 37, 68

Directgov.uk (2011) *Online driving licence applications to drive up organ donation*, http://www.direct.gov.uk/en/Nl1/Newsroom/DG_198724 [last accessed 15/09/2011]

Dolfsma, W., van der Eijk, R. & Jolink, A. (2008) On a source of social capital: Gift exchange, *Journal of Business Ethics*, 89, 315-329

Dor, F.J.M.F., Massey, E.K. et al. (2011) ELPAT's new classification for living organ donation, 15th Congress of the European Society for Organ Transplantation, 4-7 September, Glasgow

Douglas, M. (1990) No free gifts. Foreword to *The Gift, The Form and Reason for Exchange in Archaic Societies*, London: Routledge

Durlauf, S. N. and Fafchamps, M. "Social Capital." (2004) Available at: http://www.economics.ox.ac.uk/members/marcel.fafchamps/homepage/soccap handbook.pdf

Dworkin, R. (1992) Liberal Community, In *Communitarianism and Individualism*, S. Avineri & De-Shalit, A. (Eds) Oxford: Oxford University Press

Erin, C.A. & Harris, J. (2003) Janet Radcliffe Richards on our modest proposal, *Journal of Medical Ethics*, 29, 141

Etzioni, A. (1994) The Spirit of Community, New York: Touchstone

Etzioni, A. (2003) Organ Donation: A communitarian approach, *Kennedy Institute of Ethics Journal*, 13, 1-18

Farsides, T. (2007) The psychology of altruism, *The Psychologist*, 20, 474-477

Field, J. (2003) *Social Capital*, London: Routledge

Fox, R.C. & Swazey, J.P. (2004) *The courage to fail: A social view of organ transplants and dialysis (New ed)*, New York: Oxford University Press

Fukuyama, F. (1995) *Trust: The Social Virtues and the Creation of Prosperity*, London: Hamish Hamilton

Gilcrist, A (2004) T*he well connected community: A networking approach to community development*, Bristol: The Policy Press.

Goulder, A.W. (1960) The Norm of Reciprocity: A Preliminary Statement, *American Sociological Review*, 25 (2), 171

Granovetter, M. (2002 [1973]) The strength of weak ties, *American Journal of Sociology*, 78, 1360-1380
Guardian online (2010) David Cameron's 'nudge unit' aims to improve economic behaviour, *The Guardian*, http://www.guardian.co.uk/society/2010/sep/09/cameron-nudge-unit-economic-behaviour [last accessed 15/09/2011]
Hall, L., Callender, C., Yeager, C., Barber, J., Dunston, G. & Pinn-Wiggins, V. (1991) Organ donation in Blacks: the next frontier, *Transplantation Proceedings*, 23, 2500-2504
Halpern, D. (2005) *Social Capital*, Cambridge: Polity Press
Healy, K. (2006) *Last Best Gifts: Altruism and the Market for Human Blood and Organs*, Chicago and London: The University of Chicago Press
Heffron, J. M. (2000) 'Beyond community and society: The externalities of social capital building.' *Policy Sciences* 33: 477-494.
Hofstede, G. (2011) *United Kingdom* http://geert-hofstede.com/united-kingdom.html [last accessed 19/12/2011
Homans, G. (1950) *The human group*, New York: Harcourt
Komter, A.E. (2005) *Solidarity and sacrifice: An analysis of contemporary solidarity*, In L.M. Stoneham (Ed.), *Advances in Sociology*, Volume 2, New York: Novascience Publishers
Komter, A.E. (2006) *Social solidarity and the gift*, Cambridge: Cambridge University Press
Lam, W.A. & McCullough, L.B. (2000) Influence of religious and spiritual values on the willingness of Chinese-Americans to donate organs for transplantation, *Clinical Transplantation*, 14, 449-456
Lawson, A. (2008) Presumed consent for organ donation in the UK, *The Intensive Care Society*, 9 (2), 116-117
Le Grand, J. (1997) Knights, Knaves or Pawns? Human Behaviour and Social Policy, *Journal of Social Policy*, 26, 149-169
List, J. (2007) On the interpretation of giving in dictator games, *Journal of Political Economy*, 115 (31), 482-494
Mauss, M. (1923) *The Gift: Forms and Function of Exchange in Archaic Societies*, London
Misztal, B.A. (2000) *Informality: social theory and contemporary practice*, London: Routledge
Mohan, J., Barnard, S., Jones, K. & Twigg, L. (2004) *Social Capital, place and health: creating, validating and applying small-area indicators in the modelling of health outcomes*, NHS: Health Development Agency
Molm, L.D., Collett, J.L. & Schaefer, D.R. (2007) Building Solidarity through Generalised Exchange: A Theory of Reciprocity, *American Journal of Sociology*, 113 (1), 205-242
Morgan M, Hooper R, Amblin M, & Jones R. (2006) Attitudes to kidney donation and registering as a kidney donor among ethnic groups in the UK, *Journal of Public Health*, 28 (3), 226-234
Moseley, A. & Stoker, G. (2010) *Encouraging civic behaviour: A randomised control trial of interventions to influence organ donor registration*, Political studies association conference, Edinburge, 29 March - 1 April.
Nahapiet, J. & Ghoshal. S. (1998) Social Capital, Intellectual Capital, and the Organizational Advantage, *Academy of Management Review* 23(2)
Narayan, D. & Cassidy, M.F. (2001) A dimensional approach to measuring social capital: development and validation of a social capital inventory, *Current Sociology*, 49, 59-102.
Newton, K. (1999) Social and political trust, in *Critical Citizens: Global Support for Democratic Government*, P. Norris (ed.), Oxford: Oxford University Press
NHSBT (2011) NHSBT Strategic Plan 2011-2014
Nuffield Bioethics Online (2011) http://www.nuffieldbioethics.org/solidarity/solidarity-why-solidarity [last accessed 15/09/2011]

Organ donation online (2011a) *Campaigns,*
http://www.uktransplant.org.uk/ukt/campaigns/other_campaigns/detail.jsp?id=3 [last accessed 15 September 2011]

Organ donation online (2011b) *Black and Asian organ donation campaign*
http://www.uktransplant.org.uk/ukt/campaigns/other_campaigns/black_and_asian/index.jsp [last accessed 15 September 2011]

Organ Donation Taskforce (2008)
http://www.dh.gov.uk/en/Publicationsandstatistics/Publications/PublicationsPolicyAndGuidance/DH_082122 [last accessed 10 September 2011]

Poder, T.G. (2011) What is Really Social Capital? A Critical Review, *The American Sociologist.*

Portes, A. (1998) Social capital: its origins and applications in modern sociology, *Annual review of sociology*, 24, 1-24

Pratt, J. (2006) 'Citizenship, Social Solidarity and Social Policy' in Lavalette M. and Pratt A. (eds) (2006) Social Policy: Concepts, Theories and Issues (Sage).

Putnam, R. (1995) Bowling alone: America's declining social capital, *Journal of Democracy,* 6 (1), 65-78

Putnam, R. (2000) *Bowling Alone: The Collapse and Revival of American Community,* New York: Simon and Schuster

Putnam, R. (2011) 'Big society' raises questions over immigration, but gives wrong answers, http://www.guardian.co.uk/politics/blog/2011/may/31/big-society-raises-questions-immigration [last accessed 16/09/2011]

Putnam, R.D., Leonardi, R. & Nanetti, R.Y. (1993) *Making democracy work: Civic tradition in modern Italy,* New Jersey: Princeton University Press

Putnam, R.D., Leonardi, R., Nanetti, R. & Pavoncello, F. (1983) Explaining institutional secrets: the case of Italian regional government, *The American Political Science Review,* 77 (1), 55-74

Radcliffe-Richards, J., Daar, A.S., Guttman, R.D. et al (1998) The case for allowing kidney sales, *Lancet,* 351, 1950

Randhawa, G. (1998) An exploratory study examining the influence of religion on attitudes towards organ donation among the Asian population in Luton, UK, *Nephrology, Dialysis and Transplant*, 13, 1949-1954

Rapport, F.L. & Maggs, C.J. (2002) Titmuss and the gift relationship: Altruism revisited, *Journal of Advanced Nursing,* 40, 495-503

Reubsaet, A., van Hooff, H.P. & Schaeken, E.H.M. (2011) *A school-based organ donation education program to encourage organ donation registration and to change public attitudes related to organ donation*, ESOT Conference, 4-7 September, Glasgow

Rose, H. (1981) Rereading Titmuss: The sexual division of welfare, *Journal of Social Policy*, 4, 477-502

Rushton, J.P. (1980) *Altruism, socialisation and society*, Englewood Cliffs, NJ: Prentice Hall

Ryan, L., Sales, R., Tilki, M. & Siara, B. (2010) Social networks, social support and social capital: the experiences of recent polish migrants in London, *Sociology: The Journal of the British Sociological Association*, 42 (4), 672-690

Sahlins, M.D. (1978) *Stone Age Economics,* London: Routledge

Scheper-Hughes N (2007) The tyranny of the gift: sacrificial violence in living donor transplants *American Journal of Transplantation* 7: 507–11.

Schuller, T., Baron, S. and Field, J. (2000), Social Capital: a review and critique, pp. 1-38 in Baron, S., Field, J., and Schuller, T. (eds.) *Social Capital: critical perspectives*, Oxford University Press, Oxford

Sibeon, R. (1997) *Contemporary sociology and public policy analysis: the new sociology of public policy*, Tudor Business Publishing

Siisiäinen, M. (2000) Two concepts of social capital: Bourdieu vs. Putnam, Paper presented at ISTR Fourth International Conference, 'The Third Sector: For what and for whom?', Trinity College, Dublin, Ireland, July 5-8.

Siminoff, L. & Chillag, K. (1999) The fallacy of the 'gift of life', *Hastings Centre Report*, 29 (6), 34-41

Smith, A. (1995) An analysis of altruism: a concept of caring, *Journal of Advanced Nursing*, 22, 785-790

Smith, N. (2007) *Religion, altruism and social capital*, SSSR Conference in Tampa, Florida, November 2-4

Social Capital Blog (2011) *U.S. Government expands social capital measures* http://socialcapital.wordpress.com/2011/11/30/government-expands-social-capital-measures/ [last accessed 19/12/2011]

Sque, M. & Payne, S. (1994) Gift exchange theory: A critique in relation to organ transplantation, *Journal of Advanced Nursing*, 19, 45-51

Sygora (2009) Altruism in Medical Donations Reconsidered: the Reciprocity approach. In Steinmann, M., Sykora, P. & Wiesing, U. *Altruism Reconsidered: Exploring New Approaches to Property in Human Tissue,* Surrey: Ashgate

Sztompka, P. (1999) *Trust: A sociological theory*, Cambridge: Cambridge University Press

Thaler, R.H. & Sunstein, C.R. (2008) *Nudge: Improving decisions about health, wealth and happiness*, London and New Haven: Yale University Press

Titmuss, R. (1970) *The Gift Relationship: From Human Blood to Social Policy,* New Press

Tonkiss, F. & Passey, A. (1999) Trust, confidence and voluntary organisations: between values and institutions, *Sociology*, 33 (2), 257-74

Trivers, R. L. (1971). The Evolution of Reciprocal Altruism, *The Quarterly Review of Biology*, 46 (1), 35–57

Uphoff, N. (1999) "Understanding social capital: Learning from the analysis and experience of participation." Pp. 215-253 in *Social Capital: A multifaceted perspective*, edited by Ismail Serageldin. Washington, DC: World Bank

Uphoff, N. (2000) Understanding Social Capital: Learning from the Analysis and Experience of Participation, in *Social Capital: A Multifaceted Perspective*, P. Dasgupta and I. Serageldin (Eds), Washington D.C.: The World Bank

Vinokur, A.D., Merion, R.M., Couper, M.P., Jones, E.G. & Dong, Y. (2006) Educational web-based intervention for high school students to increase knowledge and promote positive attitudes toward organ donation, *Health education and behaviour*, 33 (6), 773-786

Whitelaw, B. (2011) Transplanting a culture of organ donation, Guardian online, http://www.guardian.co.uk/healthcare-network/2011/jul/12/communications-strategy [last accessed 12 September 2011]

Woolcock, M. (2001) The place of social capital in understanding social and economic outcomes, *Isuma: Canadian Journal of Policy Research*, 2 (1), 1-17

World Values Survey (2006) *Interpersonal Trust* http://www.jdsurvey.net/jds/jdsurveyMaps.jsp?Idioma=I&SeccionTexto=0404&NOID=104 [last accessed 19/12/2011]

9

Live Donor Kidney Transplants: Psychological Aspects of the Donor-Receiver Relationship

Elisa Kern de Castro[1],
Evelyn Soledad Reyes Vigueras[2] and Caroline Venzon Thomas[2]
[1]Sinos Valley University
[2]Catholic University of Rio Grande do Sul
Brazil

1. Introduction

A live donor kidney transplant is a therapeutic option for treating chronic kidney diseases widely used in several countries, frequently due to the scarcity of donors who have died. As is the case in non-living donor kidney transplants, the patient who is submitted to this type of surgery has already undergone a long period of chronic illness and dialytic treatment, which causes both physical and emotional damage. Thus, the suffering produced by the irreversible chronic illness associated with the anguish of waiting for a donor for the transplant affects not only the patient, but also his or her family and all those involved.

The live donor is usually someone who is known to and emotionally involved with the receiver. The choice of the donor is a complex task, as it involves a series of clinical evaluations which include, besides the physical, laboratory, immunological and image examinations, the evaluation of the emotional conditions and motivation of the candidate to be a donor before undergoing the operation (Burroughs et al 2003; Dew, 1997).

Thus, in donating organs with a live donor there are apparent and latent psychological aspects which affect the decision to donate and that are closely related to the psychological dynamics of the donor and his or her relationship with the receiver (Lima et al., 2006). For the donor, the decision can be very difficult, as the obvious reasons for the donation are predominantly altruistic and aim at the receiver being able to stop having dialysis and have an improved condition of life. Nevertheless, the donation involves self-mutilation and evokes the fear of death, which occurs in the donor through the apprehension of not coming out of anesthesia or of being impaired after the donation (Jordan et al., 2004).

Thus, regarding the reality of the suffering caused by chronic kidney disease, the transplant is often the only possibility of having a life with greater quality. Therefore, the possibility of having a transplant generates expectations both in patients and all the family group. As a result, donating organs with a live donor can cause ambivalent and contradictory feelings in both the donor and the receiver. That is why being aware of the psychological aspects of the donor and receiver is important for the team to deal better with the patient and his or her family, and for planning the psychosocial interventions required throughout the transplant process (Santos & Massarollo, 2005).

Thus, the present chapter aims to present a review of the literature about the experience of live donor kidney transplants from the point of view of donors and receivers, seeking to understand some of the psychological aspects involved in the process of donating organs. Therefore, first the psychological effects of live donor kidney transplants will be looked at, and then the psychological aspects of the donation and donor-receiver relationship will be discussed.

2. Live donor transplants and their psychological effects

Live donor transplants can be performed with blood relations and members of the same family up to the fourth degree, although the donors are usually close relatives. The operation is usually performed by choice with the donor available or, preferably, with the one with best compatibility concerning the antigens of the HLA complex (Manfro & Carvalhal, 2006).

The option for the transplant usually arises from the chronically ill person seeking a better quality of life. Upon opting for the transplant, the patient needs to enroll in a transplant center, where he or she undergoes a process of evaluation and preparation. The pre-transplant evaluation of both receivers and live donors is extensive and detailed. It aims to check the health conditions of both and the presence of any co-morbidity which might lead to an adverse result in the transplant. During this period, the patient undergoes several examinations and is sent to different specialists, which frequently also includes a psychological examination. At the end, and provided that there are no medical contraindications, the patient with the live donor has his or her operation scheduled and the patient with the dead donor is enrolled on the waiting list for the organ (Lage & Monteiro, 2007; Mendes & Shiratori, 2002).

Although the transplant process creates a series of emotions coming from the suffering of the patient who has a chronic disease, the doubts and fear related to the transplant and the apprehension of submitting a healthy person - possible donor - to a very large operation, on the other hand there is the hope that someone close can be the compatible donor. There is the euphoria and ecstasy because the disease can be treated - the transplant - and, simultaneously there is the despair and fear concerning the result of the procedure. Patients and those close to them are continually confronting finiteness and death, which launches them into an emotional spiral which causes accentuated psychological wear.

In the case of live donor organ transplants, the fact of injuring a physically healthy person to benefit another is an aspect which merits care and discussion among all those involved: patient, family and health team. Although it is small, there is a risk of death for the organ donor. He or she will also undergo a period of intense stress due to the operation, and will have to deal with the loss of a vital organ. The patient, on the other hand, can also undergo states of intense suffering and will have to adapt to his or her new condition of transplantee, which includes limitations in his or her daily life and care with food, medicaments, etc. In this context, reactive psychopathological states can appear in both the patient and the donor, which can be unleashed by the disease, the clinical examinations, the hospitalization and the transplant.

According to Garcia, Souza and Holanda (2005), in the psychological evaluation of the candidate to be a donor, it is important to check the feelings and beliefs related to the donation, provide clarification concerning the surgical process and recovery, and prepare him or her for a possible rejection of the graft by the receiver. The decision to be a donor encompasses, besides the family pressures and expectations, emotional issues, ambivalence in wanting and not wanting to donate and the fears and conflicts unleashed by the situation (Quintana & Muller, 2006).

Frequently, in the pre-transplant period the patient expresses his or her desire to be cured of the disease (Walter et al. 2007). He or she often believes that the transplant is an opportunity to be reborn and have a life equal to the one enjoyed before falling ill. It is not rare, that upon being informed about the characteristics of the transplant and the limitations and care entailed for the rest of his or her life, the patient and family react with a selective shield, i.e., only storing some of the information provided by the team and thereby preserving the idea of a total cure for his or her problem. Together with this there is the great quantity of information which the patient and his or her family receive about the procedure. Sometimes, it is information which is difficult to be understood, technical names hitherto unknown, which makes understanding difficult because until then it was not part of their daily lives.

Some patients are proactive concerning the disease and seek information from the health team, in books, on the Internet and from other patients about the disease and the transplant. On the other hand, there are those who avoid asking about the disease or who use rationalization and simplification of the process to handle the anxiety generated by the situation. In any case, it is known that information is a key element for the patient to have a realistic perception of the disease and, consequently, be able to face the transplant in a suitable manner. Avoidance and flight are inappropriate strategies for dealing with these situations, as they defer being aware of the disease and can affect adhering to the medical treatment prescribed.

Regarding the selection of the donor, frequently the patient's family, upon arriving at the doctor to speak about the matter, has already chosen this person due to its dynamics of functioning and the roles which each of the members can assume. Upon other occasions, the potential donor is chosen in an arbitrary way, by means of the compatibility of the blood type discovered by several members undergoing the relevant examination. Frequently, nevertheless, the potential donor is a volunteer in this process, i.e., it is someone who is motivated to give his or her kidney to the person who is close that is suffering. This occurs regardless of the time of dialytic treatment of the receiver and the gravity of his or her situation. The patient rarely requests the organ from somebody who is close. The donor is usually one of the parents, children, spouses, or a person with a strong affective link with the receiver and attained indirectly by his or her disease (Ismael, 2005).

Some patients can come to show the team clearly their fear of bringing losses to the donor, and owing the donor something in exchange for the organ. The conflicts, doubts and even the pressures of which the donor can be the target are exposed in the psychological evaluation course (Fukunishi et al. 2002; Walter et al., 2002).

In recent years there has been much discussion about the ethical issues involved in using psychosocial criteria in evaluating candidates for transplants, especially of vital organs for the survival of the individual. If on one hand, the psychological evaluation is important for being aware of the emotional resources of the patient and family to face the process of the patient's transplant and rehabilitation, on the other hand, the identification of psychological or psychiatric disorders prior to the operation can be an indicator of risk for adhering to the ensuing treatment (Caiuby et al. 2004; Mendes & Shiratori, 2002).

Thus, there arises the conception that psychosocial factors can have a significant impact on the adaptation to the transplant and adhering to the treatment, but on the other hand it can be questioned up to what point these same criteria can be capable of preventing the indication of a patient for the procedure. It is agreed, however, that the psychological evaluation will be able to make an important contribution to helping the team to deal with the patient in the pre-, peri- and post-transplant phases, and also to viewing the patient's prognosis concerning caring for his or her health (Jordan et al., 2004).

3. Psychological aspects of the donation and the donor-receiver relationship

The wait for an organ, often long, is an extremely stressing period owing to the anxiety and fear of the transplant and the possible worsening and death due to complications of the patient's state of health. The disease and its consequences, therefore, can unleash psychological disturbances and symptoms in the patient and in members of his or her family. That is why, when the receiver or donor - in the case of an organ transplant with a related live donor - is evaluated in the pre-transplant period by a mental health professional, this evaluation must include and examine some risk factors for their handling the situation and ensuing mental health, as the presence of psychiatric disorders (especially anxiety and depression), understanding and beliefs about the disease, level of schooling and socioeconomic level.

As the transplant of organs is a procedure which has great emotional impact, due to the receiver having to take as his or her own an organ which belonged to another person, some emotional conflicts can be observed in the receiver regardless of the type of donation - whether the donor is living or dead: guilt related to waiting for somebody to die to benefit, or the removal of the part of someone, in his or her benefit (Achille et al., 2007).

The concern about possible losses to the donor's health is often reported by the patients. The donation involves self-mutilation and evokes the fear of death, which appears in the donor through the apprehension of not coming out of anesthesia or of having an impaired life after the donation.

It is common for there to be difficulties in the relationship between live donors and receivers. According to Walter et al.[14], the introduction of the transplant with a live donor was responsible for new and important psychological conflicts emerging in the transplant process, as for example the debt for life felt by the receiver towards the donor.

The psychological disorders are more frequent in the receivers than in the donors of organ transplants. Nevertheless, there can be differences in the significance of donating an organ such as a kidney or a liver. Whereas the kidney donor will continue his or her life with only one kidney functioning and, therefore, loses a vital organ, in donating the liver the mutilation is only temporary, as this organ is regenerated. In this respect, the donation of the kidney has much more serious implications for the donor's physical health, which can also have greater psychological implications than in donating the liver.

Currently, reactive psychiatric disorders of several degrees have been found in both receivers and donors even when the transplant is successful, without rejection of the graft or any other medical complication. This paradoxical psychiatric syndrome is often found in adult receivers, especially in those where the transplant was a related live donor, and includes major depression, somatization disorder, adjustment disorder and conversion disorder (Caiuby, 2004).

As in any large surgical procedure, the transplant may not have the functioning expected. In these cases, when the donation was made by a living donor, the failure of the kidney transplant can cause adverse emotional reactions in the donors due to the effort having been made in vain, as anxiety, regret, depression and reduced self-esteem. In spite of positive attitudes concerning the transplant predominating, in situations of the graft not functioning it is possible to observe regret and guilt in the donor-receiver pair. For the receiver, the immediate clinical intercurrences regarding the loss of the graft do not weigh so heavily as the perspective of returning to the hemodialysis machine: in it the loss of hope and the meeting with death are projected. For the donor, frequently after the operation he or she becomes of secondary importance, as all the attention is turned towards the receiver and his or her kidney function, which can cause the donor to be resentful.

Generally speaking, the studies indicate that donating a liver allows wellbeing and an increased self-esteem of the donor[19,20]. Attention should be paid, nevertheless, to the fact that this situation does not necessarily lead to the relationship of the receiver-donor pair being strengthened. The receiver's attention reverts to the functioning of the graft, whereas the donor has already achieved his or her function and can be forgotten in this period.

4. Final considerations

Due to that set out above, live donor kidney transplants generate great psychological impact on both the donor and the receiver, generating changes in the relationship established between them. The debt for life which the receiver will have for ever is a factor which, at the same time that it can bring him or her emotionally nearer to the donor, can also make him or her more distant owing to possible feelings of guilt for having interfered with the state of health of a healthy person.

In this respect, the evaluation of the mental health of the donor and receiver becomes of paramount importance within the pre-transplant evaluation in order to provide guidance about the aspects which interfere with the desire to donate and in the interference of the donation and transplant in the ensuing relationship of the donor-receiver pair. The psychosocial evaluation of donors (pre- and post transplant) is advocated; however, there is a paucity of data on the process and content of psychosocial evaluations (Hardeveld & Tong,2010). There are no set standards regarding who should conduct psychosocial evaluations, whether evaluations should be mandatory, at what stage of the work-up evaluations should be conducted, at what time interval repeat evaluations should be performed and what criteria need to be met (Hardeveld & Tong, 2010). Also, there is no consensus about how the pre-transplant psychological evaluation should be done in donors and recipients. In all world, there is a lot of differences in the procedures used among different centers; in others, there is no psychological evaluation (Sajjad, Baines, Salifu & Jindal, 2007). In this sense, it is recommended that the psychosocial evaluation in kidney candidates, to examine the undestanding of the candidates about the donation process, risk and benefits envolved. Moreover, it will furnish greater awareness of them both, which will aid in future interventions which aim to help them in maintaining and adhering to the post-transplant treatment.

5. References

Achille M. Soos F.M.C; Pâquet M.; Hérbert M.J. (2007) Differences in psychosocial profiles between men and women living kidney donors. Clin Transplant, 21, 314-20.

Burroughs TE, Waterman AD, Hong BA. (2003). One organ donation, three perspectives: experiences of donors, recipients, and third parties with living kidney donation. Prog Transplant, 13,142-50.

Caiuby, AV; Lefreve, F.; Silva, AP. (2004). Análise do discurso dos doadores renais - abordagem da psicologia social [Speech Analysis of Kidney Donors - Social Psychological Approach]. Jornal Brasileiro de Nefrologia, 26.

Dew, MA. (1997) Does Transplantation Produce Quality of Life benefits? A Quantitative Analysis of the Literature, Clin Transp., 9, 1261-1273.

Fukunishi I, Sugawara Y,Takayama T et al. (2002). Association between pretransplant psychological assessments and postransplant psychiatric disorders in living-related transplantation. Psychosomatics, 43, 49-54.

Garcia M.L.P; Souza A.M.A; Holanda T.C.(2005). Intervenção Psicológica em uma Unidade de Transplante Renal de um hospital Universitário [Psychological assistance of the renal transplantation departament at a university hospital]. Psicologia, Ciência e Profissão; 25, 472-483.

Gouge, F; Moore JT, J; Bremer, B,A; Mccauly, C,R; Johnson, J.P. (1990). The quality of life of donors, potential donors, and recipients of living-related donor renal transplantation. Transpl Proc. , 5, 2049-2413.

Ismael, S. (2005). A prática psicológica e sua interface com as doenças. São Paulo: Casa do Psicólogo.

Jordan J.; Sann U.; Janton A.; Gossmann J.; Kramer W.; Kachel HG.; Wilhelm A.; Scheuermann E. (2004). Living kidney donors' long-term psychological status and health behavior after nephrectomy - a retrospective study. J Nephrol, 17, 728-35.

Lage, A. M.V.; Monteiro, K.C.C. (2007). Psicologia Hospitalar. Teoria e práticas em hospital universitário.Fortaleza: UFC.

Lima DX, Petroianu A, Hauterr HL. (2006) Quality of life and surgical complications of kidney donors in the late post-operative period in Brazil. Nephrol Dial Transplant. 21, 3238-42.

Manfro, R.C.; Carvalhal, G.F. (2003). Simpósio sobre transplantes [Symposium about Transplantation]. Rev Amrigs. 47, 14-9.

Mendes, CA.; Shiratori, K. (2002). As percepções dos pacientes de transplante renal [The perception of a patient carrying a kidney disease regarding the kidney transplant]. Nursing, 4, 15-22.

Quintana AM, Muller AC. (2006). Da saúde à doença: representações sociais sobre a insuficiência renal crônica e o transplante renal [From Sickness To Health: Social Representations About Chronic Renal Insufficiency And Kidney Transplantation]. Psicol argum, 24, 73-80.

Sajjad, I., Baines, L. S., Salifu, M., & Jindal, R. M. (2007). The dynamics of recipient-donor relationships in living kidney transplantation. Am. Journal kidney Diseases, 50(5), 834-854.

Santos M.J.: Massarollo , M. (2005). Processo de doação de órgãos: percepção de familiares de doadores cadáveres [Organ donation process: perception by relatives of cadaverous donors]. Revista Latino Americana de Enfermagem.13, 382-7

Walter M, Moyzes D, Rose M et al. (2002). Psychosomatic interrrelations following liver transplantation. Clin Transplant. 16, 301-305.

Part 2

Clinical Issues in Transplantation

10

Posttransplant Lymphoproliferative Disorders Following Solid Organ Transplantation

Laura Rodriguez and Angela Punnett
University of Toronto/Hospital for Sick Children
Canada

1. Introduction

Posttrasplant lymphoproliferative disorders (PTLD) represent a wide spectrum of pathologic and clinical manifestations that occur in the setting of depressed T-cell function and altered immune surveillance, such as is observed in the setting of solid organ transplantation (SOT). PTLD is a major contributor to long-term morbidity and mortality in this population and is the most common cancer observed in children following SOT. (Webber et al., 2006) Many cases are associated with Epstein-Barr virus (EBV) infection and most, but not all, are of host origin. (Petit et al., 2002, Taylor et al., 2005) This article reviews the pathology, epidemiology, risk factors, and clinical aspects of PTLD, and identifies the need for ongoing systematic study of complex biologic and therapeutic questions.

2. Pathology

PTLD encompasses a remarkable diversity of pathologic conditions. The most commonly used pathologic classification scheme is the World Health Organization (WHO) categorization, outlined in Table 1. (Swerdlow et al., 2008) Pathologic evaluation requires assessment of tissue architecture and cytologic features including immunophenotype; excisional biopsies are preferred and tissue samples should be submitted fresh rather than in formalin. It must be established if the PTLD is EBV-associated disease, for example by EBV-encoded RNA in situ hybridization (ISH) testing of diagnostic tissues. Cytogenetic studies assist with determination of clonality (immunoglobulin heavy [IgH] gene rearrangement; T-cell receptor gene rearrangement) and identify disease-associated chromosomal abnormalities. It is important to exclude other diagnoses including infection, inflammatory processes or rejection. Characteristics that suggest but are not pathognomonic of PTLD include enlarged nodules, mass lesions, lymphoid atypia, a very B cell rich infiltrate, extensive necrosis in the infiltrate and numerous EBV+ cells. (Dharnidharka, 2010) PTLD may be observed simultaneously at different sites in a patient, and a patient may have two different types of PTLD simultaneously or subsequently. (Blaes & Morrison, 2010)

3. Epidemiology and risk factors

The overall incidence of lymphoproliferative disease varies from 1 to 20% depending on the type of transplant and other risk factors. (Vegso et al., 2010) The frequency of PTLD is higher in childhood; regardless of the transplanted organ the incidence is 2 to 3-fold compared to adults. The principal risk factors in the development of PTLD are the degree of immunosuppression and the EBV serostatus of the recipient. (Dharnidharka et al., 2001; McDonald et al., 2008; Opelz & Dohler, 2004) Similarly, younger age at transplant is a strong risk factor for PTLD, but likely reflects the proportion of recipients who are EBV-seronegative. Other risks described include past history of malignancy, the degree of HLA-compatibility and the occurrence and severity of acute rejection, the type of the transplanted organ, and the immunosuppressive drugs used. (Bakker et al., 2005b; Taylor et al., 2005; Tsao & Hsi, 2007)

3.1 Pathogenic mechanism of EBV

EBV is a polyclonal stimulator of B-cell proliferation. More than 90% of the world's population is infected with EBV and infected individuals remain lifelong carriers of the virus. (Rickinson & Kieff, 1996) The life cycle of EBV is outlined in Fig. 1. Primary infection occurs through the oropharynx, where the virus infects resting B cells. The expression of viral proteins induces polyclonal proliferation of infected B-cells and some of these differentiate into memory cells which carry the virus in a latent form. (Thorley-Lawson, 2001) Among immunocompetent hosts, control of virus spread and of unrestrained infected B-cell proliferation is maintained by the development of a specific immune response.

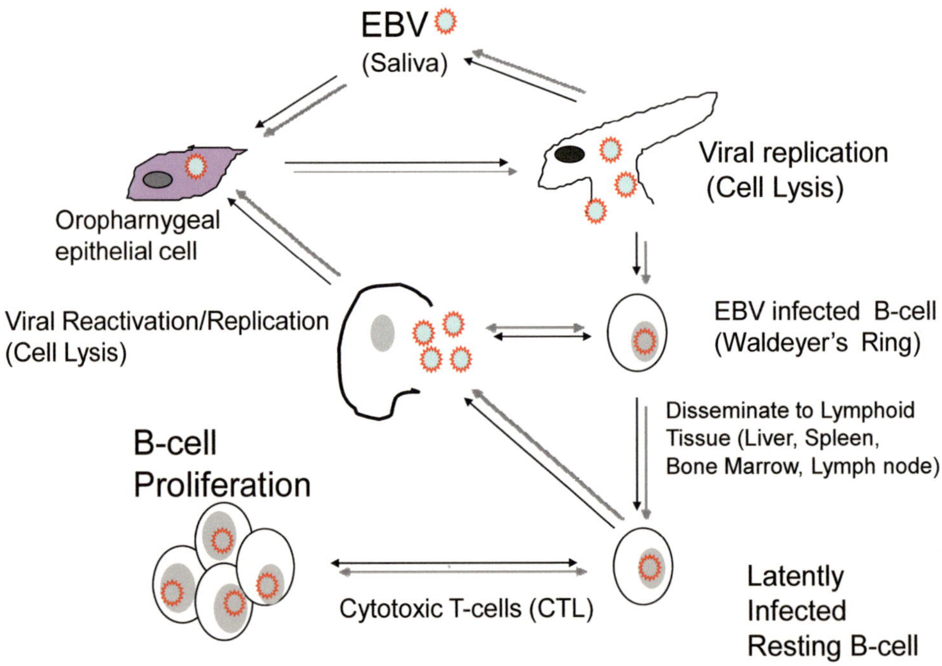

Fig. 1. EBV Life Cycle. (Courtesy of Dr. Thomas G. Gross)

Pathologic Categories of PTLD	
Category	**Description**
Early lesions • *Reactive Plasmatic Hyperplasia* • *Infectious mononucleosis-like*	• Lymphoid proliferations with preservation of normal tissue architecture. • In some cases just prominent follicular hyperplasia is seen. • Most of these early PTLD cases occur within a relatively short time after transplantation. • Polyclonal B cells. • More frequently in previously EBV-naive SOT recipients. • EBV often positive. (Swerdlow et al., 2008).
Polymorphic	• Morphology shows destruction of the underlying architecture of the tissue with perineural and blood vessel invasion. • Heterogeneous population with a full range of B-cell maturation and includes areas that seem more monomorphic, suggesting a continuum between polymorphic and monomorphic disease. • EBV often positive. • Monoclonal B cells, nonclonal T cells. • BCL6 somatic hypermutations may be seen. (Swerdlow et al., 2008).
Monomorphic ***B-cell neoplasms*** • *Diffuse large B-cell lymphoma* • *Burkitt lymphoma* • *Plasma cell myeloma* • *Plasmacytoma-like lesion* • *Other* ***T-cell Neoplasms*** • *Peripheral T-cell lymphoma, not otherwise specified* • *Hepato-splenic* • *Other*	• Classified according to the B-cell or T/natural killer (NK)-cell neoplasms described in the immunocompetent host. • Architectural effacement usually seen. • EBV +/-. • Clonal B cells or T cells. • Markers of oncogenes and tumor suppressor genes (eg, C-myc, N-ras, and p53) may be used to facilitate diagnosis in more complex cases. • Recurrent chromosomal abnormalities have been reported in some series of B-cell PTLD and may portend a worse prognosis. (Chadburn et al., 1997; Djorkic et al., 2006; Maecker et al., 2007; Swerdlow et al., 2008).
Classical Hodgkin lymphoma	• Primarily among renal transplant recipients. • Should fulfill the criteria for classical Hodgkin lymphoma recognized in the immunocompetent host as, Reed-Sternberg-like cells may be seen in early, polymorphic, and some monomorphic PTLD. • The expression pattern of EBV proteins (EBV-latency pattern) may aid in the diagnosis of cHL. • Architectural effacement usually seen. • EBV almost always positive. • IgH not easily demonstrated. (Pitman et al., 2006; Ranganathan et al., 2004; Rohr et al., 2008; Swerdlow et al., 2008).

Table 1. WHO classification of PTLD.

In a persistent infection, EBV antigen-specific T cells are maintained at a frequency of 1% to 5% of peripheral blood T cells to immune survey and eliminate reactivating/ proliferating infected B cells when they express the growth program. (Steven et al., 1996) T cell–mediated responses to the immunogenic proteins prevent outgrowth of EBV-infected B cells. In contrast, when T cell–mediated responses are impaired, uncontrolled proliferation of EBV-infected B cells will lead to the development of EBV-associated lymphoproliferative diseases. The disease is polyclonal in the beginning, however infected cells may then acquire genetic alterations that promote monoclonal lymphoma formation. The existence of EBV-unrelated PTLD supports the theory of a pathologic interaction between genetic aberration, viral oncogenes, impaired immunity and chronic antigen stimulation. (Nourse et al., 2011)

3.2 EBV+ vs EBV-

In children PTLD is usually induced by primary EBV infection which may occur via transmission from the allograft or the natural route via salivary secretion. Pediatric patients in particular are often EBV-seronegative, but around 90% will be positive at 6 months post-transplant. (Newell et al., 1996) However not all EBV-seronegative SOT recipients develop PTLD. (Guthery et al., 2003; Tsao & Hsi, 2007) In one pediatric report of pediatric liver transplant recipients, it was found that no seropositive patients developed PTLD following liver transplant; but 10.5% of patients who were seronegative prior to transplant developed PTLD. (Ho et al., 1988) The EBV status of the donor and the recipient is a relevant factor; the risk of PTLD increases 10 to 50-fold when the recipient is EBV-seronegative and the donor is EBV-seropositive. (McDonald et al., 2008, Tsao & Hsi, 2007) Of note, EBV cannot be detected in 15%–40% of cases of PTLD. PTLD was historically considered an early phenomenon with most cases reported within the first year following transplant and attributed to the more intense immunosuppression used for induction therapy or exposure of the EBV-seronegative host to the virus. (Faull et al., 2005; Webber et al., 2006).More recent data suggest that the median time is later, at approximately 3 years after SOT. (Evens et al., 2010; Ghobrial et al., 2010; Knight et al., 2009; Maecker et al., 2007) This is partly due to an increase in the diagnosis of EBV-unrelated disease. Multiple reports have shown that EBV-unrelated PTLD occurs later after SOT, most commonly after 3 to 5 years. (Dotti et al., 2002; Mamzer-Bruneel et al., 2000) The incidence of EBV-unrelated PTLD has been increasing and may be explained by changing immunosuppressive regimens, longer survival after SOT, and an improvement in the diagnosis. (Nelson et al., 2000) EBV-related and EBV-unrelated PTLD usually have different clinical manifestations. EBV-unrelated PTLD is usually a monomorphic disease with late manifestation and has historically carried a poor prognosis. (Dotti et al., 2002; Leblond et al., 1998; Nelson et al., 2000; Taylor et al., 2005) Recent data shows an improved response to treatment, which could be explained both by improvements in treatment strategies of the tumors and by improved supportive care. (Elstrom et al., 2006; Evens et al., 2010; Knight et al., 2009; Maecker et al., 2007)

3.3 Immunosuppression

In the absence of a reliable and reproducible method to measure intensity of immunosuppression, it is difficult to assess the effect of individual immunosuppressive agents on the risk of developing PTLD. In addition there is often a learning curve with new agents, such that the incidence of PTLD may be higher when an agent is first introduced to clinical care. (Nourse et al., 2011; Webster et al., 2005) It does appear that increasing T cell–specificity of immunosuppression is associated with a higher incidence of PTLD. The use of antibody preparations that deplete T cells has been identified as a risk factor for PTLD in early studies by both univariate and multivariate analyses. (Faull et al., 2005; Kirk et al., 2007; Opelz & Dohler, 2004; Yang et al., 2008) However, data from multiple transplant registries have demonstrated mixed results regarding a direct association between the use of Thymoglobulin and the risk of developing PTLD. (Marks et al., 2011) Quinlan et al. in a retrospective cohort study among 156,740 kidney transplant recipients reported that the use of antibody induction or antirejection therapies was not associated with PTLD risk, even when restricted to T-cell-based therapies, in contrast to earlier reports where there was an association between antibody induction therapy and risk of early onset PTLD. (Caillard et al., 2005; van Leeuwen et al., 2009) This difference may be related to different eras of treatment and increasing experience with antibody-based induction therapies, leading to an attenuation of associated PTLD risks. (Quinlan et al., 2011)

In contrast, PTLD occurred 2 to 3-fold more frequently after receipt of OKT3 than with other drugs. (Opelz & Dohler, 2004; Taylor et al., 2005) Gajarski et al. report that as induction agents thymoglobulin and IL-2R antagonists had the lowest associated PTLD rates compared to OKT3, attributing this to its long-lasting depletional effects on CD-3 positive T-lymphocytes. (Gajarski et al., 2011) IL-2 receptor inhibitor antibodies (daclizumab, basiliximab) which specifically target activated T cells and are non-depleting, do not increase PTLD risk. Induction with alemtuzumab (anti-CD52 antibody), which depletes both T and B lymphocytes, was also not found to be associated with PTLD. (Caillard et al., 2005; Kirk et al., 2007; Opelz &Dohler, 2004) Shapiro et al. reported a small series using alemtuzumab as pre-conditioning with tacrolimus monotherapy in pediatric renal transplantation, with no cases of PTLD after a median time of follow up of 25 months. (Shapiro et al., 2007)

There are some controversies regarding the risk with the use of calcineurin inhibitors, which at this point in time continue as the pillars of maintenance regimens. Although early studies suggested the use of tacrolimus increases the risk of PTLD two to fivefold compared to cyclosporine, more recent studies suggest that if serum levels are monitored closely, there is no difference in risk of PTLD. (Dharnidharka et al., 2001; Guthery et al., 2003; Opelz & Dohler, 2004; Russo et al., 2004; Webster et al., 2005) Several groups have shown an increased risk of PTLD in kidney transplant recipients receiving tacrolimus compared with cyclosporine if they had not received antibody induction, but no difference in the recipients that had received induction. (Stojanova et al., 2011) In a recent report patients treated with tacrolimus after heart transplantation were at increased risk for the development of PTLD compared with patients treated with cyclosporine. (Dayton et al., 2011) Cyclosporine increases the risk mainly in higher doses (>6.6 mg/kg per day). (Boubenider et al., 1997) Both cyclosporine and tacrolimus inhibited apoptosis in a lymphoblastoid cell line, but it has been suggested that a difference in the risk could be due to a higher level of immunosuppression with tacrolimus compared to cyclosporine. (Stojanova et al., 2011)

Some studies have reported that sirolimus may decrease the incidence of PTLD. (Kauffman et al., 2005; Yakupoglu et al., 2006) Conflicting data from the UNOS registry study suggest that sirolimus is strongly associated with PTLD in kidney transplant recipients. The highest risk was limited to EBV-seronegative recipients with the clinical implication that sirolimus should probably be avoided in this population, especially in those who are already at higher risk for PTLD. (Kirk et al., 2007) Nee et al. also noted the same higher risk of PTLD with sirolimus, in a retrospective cohort of 53,719 kidney transplant recipients. (Nee et al., 2011)

It seems that antimetabolites such as azathioprine and mycophenolate mofetil used primarily as adjunct therapy alongside calcineurin inhibitors for preventing allograft rejection, are associated with a lower or not increased risk of PTLD. (Caillard et al., 2005; Kauffman et al., 2005) Mycophenolate mofetil may reduce PTLD risk by allowing the use of lower-dose calcineurin inhibitors. (Gajarski et al., 2011) Belatacept, is a new immunosuppressive agent that selectively blocks T-cell co-stimulation. In a recent study belatacept was associated with a greater risk of PTLD in the central nervous system (CNS) when compared with cyclosporine, especially in EBV-seronegative recipients and when used at more intensive doses. (Grinyo et al., 2010)

In addition to the type of the immunosuppressive drugs, the dosage, the combinations and the length of aggressive treatment influence the risk of PTLD, so the total immunosuppression exposure rather than induction alone may be a more accurate determinant of PTLD risk, and may be modified by choice of induction agent. (Gajarski et al., 2011)

3.4 Type of transplant

Most analyses suggest that the risk of PTLD is associated with the type of organ transplanted. The risk is lowest (1% to 3%) following renal and liver transplantation, moderate (1% to 6%) after heart transplantation, and highest after lung (4% to 10%), small intestine and multivisceral transplantation (>10% and may be as high as 20% for intestinal transplants). (Swerdlow et al; 2008) The reasons for these observed differences in incidence of PTLD include recipient factors, such as age and EBV serostatus, but also allograft factors, such as differing risk of transmitting EBV-infected B cells (in associated lymphoid tissue) with intestine and lung transplants compared with liver, heart, and kidney transplants, and the amount of immunosuppression required to prevent rejection. (Opelz & Dohler, 2004; Petit et al., 2002; Tsao & Hsi, 2007; Taylor et al., 2005) Among the differences regarding the type of organ transplanted is the time of presentation. Early-onset presentation of PTLD is characteristic for heart and lung transplantation, with nearly half of the cases appearing in the first year. In contrast among kidney transplant recipients, late-onset presentation is more common. This difference is due to higher doses of immunosuppression and induction treatment required following heart and lung transplantation. (Quinlan et al., 2011; Taylor et al., 2005) Another difference noted is the origin of the PTLD in renal transplantation-- PTLD of donor origin has been described. (Olagne et al., 2011)

3.5 Other risks

There are several other risks related to PTLD. A recent study reported that African American kidney transplant recipients are at lower risk for PTLD, irrespective of the recipient EBV serostatus. (Nee et al., 2011) Quinlan et al. found that non-Hispanic whites were at significantly higher risk of early-onset and late-onset PTLD than other racial or ethnic groups. (Quinlan et al., 2011) In the same study it was also demonstrated that CMV-seronegativity was associated with increased early-onset PTLD risk. (Quinlan et al., 2011) However, it seems that the role of CMV and HCV as risk factors for PTLD is controversial, as is that of herpes simplex or simian virus infections. (Nee et al., 2011; Tsao & Hsi, 2007) An increase in the risk of PTLD has been described in the presence of specific cytokine gene polymorphisms. (Taylor et al., 2005; Tsao & Hsi, 2007) Malignancy and autoimmunity are also associated with PTLD. Patients with PTLD are more likely to have a history of pre-transplant malignancy than those without PTLD. (Caillard et al., 2005; Nee et al., 2011) Transplantation due to autoimmune hepatitis and primary biliary cirrhosis carries a higher risk of PTLD likely related to chronic immunologic stimulation. (Shpilberg et al., 1999). Transplantation due to cystic fibrosis and Langerhans-cell histiocytosis carries a higher risk of PTLD due to a higher incidence of refractory rejection. (Cohen et al., 2000; Newell et al., 1997) In addition, Zimmermann et al. found that liver recipients who received steroids before transplant for immunological disorders are at particularly high risk to develop PTLD. (Zimmermann et al., 2010)

The role of HLA mismatch in the risk of PTLD is controversial. Among kidney transplant recipients, HLA-B mismatches have been reported to increase the risk of lymphoma in the allograft, whereas HLA-DR locus mismatches may increase the risk of non-Hodgkin lymphoma in the allograft and the central nervous system. (Bakker et al 2005b; Opelz & Dohler 2010) Reshef et al. suggest that the HLA-A26, B38 haplotype is mainly responsible for predisposition to PTLD, at least among Caucasian recipients, as an independent risk factor. (Reshef et al., 2011) Other studies have been unable to confirm a role for HLA mismatches and an increased risk of PTLD. (Nee et al., 2011; Quinlan et al., 2011)

The assessment of risk factors for PTLD is complicated by the complex nature of the disease and the variability among studies with respect to disease definitions, immunosuppression protocols and the length of follow up. Methods of screening for and monitoring of EBV have improved over time, as well as the supportive therapy for transplant procedures and their complications. As a consequence, there is a tendency toward lower incidence of PTLD; it was observed to be less likely to develop in patients who received their allograft after 1996, than those who received allograft before 1996. (Dayton et al., 2011; Marks et al., 2011; Tsao & Hsi 2007)

4. Diagnosis

4.1 Clinical presentation

A high index of suspicion is required for a timely diagnosis of PTLD. Patients often present with relatively benign findings before developing more significant symptomatology. Rarely, SOT recipients may present with so-called fulminant PTLD. Other EBV-associated diseases must be differentiated from PTLD, although the initial management is similar. (Gross, 2009) There are two forms of presentation: early-onset and late-onset PTLD. Early-onset PTLD occurring within 2 to 3 years of transplantation is more common among pediatric SOT recipients because of their risk for primary EBV infection. (Opelz & Dohler, 2004) Early-onset disease is more likely to involve the allograft and present with declining allograft function, excepting heart allografts, in which direct involvement by PTLD is rare. (Bakker et al., 2005a) The major differential diagnostic considerations include allograft rejection and infection. Later-onset disease is more likely to be EBV negative and to include T/NK-cell disease, to involve extranodal sites (especially GI sites) or to present with dissemination. (Guthery et al., 2003; Ho et al., 1988; Leblond et al., 1998; Nelson et al., 2000; Steven et al., 1996) T/NK-cell disease is rare although it may be increasing, is clinically aggressive and is more often EBV negative (two-thirds of cases). (Azhir et al., 2009; Gupta et al., 2010; Miloh et al., 2008; Williams et al., 2008; Yang, et al 2008)

Virtually no site is exempt from PTLD involvement. Outside the allograft, common areas affected include lymphoid tissues, GI tract, lung, kidney and liver. Patients may present with constitutional symptoms (fever, poor weight gain, rash), mono-type illness, lymphadenopathy, and organ dysfunction. A frequent presentation in early-onset disease is adenotonsillar involvement with associated sore throat and obstructive symptoms (new onset snoring or mouth breathing). (Allen et al., 2005) Involvement of the GI tract may present with feeding intolerance, vomiting, diarrhea, protein losses, bleeding, intussusception, or obstruction. Perforation may occur at presentation or immediately following initiation of therapy in the presence of transmural lesions. New-onset anemia or hypoalbuminemia may indicate GI involvement. (Selvaggi et al., 2006) Lung disease may result in unexplained cough, wheezing and respiratory insufficiency or asymptomatic nodules. Liver disease may present as an unexplained increase of serum transaminases, diffuse hepatitis or nodular lesions. Other signs are joint pain and auto-immune cytopenias. PTLD of the central nervous system, isolated or as part of multiorgan disease, may be as high as 30%, compared to only 1% among non-Hodgkin lymphomas of the non-transplanted population. (Maecker et al., 2007; Taylor et al., 2005) Patients may present with headache, seizures, or focal neurologic findings.

Some general comments may be made in regard to clinicopathologic correlation. The early-onset PTLD lesions are generally EBV-related and typically fall into the category of early lesions or polymorphic PTLD. In children and adults with late-onset PTLD, EBV-related early lesions or polymorphic PTLD may still be observed, but there is a greater percentage of monomorphic and EBV-unrelated diseases, especially in adults. (Allen, 2010) However, Quinlan et al. in a retrospective cohort study of kidney transplant recipients, reported that early-onset PTLD was more likely to be monomorphic than polymorphic (48.2% vs. 41.6%, with 10.2% of unknown), and late-onset PTLD was even more likely to be of monomorphic pathology (55.9% vs. 31.4%, 12.7% unknown). Early onset PTLD was predominantly of B-cell origin, late-onset PTLD showed a slightly higher proportion of T-cell PTLD (64.3% B-cell vs. 9.7% T-cell, 25.9% unknown). (Quinlan et al., 2011)

4.2 Clinical evaluation

Initial assessment includes a full physical examination with meticulous assessment for lymphadenopathy, and a risk adapted approach to the selection of screening evaluations and EBV-specific monitoring.

4.2.1 Screening tests

Screening tests include a complete blood count with differential, chemistry panel to assess for tumor lysis syndrome, allograft function screening, CMV by PCR and other viruses (human immunodeficiency virus type 1 & 2, hepatitis B, hepatitis C). Imaging evaluation is essential and is directed initially by the location of suspected lesions and prior radiographic studies of each patient. Ultrasound is effective for initial imaging in patients with suspected abdominal/pelvic or soft-tissue PTLD. CT is used in evaluation for neck and chest disease and in staging with a suspected or confirmed diagnosis. Head CT or MRI should be included to assess relevant symptoms and in staging evaluations. In patients with abdominal symptoms, upper and lower endoscopy should be considered early as lesions may be missed on routine imaging. (Allen, 2010) The role of [18F]2-fluoro-2-deoxyglucose (FDG)-positron emission tomography (PET) in the diagnosis of equivocal lesions, staging, and response assessment of PTLD is currently being defined. (von Falck, et al 2007) Bakker and colleagues demonstrated additional extranodal sites on PET not appreciated on computed tomography (CT) in 50% of patients and concordance of PET response with outcome. (Bakker et al., 2006) However, false positives have been described when PET is used for disease monitoring in children and for the evaluation of lung lesions. (McCormack et al., 2006; Rhodes et al., 2006) Recommended diagnostic procedures are similar to other non-Hodgkin lymphoma patients, and staging is completed using the Ann Arbor staging system. Diagnosis must be confirmed by biopsy. See Fig. 2

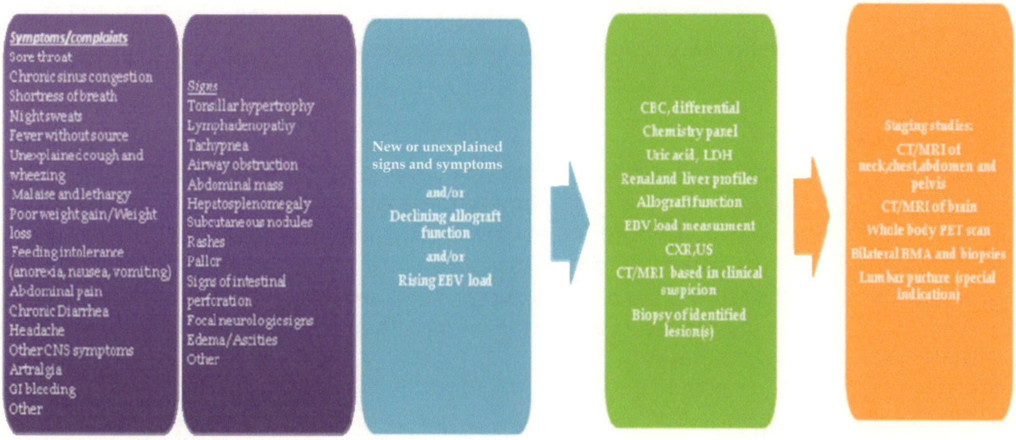

Fig. 2. Diagnostic and staging procedures for PTLD.

4.2.2 EBV-specific tests

Serology is critical to categorize the serostatus of the donor and recipient at the time of transplant. Serology following SOT is unreliable as a diagnostic test in immunocompromised patients as they have marked delay in their humoral response. Primary EBV infection, rather than EBV reactivation, is responsible for the majority of PTLD cases in children, and early diagnosis may be prompted by serial measurements of EBV DNA in peripheral blood after transplant. An increasing EBV DNA load may be an early sign of PTLD, requiring further evaluation and closer monitoring. (Allen, 2010)

EBV-DNA may be measured in the plasma, peripheral blood mononuclear cells (PBMC) and in the whole blood by quantitative PCR assays. Testing done with plasma measures the cell-free fraction only and may lead to an underestimation; however the detection of plasma EBV-DNA is a highly specific test with a high positive predictive value (100%). One possible explanation is that free viral DNA is released from latently infected cells, but most notably tumor cells undergoing apoptosis. Tsai et al. found EBV-DNA measured in plasma had comparable sensitivity and improved specificity compared to whole blood for diagnosis of EBV-related PTLD. (Tsai et al., 2008) Measuring intracellular EBV (PBMC) is considered to be less specific, due to the high rate of false positivity. In patients with infectious mononucleosis viral DNA is detectable in serum for only 7 days after symptom onset and then remains detectable in the cellular fraction. Whole blood assays detect EBV-DNA present in the cells and in the plasma. Whole blood assays may be better used when screening for PTLD, and plasma assays may be better for the evaluation after therapy of PTLD. The time intervals for routine monitoring and duration of monitoring may vary depending on the type of transplant and individual risk factors. Clinicians must be aware that PTLD may be EBV-unrelated, and that EBV-related disease may develop or recur in the absence of an increasing EBV-DNA load. (EBV Work Group, Cincinnati Children´s Hopsital Medical Center, 2011; Tsai et al., 2008) Adjunctive tests to assess the resiliency of the immune system have been investigated, including T-cell restoration or EBV-specific T-cell response. Low T-cell response and high EBV-DNA load indicates high degree of immunosuppression and an increased PTLD risk, which have to lead a modification of immunosuppression and further examination of the patient. Testing of EBV in the CSF is often used to assist in the diagnosis of CNS PTLD and avoid the need for more invasive biopsy procedures. (Preiksaitis, 2009)

5. Treatment

Treatment strategies for PTLD must be tailored to individual clinical contexts and require input from an interdisciplinary team including a transplant specialist, an oncologist and an infectious disease specialist. Decisions are based on multiple factors including disease presentation, EBV status, patient comorbidities and performance, risk of rejection, type of organ graft, and the drugs used for immunosuppressive therapy. Where impairment of the transplanted organ can lead to the death of the patient, the protection of the organ graft is a critical factor in planning therapy.

5.1 Primary prevention

5.1.1 Donor EBV serologic status

Avoiding EBV-positive donors in EBV-naive recipients to limit primary infection may prevent PTLD. However, only a very small proportion of donors are EBV negative and this approach cannot be applied universally. (Lazda, 2006)

5.1.2 Antiviral therapy

Increased attention is focused on the prevention of EBV-related PTLD through the use of antiviral therapy. Antiviral agents, such as acyclovir and ganciclovir, are nucleoside analogues that act by inhibiting the replication of EBV DNA through inhibition of viral DNA polymerase. Their activity is dependent on intracellular phosphorylation by virally encoded thymidine kinase. Ganciclovir seems to be more potent and to have a prolonged effect. Antiviral therapy may help prevent PTLD in EBV seronegative SOT recipients. Cells that are latently infected with EBV and cells of EBV-driven lymphomas do not express thymidine kinase. Therefore, these agents would not be expected to be effective in EBV-positive PTLD; however, they do limit the lytic replication of EBV-infected cells, reduce the viral load, and prevent infection of memory B cells and germinal center cells. (Taylor et al., 2005)

Limited evidence is available to address the efficacy of this therapy in the prevention of PTLD and most studies are retrospective, with inherent limitations and contradicting results. Prophylactic intravenous ganciclovir after liver transplant in children has been associated with decreased incidence of PTLD, perhaps due to reduction in the number of latently infected B lymphocytes. (Thorley-Lawson & Gross 2004) Marks et al. report that the overall incidence of PTLD was significantly lower when antiviral prophylaxis was used than when it was not used or not reported. They suggest that antiviral drug therapy may affect PTLD risk, even when the primary purpose is prevention of CMV infection, as prophylaxis may also inhibit EBV reactivation and primary infection, or progression to B-cell transformation and PTLD. (Marks et al., 2011) A retrospective study of 3,393 heart transplant recipients demonstrated that PTLD incidence did not increase after OKT3 or ATG induction therapy when acyclovir or ganciclovir were administered prophylactically. (Crespo-Leiro et al., 2007) However, Opelz et al. found in a retrospective study of 44,828 kidney transplant recipients that ganciclovir or acyclovir had no impact on the development of PTLD. (Opelz et al., 2007)

There have been small studies that have attempted to use arginine butyrate, an amino acid derivative, which induces EBV thymidine kinase expression in latently infected B cells, in conjunction with antivirals in the therapy of PTLD. (Oertel & Riess 2002; Perrine et al., 2007) This therapy is currently only available in clinical trials.

5.1.3 Passive and active immunization

An absence of antibody against at least one of the Epstein-Barr nuclear antigens (EBNA) in EBV-seropositive organ transplant recipients has been associated with the subsequent development of PTLD. There are also many patients that undergo primary EBV infection following transplantation and fail to develop anti-EBNA antibodies. Thus, the absence of anti-EBNA antibodies appears to correlate with an increased risk of developing PTLD. Increasing levels of anti-EBNA antibodies, including those introduced through transfusion, have correlated with decreasing EBV load. All of these data suggest a potential role for antibody in controlling EBV infected cells. (Green, 2010) The potential prophylactic benefit of CMV-IVIG against the development of EBV-related PTLD in pediatric liver transplant recipients has been evaluated in a randomized multicenter trial. Statistically significant differences were not observed, but rates of EBV disease and PTLD were somewhat lower in recipients of CMV-IVIG than in those who received placebo. (Green et al., 2006) One study found that anti-CMV immunoglobulin was effective in the prevention of early-onset PTLD in kidney transplant patients, but not in the prevention of late-onset PTLD. (Opelz et al., 2007)

EBV vaccination may be effective in PTLD prevention, especially in EBV-seronegative pediatric transplantation candidates, but the vaccines to date have had no reliable effects on the development of cell-mediated immunity. The role of this therapy is still controversial, and it is not commercially available. (Posfay-Barbe & Siegrist 2009)

5.2 Secondary prevention

5.2.1 Intervention after rising EBV-DNA load

Development of EBV-associated PTLD is usually preceded by increased levels of EBV-DNA load in peripheral blood, typically from 2 to 16 weeks before diagnosis. (Rowe et al., 2001; Schubert et al., 2008) EBV-DNA load is higher among SOT recipients subsequently diagnosed with PTLD than those who remain disease free.(Bingler, et al 2008; Webber et al., 1999) There is a trend towards higher EBV loads following primary infection compared with reactivation (Kenagy et al., 1995), consistent with the clinical observation of higher risk of PTLD following primary infection. (Allen et al., 2005; Ho et al., 1988) Between 60% and 80% of EBV-negative children seroconvert within 3 months of transplant (Green & Webber, 2007) and a small population maintain high viral loads after primary EBV infection or EBV-associated PTLD. (Bingler et al., 2008; Green & Webber, 2007) It is common practice to perform biweekly or monthly EBV-DNA load monitoring by quantitative PCR and/or immune function monitoring in the immediate post transplantation period with varying clinical practice for reduction of immunosuppression (RI), use of antiviral agents, use of monoclonal anti-CD20 (Rituximab) or cellular therapy in the event of rising EBV-DNA load. Which form of pre-emptive therapy is best to prevent PTLD is unclear at this time.

In pediatric liver transplant recipients, monitoring EBV-DNA loads in the first 6 months after transplant with RI and initiation of ganciclovir at the time of rise in EBV-DNA load resulted in a 50% reduction in the incidence of PTLD. (McDiarmid et al., 1998; Stevens, et al., 2002) In 73 pediatric liver transplant patients treated during 2001- 2004, the incidence of PTLD was reduced from 16 to 2% by RI in individuals with a high EBV load. (Lee, et al 2005) Series of pediatric intestinal transplant recipients reported similar results. (Green et al., 2000; Krieger, et al 2000) Rituximab is generally well tolerated and rapidly induces the depletion of mature B-lymphocytes, reducing the compartment of EBV infected cells, with an associated normalization of the viral load. It has been successfully used as a preemptive treatment for PTLD, specifically in the HSCT population. (Comoli et al., 2007; Styczynski et al., 2009) A preliminary report of adult cardiac recipients given rituximab as pre-emptive therapy, showed that only one patient (n=251) developed PTLD. (Choquet et al., 2011) This approach merits further evaluation for widespread application.

5.2.2 Cellular therapy

Recognizing the critical role of EBV-specific cytotoxic T-cells (CTLs) in immune surveillance, cellular therapy is considered both a preventive and therapeutic strategy with initial experience in EBV-related PTLD following HSCT. (Rooney et al., 1998) The implementation of this therapy in SOT it is more problematic where PTLD is primarily of recipient origin and often occurs in patients who are EBV seronegative prior to transplant. Some of the problems with the use of individual-based EBV-specific CTLs are the cost and the processing time required to generate the cells. Moosmann et al. recently reported a system that allowed the rapid isolation and generation of clinical-grade EBV-specific CTLs for the treatment of HSCT-related PTLD. (Moosmann et al., 2010) An alternative is to use allogeneic CTLs closely matched with human leukocyte antigen (HLA) from donors who are EBV seropositive. In a phase II multicenter clinical trial, relapsed and refractory PTLD patients were treated by weekly intravenous allogeneic CTL infusions for 4 weeks. No adverse effects were observed and the response rate was 64% at 5 weeks and 52% at 6 months in 33 patients. (Haque et al., 2007) Commercial banks of EBV specific CTLs generated from the peripheral blood of EBV-positive blood donors are in development. In the SOT setting, there is often the need to continue immunosuppression and this impairs the efficacy of adoptive T-cell therapy. In a effort to solve this problem, two groups have generated EBV-based CTLs resistant to calcineurin inhibitors and have shown efficacy of this approach without requiring a reduction in immunosuppression. (Brewin et al., 2009; Haque et al., 2007) EBV specific CTL therapy is now recommended for persistent or progressive EBV driven polymorphic or monomorphic PTLD. (NCCN Guidelines Version 4.2011)

5.3 Therapy

5.3.1 Reduction in immunosuppression (RI)

The initial approach to managing patients with PTLD is RI, which might restore CTL function and elicit a favorable response in EBV-positive PTLD. The dosage of immunosuppressive drugs must be reduced by 25%-50% of the normal therapeutic whole blood level. This approach is most effective for early lesions and polymorphic disease and for those patients diagnosed early following transplantation. (Cheema et al., 2008; Nelson et al., 2000; Taylor et al., 2005) The long term remission rate of early lesions and polymorphic PTLD treated with RI is 40%-86% in children but considerably lower in adults. (Carbone, et al 2008, Green, et al 1999; Taylor et al., 2005) In many cases additional therapy is required

(Reshef R et al., 2009). Lack of response to RI has been associated with elevated LDH at presentation, organ dysfunction, late-onset PTLD, and multiorgan involvement. The median time to response of RI is 2 to 4 weeks; patients with aggressive disease or high tumor burden often warrant more immediate treatment. The risk of graft rejection must be considered before RI. (Caillard, et al 2005) The risk of acute rejection may be reduced by the administration of corticosteroids, which are also important components of most chemotherapy regimens for PTLD. (Taylor et al., 2005) RI is generally well tolerated among liver and renal transplant recipients with non-invasive screening available for detection, and decreased risk and relative tolerability, of organ rejection; indeed complete withdrawal of immunosuppression may be possible in selected liver transplant recipients. (Londono et al., 2010; Tsai et al., 2001) RI strategy is not standardized. Differences of aggressiveness and duration of RI, amount of time to evaluate response prior to initiating second-line treatment, and patient factors (type of transplant, extent of disease, time from transplant and immunosuppression history), may explain reported differences in outcomes.

5.3.2 Chemotherapy and rituximab

Chemotherapy and/or rituximab are commonly used when RI fails to control the disease, and as an initial therapy for aggressive, monoclonal PTLD. Low dose chemotherapy may decrease toxic complications seen in immunosuppressed patients, but may lead to higher relapse rates. (Gross, et al 2005) The use of anti-CD20 antibody therapy (rituximab) as a single agent has been associated with overall response rates of 37–69% and is potentially beneficial and less toxic than systemic chemotherapy. (Blaes et al., 2005; Orjuela, et al 2003) Rituximab/chemotherapy (R/C) combination has been examined in an attempt to improve response rates. (Evens et al., 2010) Gupta et al., reported an overall response rate of 100% in the patients treated with R/C combination (low dose of chemotherapy) with a recurrence rate of only 12% and 2-year failure free survival of 80%. (Gupta et al ., 2010) Orjuela et al., in a pilot multi-center study of pediatric patients treated with cyclophosphamide, prednisone and rituximab, report an overall response rate of 100% (five complete response [CR] and one partial response) with a median follow-up of 12.5 months. (Orjuela, et al 2003) A recent single-center study reported a two year OS and EFS of 85.7% and 57%, respectively, with a combination of rituximab and a milder chemotherapy regimen. (Gallego et al., 2010) Trappe et al have recommended a risk stratified approach based on upfront response to 4 weekly doses of rituximab: patients with a complete response (CR) to rituximab continued to receive an additional 4 doses of rituximab alone whereas patients with less than a CR subsequently received rituximab plus CHOP chemotherapy for four cycles with growth factor support. Using this approach, the overall response rate was 89%. (Trappe et al., 2009) Rituximab as a single agent is a consideration for many patients, with the use of combination chemotherapy for progressive or relapsed disease or for patients with concomitant allograft rejection.

Some groups have tried to identify at diagnosis patients likely to have a poor response to rituximab monotherapy. One study suggested that good response in late PTLD was only seen when rituximab was used after either surgical resection or radiotherapy (Dotti et al, 2001) and, in another, EBV-negative PTLD did not respond to rituximab and subsequently required chemotherapy (Oertel et al, 2005). The recommendation of the British Committee for Standards in Haematology (BCSH) and the British Transplantation Society (BTS) guidelines for adults is that rituximab plus chemotherapy should be used for patients who fail to respond within 8 weeks of rituximab plus RI and it should be considered immediately at any stage following diagnosis for patients with clinically aggressive disease or those with critical organ compromise (Parker et al, 2010).

Chemotherapy is used as a first line therapy for Burkitt lymphoma, T-cell disease and for most cases of Hodgkin lymphoma. Burkitt lymphoma seems to respond well to immediate aggressive chemotherapy. (Picarsic et al., 2010) Hodgkin disease is often associated with EBV and responds well to standard therapy. (Bierman et al., 1996) Available literature suggests that T -cell PTLD is clinically aggressive and may be associated with a poor prognosis. (Azhir et al., 2009; Gupta et al., 2010, Miloh et al., 2008; Williams et al., 2008; Yang, et al 2008)

5.3.3 Isolated CNS PTLD

CNS disease has been associated with significantly inferior survival, compared with non-CNS PTLD. (Buell et al., 2005; Knight et al., 2009; Maecker et al., 2007) It is more commonly associated with EBV. (Choquet et al., 2008) The optimal therapy for CNS PTLD is not known and proposed treatment approaches include high-dose methotrexate-based therapy, intrathecal chemotherapy and intrathecal rituxumab. (Bonney et al., 2011; Choquet et al., 2008; Taj et al., 2008; van de Glind et al., 2008)

5.3.4 Surgery and radiation

Resection of a total solitary lesion may be curative, but is usually combined with RI. (Allen, et al 2001) Radiation is rarely used but may be considered when rapid local responses are required (eg. airway compression) and in some cases of CNS PTLD.

5.3.5 Relapsed/refractory disease

There is no standard recommendation for relapsed or refractory PTLD. Trappe et al. have shown that rituximab may still lead to response in patients who fail chemotherapy, and chemotherapy might lead to response in patients with failure after rituximab. (Trappe et al., 2007a, 2007b) In addition, autologous hematopoietic stem cell transplantation has been reported as a viable treatment option for relapsed PTLD. (Amar et al., 2006) The role for cellular therapy in this context was reviewed above.

6. Prognosis

Although there has been improvement over time for patient and graft survival, outcomes after PTLD remain suboptimal. Survival after PTLD differs by recipient age and allograft type. Outcomes for children with PTLD are much better than for adults. (Dharnidharka, 2010) Outcomes are highest for recipients of renal and liver allografts, with survival rates for children reported at 89% and 80% respectively (Fernandez et al., 2009; McDonald et al., 2008), but significantly lower for other types of transplant, 67% at five years in heart transplant recipients, 54% and 42% at 3 and 5 years respectively in lung transplant recipients. (Cohen et al., 2000; Webber et al., 2006) Further, the overall survival according to stage is 80% for stages I/II, 61% for stage III, 20% for CNS involvement and less than 20% for BM involvement. The overall survival success for mild to moderate PTLD cases seemed similar across the various treatment options. (Maecker et al., 2007)

7. Conclusions

Patients with PTLD present a multifaceted clinical challenge balancing cure, allograft function and other co-morbidities. The epidemiology of PTLD appears to be changing with the median time of presentation trending later and the percentage of monomorphic and EBV negative disease increasing concomitant with changing immunosuppression practices, improved identification of patients at risk, and early introduction of RI. Even with these advances some patients have a good initial response to therapy without a long remission, and the mortality rates remain high. There is an ongoing need for coordinated care programs and clinical practice guidelines for a consistent approach to care and to further research programs. Novel therapeutic approaches aimed at restoration of immune surveillance should continue to be examined.

8. References

Allen, U., et al. (2001). Epstein-Barr virus-related post-transplant lymphoproliferative disease in solid organ transplant recipients, 1988-97: a Canadian multi-centre experience. *Pediatr Transplant,* 5,3, (June 2001), pp. (198-203), 1397-3142.

Allen, U.D., et al. (2005). Risk factors for post-transplant lymphoproliferative disorder in pediatric patients: a case-control study. *Pediatr Transplant,* 9,4, (July 2005), pp. (450-455), 1397-3142.

Allen, U.D. (2010). Clinical Features and Diagnostic Evaluation of Posttransplant Lymphoproliferative Disorder, In: *Post-Transplant Lymphoproliferative Disorders,* Vikas R. Dharnidharka, Michael Green , Steven A. Webber., pp. (69-97) Springer Verlag, Berlin.

Amar, S., Sekhon, SS., Roy, V. (2005). Autologous hemopoietic stem cell transplantation is a viable treatment option for post liver transplant lymphoproliferative disorder: a case report. *Blood* 108(11), (2006) (Abstract 5447).

Azhir, A., et al. (2009). Post transplant anaplastic large T-cell lymphoma. *Saudi J Kidney Dis Transpl,* 20, 4 (July 2009), pp.(646-651), 1319-2442.

Bakker, N.A., et al. (2005a). Early onset post-transplant lymphoproliferative disease is associated with allograft localization. *Clin Transplant,* 19,3, (May 2005), pp. (327-334), 0902-0063.

Bakker, N.A., et al. (2005b). HLA antigens and post renal transplant lymphoproliferative disease: HLA-B matching is critical. *Transplantation,* 80,5, (September 2005), pp.(595-599), 0041-1337.

Bakker, N.A., et al. (2006). PTLD visualization by FDG-PET: improved detection of extranodal localizations. *Am J Transplant,* 6,8 (August 2006), pp. (1984-1985), 1600-6135.

Bierman, P.J., et al. (1996). Hodgkin's disease following solid organ transplantation. *Ann Oncol,* 7,3, (March 1996), pp.(265-270) 0923-7534.

Bingler, M.A., et al. (2008). Chronic high Epstein-Barr viral load state and risk for late-onset posttransplant lymphoproliferative disease/lymphoma in children. *Am J Transplant,* 8,2, (January 2008), pp.(442-445) 1600-6143.

Blaes, A.H., et al. (2005). Rituximab therapy is effective for posttransplant lymphoproliferative disorders after solid organ transplantation: results of a phase II trial. *Cancer,* 104,8,(September 2005), pp.(1661-1667), 0008-543X.

Blaes, A.H. & Morrison, V.A. (2010) Post-transplant lymphoproliferative disorders following solid-organ transplantation. *Expert Rev Hematol,* 3,1, (November 2010), pp.(35-44) 1747-4094.

Bonney, D.K., et al. (2011). Sustained response to intrathecal rituximab in EBV associated Post-transplant lymphoproliferative disease confined to the central nervous system following haematopoietic stem cell transplant. *Pediatr Blood Cancer,* (May 2011), 1545-5017

Boubenider, S., et al. (1997). Incidence and consequences of post-transplantation lymphoproliferative disorders. *J Nephrol,* 10,3 (May 1997), pp.(136-145),1121-8428.

Brewin, J., et al. (2009).Generation of EBV-specific cytotoxic T cells that are resistant to calcineurin inhibitors for the treatment of posttransplantation lymphoproliferative disease. *Blood,* 114,23, (September 2009), pp.(4792-4803), 1528-0020.

Buell, J.F., et al. (2005). Posttransplant lymphoproliferative disorder: significance of central nervous system involvement. *Transplant Proc,* 37,2, (April 2005), pp.(954-955), 0041-1345.

Caillard, S., et al. (2005). Posttransplant lymphoproliferative disorders after renal transplantation in the United States in era of modern immunosuppression. *Transplantation,* 80,9, (May 2005), pp.(1233-1243), 0041-1337.

Carbone, A., et al. (2008). EBV-associated lymphoproliferative disorders: classification and treatment. *Oncologist,* 13,5, (June 2008), pp.(577-585), 1083-7159.

Cohen, A.H., et al. (2000). High incidence of posttransplant lymphoproliferative disease in pediatric patients with cystic fibrosis. *Am J Respir Crit Care Med,* 161,4, (April 2000), pp.(1252-1255), 1073-449X.

Comoli, P., et al. (2007). Preemptive therapy of EBV-related lymphoproliferative disease after pediatric haploidentical stem cell transplantation. *Am J Transplant,* 7,6, (June 2007), pp.(1648-1655), 1600-6135.

Crespo-Leiro, M.G., et al. (2007). Influence of induction therapy, immunosuppressive regimen and anti-viral prophylaxis on development of lymphomas after heart transplantation: data from the Spanish Post-Heart Transplant Tumour Registry. *J Heart Lung Transplant,* 26,11, (November 2007), pp.(1105-1109), 1557-3117.

Chadburn, A., et al. (1997). Molecular pathology of posttransplantation lymphoproliferative disorders. *Semin Diagn Pathol,* 14,1, (February 1997), pp.(15-26).

Cheema, P., Zadeh, S., Ross, H., et al. (2008). Post-Transplant Lymphoproliferative Disorder: Evaluation of Effectiveness of Reduction of Immunosuppression or Systemic Chemotherapy. *Blood* 2008; 112, 229.

Choquet, S.O., Anagnostopoulos, I., et al. (2008). Results of the largest study on post-transplantlymphoproliferations (PTLDs) of the central nervous system (CNS) in the rituximab era: a surprising overrepresentation of kidney transplantations, key importance of methotrexate, cytarabine and radiotherapy for long term survival and low impact of rituximab. *Blood,* (ASH Annual Meeting Abstracts) 2008, 3614.

Choquet, S., Varnous, S., Deback, C., et al. (2011). Adapted management of EBV reactivation after solid organ transplantation: An effective prevention of post transplantation lymphoproliferative disorders (PTLD). Results of the largest prospective stududy on 251 patients. *Blood,* (ASH Annual Meeting Abstracts). 2011, 592.

Cohen AH, Sweet SC, Mendeloff E, et al. (2000). High incidence of posttransplant lymphoproliferative disease in pediatric patients with cystic fibrosis. *Am J Respir Crit Care Med.* 161,4, (April 2000), pp.(1252–1255) 1076-4320.

Dayton, J.D., et al. (2011). Role of immunosuppression regimen in post-transplant lymphoproliferative disorder in pediatric heart transplant patients. *J Heart Lung Transplant,* 30,4, (April 2011), pp.(420-425), 1557-3117.

Dharnidharka, V.R., et al. (2001) Risk factors for posttransplant lymphoproliferative disorder (PTLD) in pediatric kidney transplantation: a report of the North American Pediatric Renal Transplant Cooperative Study (NAPRTCS). *Transplantation,* 71,8, (May 2001), pp.(1065-1068), 0041-1337.

Dharnidharka, V.R. (2010). *Epidemiology of PTLD,* In: *Post-Transplant Lymphoproliferative Disorders.* Dharnidharka, V., Green, M., Webber, Stevan A., pp. (17-28), Springer Verlag, Berlin.

Djokic, M., et al. (2006). Post-transplant lymphoproliferative disorder subtypes correlate with different recurring chromosomal abnormalities. *Genes Chromosomes Cancer,* 45,3 (March 2006), pp.(313-318), 1045-2257.

Dotti, G., Rambaldi, A., Fiocchi, R., et al. (2001). Anti-CD20 antibody (rituximab) administration in patients with late occurring lymphomas after solid organ transplant. *Haematologica,* 86,6, (June 2006), pp.(618–623), 1141-8370

Dotti, G., et al. (2002). Lymphomas occurring late after solid-organ transplantation: influence of treatment on the clinical outcome. *Transplantation,* 74,8, (October 2002), pp.(1095-1102), 0041-1337.

EBV Work Group, (2011). Cincinnati Children´s Hospital Medical Center: Evidence-based clinical care guideline for Management of EBV-Associated Post-Transplant Lymphoprofeliferative Disease in Solid Organ Transplant. *Guideline 18,*(June 2011) pp.(1-18).

Elstrom, R.L., et al. (2006). Treatment of PTLD with rituximab or chemotherapy. *Am J Transplant,* 6,3, (March 2006), pp.(569-576), 1600-6135.

Evens, A.M., et al. (2010). Multicenter analysis of 80 solid organ transplantation recipients with post-transplantation lymphoproliferative disease: outcomes and prognostic factors in the modern era. *J Clin Oncol,* 28,6, (February 2010), pp.(1038-1046), 1527-7755.

Faull, R.J., et al. (2005). Lymphoproliferative disease after renal transplantation in Australia and New Zealand. *Transplantation,* 80,2 (July 2005), pp.(193-197)0041-1337.

Fernandez, M.C., et al. (2009). Post-transplant lymphoproliferative disorder after pediatric liver transplantation: characteristics and outcome. *Pediatr Transplant,* 13,3 (May 2009),pp.(307-310), 1339-3046.

Gajarski, R.J., et al. (2011). Infection and malignancy after pediatric heart transplantation: the role of induction therapy. *J Heart Lung Transplant,* 30,3 (March 2011), pp.(299-308), 1557-3117.

Gallego, S., et al. (2010). Post-transplant lymphoproliferative disorders in children: the role of chemotherapy in the era of rituximab. *Pediatr Transplant,* 14,1 (February 2010), pp.(61-66), 1399-3046.

Green, M., et al. (1999). The management of Epstein-Barr virus associated post-transplant lymphoproliferative disorders in pediatric solid-organ transplant recipients. *Pediatr Transplant*, 3,4 (Novemeber 1999), pp.(271-281), 1397-3142.

Green, M., et al. (2000). Predictive negative value of persistent low Epstein-Barr virus viral load after intestinal transplantation in children. *Transplantation*, 70,4 (August 2000), pp.(593-596), 0041-1337.

Green, M., et al. (2006). CMV-IVIG for prevention of Epstein Barr virus disease and posttransplant lymphoproliferative disease in pediatric liver transplant recipients. *Am J Transplant*, 6,8 (August 2006), pp.(1906-1912), 1600-6135.

Green, M. & Webber, S.A. (2007). Persistent increased Epstein-Barr virus loads after solid organ transplantation: truth and consequences? *Liver Transpl*, 13,3 (March 2007), pp.(321-322) 1527-6465.

Green, M., Michels, M. (2010). *Prevention of Epstein-Barr Virus Infection and Postransplant Lymphoproliferative Disease Following Transplantation.* In: *Post-Transplant Lymphoproliferative Disorders*. Dharnidharka, V., Green, M., Webber, Stevan A., pp. (113-144), Springer Verlag, Berling.

Ghobrial IM, Habermann TM, Maurer MJ, et al. (2005). Prognostic analysis for survival in adult solid organ transplant recipients with post-transplantation lymphoproliferative disorders. *J Clin Oncol*, 23,30 (October 2005), pp.(7574–7582), 1618-6599.

Grinyo, J., et al. (2010). An integrated safety profile analysis of belatacept in kidney transplant recipients. *Transplantation*, 90,12 (November 2010), pp.(1521-1527) 1534-6080.

Gross, T.G., et al. (2005). Low-dose chemotherapy for Epstein-Barr virus-positive post-transplantation lymphoproliferative disease in children after solid organ transplantation. *J Clin Oncol*, 23,27 (September 2005), pp.(6481-6488) 0732183X.

Gross TG. (2009). Treatment for Epstein-Barr virus-associated PTLD. *Herpes*; 15,3, (January 2009), pp.(64-67) 0969-7667.

Gupta, S., et al. (2010). Post-transplant lymphoproliferative disorder in children: recent outcomes and response to dual rituximab/low-dose chemotherapy combination. *Pediatr Transplant*, 14,7 (November 2010), pp.(896-902), 1399-3046.

Guthery, S.L., et al. (2003). Determination of risk factors for Epstein-Barr virus-associated posttransplant lymphoproliferative disorder in pediatric liver transplant recipients using objective case ascertainment. *Transplantation*, 75,7 (April 2003), pp.(987-993), 0041-1337.

Haque, T., et al. (2007). Allogeneic cytotoxic T-cell therapy for EBV-positive posttransplantation lymphoproliferative disease: results of a phase 2 multicenter clinical trial. *Blood*, 110,4 (August 2007), pp.(1123-1131), 0006-4971.

Ho, M., et al. (1988). The frequency of Epstein-Barr virus infection and associated lymphoproliferative syndrome after transplantation and its manifestations in children. *Transplantation*, 45, 4 (April 1988), pp.(19-727), 0041-1337.

Kauffman, H.M., et al. (2005). Maintenance immunosuppression with target-of-rapamycin inhibitors is associated with a reduced incidence of de novo malignancies. *Transplantation*, 80,7, (Octuber 2005), pp.(883-889), 0041-1337.

Kenagy, D.N., et al. (1995). Epstein-Barr virus DNA in peripheral blood leukocytes of patients with posttransplant lymphoproliferative disease. *Transplantation,* 60,6 (September 1995), pp.(547-554), 0041-1347.

Kirk, A.D., et al. (2007). Dissociation of depletional induction and posttransplant lymphoproliferative disease in kidney recipients treated with alemtuzumab. *Am J Transplant,* 7,11 (November 2007), pp.(2619-2625) 1600-6135.

Knight, J.S., et al. (2009). Lymphoma after solid organ transplantation: risk, response to therapy, and survival at a transplantation center. *J Clin Oncol,* 27,20, (July 2009),pp.(3354-3362),1527-7755.

Krieger, N.R., et al. (2000). Significance of detecting Epstein-Barr-specific sequences in the peripheral blood of asymptomatic pediatric liver transplant recipients. *Liver Transpl,* 6,1, (January 2000), pp.(62-66)1527-6465,.

Lazda, V.A. (2006). Evaluation of Epstein-Barr virus (EBV) antibody screening of organ donors for allocation of organs to EBV serostatus matched recipients. *Transplant Proc,* 38,10, (December 2006),pp.(3404-3405), 0041-1345.

Leblond, V., et al. (1998). Posttransplant lymphoproliferative disorders not associated with Epstein-Barr virus: a distinct entity? *J Clin Oncol,* 16,6, (June 1998),pp.(2052-2059), 0732-183X.

Lee, T.C., et al. (2005). Quantitative EBV viral loads and immunosuppression alterations can decrease PTLD incidence in pediatric liver transplant recipients. *Am J Transplant,* 5,9 (September 2005), pp.(2222-2228), 1600-6135.

Londono, M.C., et al. (2010). Minimization of immunosuppression in adult liver transplantation: new strategies and tools. *Curr Opin Organ Transplant.* (September 2010), 1531-7013.

Maecker, B., et al. (2007). CNS or bone marrow involvement as risk factors for poor survival in post-transplantation lymphoproliferative disorders in children after solid organ transplantation. *J Clin Oncol,* 25,31 (November 2007), pp.(4902-4908) 1527-7755.

Mamzer-Bruneel, M.F., et al. (2000). Durable remission after aggressive chemotherapy for very late post-kidney transplant lymphoproliferation: A report of 16 cases observed in a single center. *J Clin Oncol,* 18,21, (November 2000), pp. (3622-3632),0732-183X

Marks, W.H., et al. (2011). Posttransplantation lymphoproliferative disorder in kidney and heart transplant recipients receiving thymoglobulin: a systematic review. *Transplant Proc,* 43,5 (Novemeber 2011), pp.(1395-1404), 1873-2623.

McCormack, L., et al. (2006). How useful is PET/CT imaging in the management of post-transplant lymphoproliferative disease after liver transplantation? *Am J Transplant,* 6,7 (July 2006), pp.(1731-1736), 1600-6135.

McDiarmid, S.V., et al. (1998). Prevention and preemptive therapy of postransplant lymphoproliferative disease in pediatric liver recipients. *Transplantation,* 66,12 (December 1998), pp.(1604-1611), 0041-1337.

McDonald, R.A., et al. (2008). Incidence of PTLD in pediatric renal transplant recipients receiving basiliximab, calcineurin inhibitor, sirolimus and steroids. *Am J Transplant,* 8,5 (May 2008), pp.(984-989), 1600-6143.

Miloh, T., et al. (2008). T-cell PTLD presenting as acalculous cholecystitis. *Pediatr Transplant,* 12,6, (September 2008), pp.(717-720), 1399-3046.

Moosmann A., et al. (2010). Effective and long-term control of EBV PTLD after transfer of peptide-selected T cells. *Blood* 115,14, (April 2010), pp.(2960–2970). 1528-0020

NCCN Guidelines Version 4.2011 Post-transplant Lymphoproliferative Disorder. In: *NCCN Clinical Practice Guidelines in Oncology Non-Hodgkin's Lymphomas Version 4.2011.* National Comprehensive Cancer Network (2012), pp. PTLD-2 (www.nccn.org, accessed January 15, 2012).

Nee, R., et al. (2011). Racial variation in the development of posttransplant lymphoproliferative disorders after renal transplantation. *Transplantation,* 92,2 (July 2011), pp.(190-195), 1534-6080.

Nelson, B.P., et al. (2000). Epstein-Barr virus-negative post-transplant lymphoproliferative disorders: a distinct entity? *Am J Surg Pathol,* 24,3 (March 2000), pp.(375-385), 0147-5185.

Newell, K.A., et al. (1996). Posttransplant lymphoproliferative disease in pediatric liver transplantation. Interplay between primary Epstein-Barr virus infection and immunosuppression. *Transplantation,* 62,3, (August 1996), pp.(370-375), 0041-1337.

Newell KA, Alonso EM, Kelly SM, et al. (1997). Association between liver transplantation for Langerhans cell histiocytosis, rejection, and development of posttransplant lymphoproliferative disease in children. *J Pediatr.* 131,1, (July 1997), pp.(98–104).

Nourse, J.P., et al. (2011). Epstein-barr virus-related post-transplant lymphoproliferative disorders: pathogenetic insights for targeted therapy. *Am J Transplant,* 11,5, (May 2011), pp.(888-895), 1600-6143.

Oertel, S.H. & Riess, H. (2002). Antiviral treatment of Epstein-Barr virus-associated lymphoproliferations. *Recent Results Cancer Res,* 159, pp.(89-95), 0080-0015.

Oertel, S.H., Verschuuren, E., Reinke, P., et al. (2005). Effect of anti-CD 20 antibody rituximab in patients with post-transplant lymphoproliferative disorder (PTLD). *Am J Transplant,* 5,12, (December2005), pp.(2901–2906), 1600-6143.

Olagne, J., et al. (2011). Post-transplant lymphoproliferative disorders: determination of donor/recipient origin in a large cohort of kidney recipients. *Am J Transplant,* 11,6 (June 2011), pp.(1260-1269), 1600-6143.

Opelz, G. & Dohler, B. (2004). Lymphomas after solid organ transplantation: a collaborative transplant study report. *Am J Transplant,* 4,2, (February 2004), pp.(222-230), 1600-6135.

Opelz, G., et al. (2007). Effect of cytomegalovirus prophylaxis with immunoglobulin or with antiviral drugs on post-transplant non-Hodgkin lymphoma: a multicentre retrospective analysis. *Lancet Oncol,* 8,3, (March 2007), pp.(212-218), 1470-2045.

Opelz, G. & Dohler, B. (2010). Impact of HLA mismatching on incidence of posttransplant non-hodgkin lymphoma after kidney transplantation. *Transplantation,* 89,5, (March 2010), pp.(567-572), 1534-6080.

Orjuela, M., et al. (2003). A pilot study of chemoimmunotherapy (cyclophosphamide, prednisone, and rituximab) in patients with post-transplant lymphoproliferative disorder following solid organ transplantation. *Clin Cancer Res,* 9,10, (September 2003), pp.(3945S-3952S), 1078-0432.

Parker A, Bowles K, Bradley JA, et al. (2010). Haemato-oncology Task Force of the British Committee for Standards in Haematology and British Transplantation Society. Management of post-transplant lymphoproliferative disorder in adult solid organ transplant recipients - BCSH and BTS Guidelines. *Br J Haematol.* 149,5,(Jun 2010), pp.(693-705), 1078-0432.

Perrine, S.P., et al. (2007). A phase 1/2 trial of arginine butyrate and ganciclovir in patients with Epstein-Barr virus-associated lymphoid malignancies. *Blood,* 109,6, (March 2007), pp.(2571-2578), 0006-4971.

Petit, B., et al. (2002). Influence of host-recipient origin on clinical aspects of posttransplantation lymphoproliferative disorders in kidney transplantation. *Transplantation,* 73,2, (January 2002), pp.(265-271), 0041-1337.

Picarsic, J., et al. (2010). Post-transplant Burkitt lymphoma is a more aggressive and distinct form of post-transplant lymphoproliferative disorder. *Cancer.* (March 2010),pp.(1-11)

Pitman, S.D., et al. (2006). Hodgkin lymphoma-like posttransplant lymphoproliferative disorder (HL-like PTLD) simulates monomorphic B-cell PTLD both clinically and pathologically. *Am J Surg Pathol,* 30,4, (April 2006), pp.(470-476), 0147-5185.

Posfay-Barbe, K.M. & Siegrist, C.A. (2009). Immunization and transplantation--what is new and what is coming? *Pediatr Transplant,* 13,4 (June 2009), pp.(404-410),1399-3046.

Preiksaitis, J. (2009). *Epstein-Barr Viral Load Testing: Role in the Prevention, Diagnosis and Management of Posttranplant Lymphoproliferative Disorders.* In: *Post-Transplant Lymphoproliferative Disorders.* Dharnidharka, V., Green, M., Webber, Stevan A., pp. (45-68), Springer Verlag, Berling.

Quinlan, S.C., et al. (2011). Risk factors for early-onset and late-onset post-transplant lymphoproliferative disorder in kidney recipients in the United States. *Am J Hematol,* 86,2, (February 2011), pp.(206-209), 1096-8652.

Ranganathan, S., et al. (2004). Hodgkin-like posttransplant lymphoproliferative disorder in children: does it differ from posttransplant Hodgkin lymphoma? *Pediatr Dev Pathol,* 7,4, (Jul-Aug 2004), pp.(348-360), 1093-5266.

Reshef R, Vardhanabhuti S, Luskin MR *et al.* (2009).Reduction of immunosuppresion as initial therapy for post-transplantation lymphoproliferative disorder: analysis of efficacy, safety and prognostic factors. *Blood* 114, (2009) (Abstract 103).

Reshef, R., et al. (2011). Association of HLA polymorphisms with post-transplant lymphoproliferative disorder in solid-organ transplant recipients. *Am J Transplant,* 11,4, (April 2011), pp.(817-825), 1600-6143.

Rhodes, M.M., et al. (2006). Utility of FDG-PET/CT in follow-up of children treated for Hodgkin and non-Hodgkin lymphoma. *J Pediatr Hematol Oncol,* 28,5, (May 2006), pp. (300-306), 1077-4114.

Rickinson, A., Kieff, E. (1996). *Epstein-Barr Virus.* Field, BN., Knipe, DM., Howley, PM., et al. pp.(2397-2446), Lippincott-Raven, Philadelphia.

Rohr, J.C., et al. (2008). Differentiation of EBV-induced post-transplant Hodgkin lymphoma from Hodgkin-like post-transplant lymphoproliferative disease. *Pediatr Transplant,* 12,4, (June 2008), pp.(426-431), 1399-3046.

Rooney, M.M., et al. (1998). The contribution of the three hypothesized integrin-binding sites in fibrinogen to platelet-mediated clot retraction. *Blood,* 92,7, (October 1998), pp.(2374-2381), 0006-4971.

Rowe, D.T., et al. (2001). Epstein-Barr virus load monitoring: its role in the prevention and management of post-transplant lymphoproliferative disease. *Transpl Infect Dis,* 3,2 (June 2001), pp.(79-87), 1398-2273.

Russo, L.M. & Webber, S.A. (2004). Pediatric heart transplantation: immunosuppression and its complications. *Curr Opin Cardiol,* 19,2, (March 2004), pp.(104-109), 0268-4705.

Schubert, S., et al. (2008). Relationship of immunosuppression to Epstein-Barr viral load and lymphoproliferative disease in pediatric heart transplant patients. *J Heart Lung Transplant,* 27,1, (January 2008), pp.(100-105), 1557-3117.

Selvaggi, G., et al. (2006). Etiology and management of alimentary tract ulcers in pediatric intestinal transplantation patients. *Transplant Proc,* 38,6 (Jul-Aug 2006), pp.(1768-1769),0041-1345.

Shapiro, R., et al. (2007). Alemtuzumab pre-conditioning with tacrolimus monotherapy in pediatric renal transplantation. *Am J Transplant,* 7,12, (December 2007), pp.(2736-2738), 1600-6135.

Shpilberg O, Wilson J, Whiteside TL, Herberman RB. (1999). Pre-transplant immunological profile and risk factor analysis of post-transplant lymphoproliferative disease development: the results of a nested matched case-control study. The University of Pittsburgh PTLD Study Group. *Leuk Lymphoma.* 36,2-1, (Decemeber 1999), pp.(109–121), 10613455.

Steven, N.M., et al. (1996). Epitope focusing in the primary cytotoxic T cell response to Epstein-Barr virus and its relationship to T cell memory. *J Exp Med,* 184,5, (November 1996), pp.(1801-1813), 0022-1007.

Stevens, S.J., et al. (2002). Role of Epstein-Barr virus DNA load monitoring in prevention and early detection of post-transplant lymphoproliferative disease. *Leuk Lymphoma,* 43,4, (April 2002), pp.(831-840), 1042-8194.

Stojanova, J., et al. (2011). Post-transplant lymphoproliferative disease (PTLD): Pharmacological, virological and other determinants. *Pharmacol Res,* 63,1 (January 2011), pp.(1-7), 1096-1186.

Styczynski, J., et al. (2009). Outcome of treatment of Epstein-Barr virus-related post-transplant lymphoproliferative disorder in hematopoietic stem cell recipients: a comprehensive review of reported cases. *Transpl Infect Dis,* 11,5, (October 2009), pp.(383-392), 1399-3062.

Swerdlow, S.H., Webber, S.A.,Chadburn, A., et al. (2008). Post-transplant lymphoproliferative disorders. In: *WHO classification of tumours of haematopoietic and lymphoid tissues.* (ed. by Swerdlow, S.H., Campo, E., Lee Harris, N.), pp. (343-351.) International Agency for Research on Cancer (IARIC), Lyon (France).

Taj, M.M., et al. (2008). Efficacy and tolerability of high-dose methotrexate in central nervous system positive or relapsed lymphoproliferative disease following liver transplant in children. *Br J Haematol,* 140,2, (January 2008), pp.(191-196),1365-2141.

Taylor, A.L., et al. (2005). Post-transplant lymphoproliferative disorders (PTLD) after solid organ transplantation. *Crit Rev Oncol Hematol,* 56,1 (October 2005), pp.(155-167),1040-8428.

Thorley-Lawson, D.A. (2001). Epstein-Barr virus: exploiting the immune system. *Nat Rev Immunol,* 1,1, (October 2001), pp.(75-82), 1474-1733.

Thorley-Lawson, D.A. & Gross, A. (2004). Persistence of the Epstein-Barr virus and the origins of associated lymphomas. *N Engl J Med,* 350,13, (March 2004), pp.(1328-1337), 1533-4406.

Trappe R, Riess H, Babel N, et al. (2007). Salvage chemotherapy for refractory and relapsed posttransplant lymphoproliferative disorders (PTLD) after treatment with single-agent rituximab. *Transplantation,* 83,7, (April 2007), pp.(912–918), 0041-1337.

Trappe RU, Choquet S, Reinke P, et al. (2007). Salvage therapy for relapsed posttransplant lymphoproliferative disorders (PTLD) with a second progression of PTLD after upfront chemotherapy: The role of single-agent rituximab. *Transplantation,* 84,12, (December 2007), pp.(1708–1712), 0041-1337.

Trappe, R., Choquet, S., Oertel, SH., et al. (2009). Sequential Treatment with Rituximab and CHOP Chemotherapy in B-Cell PTLD - Moving Forward to a First Standard of Care: Results From a Prospective International Multicenter Trial. *Blood* 114, (2009) (Abstract 100).

Tsai, D.E., et al. (2001). Reduction in immunosuppression as initial therapy for posttransplant lymphoproliferative disorder: analysis of prognostic variables and long-term follow-up of 42 adult patients. *Transplantation,* 71,8, (April 2001), pp.(1076-1088), 0041-1337.

Tsai, D.E., et al. (2008). EBV PCR in the diagnosis and monitoring of posttransplant lymphoproliferative disorder: results of a two-arm prospective trial. *Am J Transplant,* 8,5, (May 2008), pp.(1016-1024), 1600-6143.

Tsao, L. & Hsi, E.D. (2007). The clinicopathologic spectrum of posttransplantation lymphoproliferative disorders. *Arch Pathol Lab Med,* 131,8, (August 2007), pp.(1209-1218), 1543-2165.

van de Glind, G., et al. (2008). Intrathecal rituximab treatment for pediatric post-transplant lymphoproliferative disorder of the central nervous system. *Pediatr Blood Cancer,* 50,4, (April 2008), pp.(886-888),1545-5017.

van Leeuwen, M.T., et al. (2009). Immunosuppression and other risk factors for early and late non-Hodgkin lymphoma after kidney transplantation. *Blood,* 114,3, (July 2009), pp.(630-637),1528-0020.

Vegso, G., et al. (2010). Lymphoproliferative Disorders After Solid Organ Transplantation-Classification, Incidence, Risk Factors, Early Detection and Treatment Options. *Pathol Oncol Res.* (December 2010), 1532-2807.

von Falck, C., et al. (2007). Post transplant lymphoproliferative disease in pediatric solid organ transplant patients: a possible role for [18F]-FDG-PET(/CT) in initial staging and therapy monitoring. *Eur J Radiol,* 63,3, (September 2007), pp.(427-435), 0720-048X.

Webber, S.A. (1999). Post-transplant lymphoproliferative disorders: a preventable complication of solid organ transplantation? *Pediatr Transplant,* 3,2, (May 1999), pp.(95-99), 1397-3142.

Webber, S.A., et al. (2006). Lymphoproliferative disorders after paediatric heart transplantation: a multi-institutional study. *Lancet,* 367,9506, (January 2006), pp.(233-239), 1474-547X.

Webster, A., et al. (2005). Tacrolimus versus cyclosporin as primary immunosuppression for kidney transplant recipients. *Cochrane Database Syst Rev,* 4, (Octubre 2005), CD003961, 1469-493X.

Williams, K.M., et al. (2008). Successful treatment of a child with late-onset T-cell post-transplant lymphoproliferative disorder/lymphoma. *Pediatr Blood Cancer,* 50,3, (March 2008), pp.(667-670), 1545-5017.

Yakupoglu, Y.K., et al. (2006). Individualization of immunosuppressive therapy. III. Sirolimus associated with a reduced incidence of malignancy. *Transplant Proc,* 38,2, (March 2006), pp.(358-361), 0041-1345.

Yang, F., et al. (2008). Pediatric T-cell post-transplant lymphoproliferative disorder after solid organ transplantation. *Pediatr Blood Cancer,* 50,2, (February 2008), pp.(415-418), 1545-5017.

Zimmermann, T., et al. (2010). Liver transplanted patients with preoperative autoimmune hepatitis and immunological disorders are at increased risk for Post-Transplant Lymphoproliferative Disease (PTLD). *Eur J Intern Med,* 21,3, (June 2010), pp.(208-215), 1879-0828.

11

Ischaemia Reperfusion Injury in Kidney Transplantation

Siddharth Rajakumar and Karen Dwyer
Immunology Research Centre
St Vincent's Hospital, Melbourne
Australia

1. Introduction

The disruption of an organ's blood supply is obligatory in clinical transplantation occurring at the time of organ procurement. During this ischaemic period complex pathophysiological changes occur within the organ that leave it primed in a pro-inflammatory state. Although the re-establishment of blood flow is essential to halt ongoing ischaemic damage, the organ incurs additional injury. This paradoxical response to reperfusion is known as ischaemia reperfusion injury (IRI).

In deceased-donor transplantation, the haemodynamic instability and cytokine release associated with brain death augment the injury induced by ischaemia, which is more pronounced when donation occurs after cardiac death. Even with donation from a living donor there is a brief period of warm ischaemia after arterial cross-clamping. Following procurement, the donor organ is stored on ice as a means of slowing ischaemic injury. Although cold storage improves organ viability, a new set of complex processes is initiated by the combined effects of ischaemia and hypothermia. These ischaemic periods not only cause hypoxic/anoxic cell injury but lay the foundation for the augmented inflammatory response that occurs during reperfusion.

IRI has a significant impact on both short and long-term transplant outcome. It is a principal cause of delayed graft function which is common in deceased-donor transplantation (Perico, Cattaneo et al. 2004). Delayed graft function occurs in up to 50% of recipients of kidneys following cardiac death of the donor and primary graft failure occurs in 10% of these transplants (Keizer, de Fijter et al. 2005). The inflammatory state incited during IRI enhances the immunogenicity of the graft leading to an increased incidence of rejection. The independent association between delayed graft function and graft loss has long been recognised and its influence is more pronounced with concomitant rejection (Halloran, Aprile et al. 1988; Shoskes and Cecka 1998).

The mechanisms which underpin kidney IRI are complex and not yet fully defined. Both necrotic and apoptotic pathways of cell death are implicated and components of the inflammatory cascade, innate immune response, cellular infiltration and activation and the coagulation system are involved. In the kidney, endothelial cells, tubular epithelial cells and infiltrating leukocytes all demonstrate specific responses during both ischaemic and reperfusion phases of injury, which amplify the tissue damage. Understanding the mechanisms that mediate IRI is a focus of significant scientific endeavour. Therapeutics based on this research would not only improve the utility of transplantation from a finite donor pool by increasing short and long-term outcomes, but may have applications in numerous other clinical settings. The appeal of therapies that ameliorate the effects of IRI is more pronounced with the increasing use of organs from donors after cardiac death.

2. Pathophysiological mechanisms in kidney IRI

2.1 Apoptosis and necrosis

Both apoptotic and necrotic cell death occur in kidney IRI. The tubular epithelial cell is particularly susceptible because of the low oxygen tension environment, the concentration of toxic substances and their high adenosine triphosphate (ATP) and oxygen requirements due to transporter activity. These factors confer greatest susceptibility to proximal tubular cells and the outer stripe of the S3 segment (outer medulla) of the kidney which has marginal basal oxygenation. More recently, the lysosomal degradation pathway of autophagy has an emerging role in kidney IRI. Tubular epithelial cells demonstrate autophagy as a response to injury but its role in reperfusion injury is still unclear (Koesters, Kaissling et al. 2010).

Necrotic cell death is initiated by ATP depletion and mitochondrial damage that leads to impaired oxidative phosphorylation and the generation of reactive oxygen species (ROS). These ROS lead to a loss of cell adhesion to other cells and the extra-cellular matrix, damage the plasma membrane and intracellular membranes, and destabilise cytoskeletal proteins. These changes are associated with an increase in intracellular calcium and activation of the calcium-dependent cysteine protease calpain (Shi, Melnikov et al. 2000).

Apoptosis, or programmed cell death, is ATP-dependent and results in the formation of apoptotic bodies by the condensation of cytoplasmic and nuclear components. These bodies induce phagocytosis of the apoptotic cell by surrounding macrophages. As opposed to necrosis which causes cell swelling, apoptosis results in shrinkage of the epithelial cells. While ATP depletion leads to necrotic cell death, the GTP (guanosine triphosphate) depletion noted in kidney IRI promotes apoptotic cell death (Kelly, Plotkin et al. 2001). Cells undergoing apoptosis but lacking the further ATP to proceed with the stages of programmed cell death may undergo secondary necrosis. This may explain why the apoptosis seen in IRI, unlike physiological apoptosis, is associated with inflammation.

Both extrinsic and intrinsic pathways of apoptosis are implicated in IRI and there is considerable cross-talk between them. In kidney IRI receptors that are known to induce extrinsic apoptosis (termed 'death-receptors'), such as the Fas receptor, are up-regulated (Del Rio, Imam et al. 2004). This signalling results in the activation of pro-caspase 8 via the formation of the death-inducing signalling complex (DISC). Caspase 8 subsequently activates caspase 3, 6 and 7 resulting in apoptosis. Inhibition of caspases is protective in IRI (Daemen, van 't Veer et al. 1999; Nicholson 2000). The intrinsic apoptotic pathway largely relates to mitochondrial function. The activation of pro-caspase 9, which triggers intrinsic apoptosis, is initiated by cytochrome C and the release of cytochrome C from mitochondria is regulated by the Bcl-2 family of proteins (Gogvadze, Robertson et al. 2004). Over-expression of the anti-apoptotic Bcl-2-like protein (BCL-xL) reduces cytochrome C release from mitochondria and is protective in IRI (Chien, Shyue et al. 2007). The tumour-suppressor protein p53 is activated during hypoxia (by hypoxia inducible factor 1-α). This amplifies the transcription of numerous pro-apoptotic genes such as caspases 6 and 7 (Yang, Kaushal et al. 2008) and Bcl-2. The p53 inhibitor pifithrin-α protects in kidney IRI (Kelly, Plotkin et al. 2003) as does intravenous siRNA treatment directed against p53 in rats (Molitoris, Dagher et al. 2009).

In kidney IRI extrinsic apoptotic, intrinsic apoptotic and regulatory pathways are activated. The outcome in terms of degree of apoptosis clearly relates to the balance between these complex and interacting systems.

2.2 Inflammation and metabolism

2.2.1 Toll-like receptors

Toll-like receptors (TLRs) are a family of pattern recognition receptors. Endogenous ligands exposed during tissue injury such as heat shock proteins, host DNA, fibronectin and hyaluran can activate some TLRs. Signal transduction from TLRs activates nuclear factor kappa-light-chain-enhancer of activated B cells (NFκB) leading to the activation of the innate immune system and the generation of pro-inflammatory cytokines. Renal tubular epithelial cells express TLR2 and TLR4 and their expression is up-regulated in IRI (Wolfs, Buurman et al. 2002). Both TLR2 and TLR4 bind heat-shock protein 60 and 70. TLR4 deficiency is protective in renal IRI and adoptive transfer experiments suggest that expression of TLR4 on renal tissue rather than bone-marrow derived cells mediates injury (Wu, Chen et al. 2007). Both deficiency and inhibition of TLR2 is protective in renal IRI models and TLR-2 mediated damage is, in part, dependent on the adapter protein MyD88 (Leemans, Stokman et al. 2005; Shigeoka, Holscher et al. 2007).

2.2.2 Cytokines and chemokines

IRI in the kidney leads to the generation of multiple pro-inflammatory cytokines such as IL-1, IL-6 and TNFα (Takada, Nadeau et al. 1997) by infiltrating and resident leukocytes and endothelial cells. The manifestations of kidney IRI can often be observed systemically and in other organs and is explained, at least in part, by the release of cytokines. Inhibition of IL-1, IL-6 and IL-8 is protective in IRI; conversely, inhibition of IL-4 and IL-10 worsens renal injury (Deng, Kohda et al. 2001).

Chemokines are a sub-family of cytokines that have an emerging role in kidney IRI. Their principal actions relate to leukocyte activation and chemotaxis. The renal expression of the CXC chemokine receptor 3 (CXCR3), which binds several chemokines, monokine, IFN-γ, IP-10 and CXCL11, is increased after IRI and mice deficient in CXCR3 were protected from an ischaemic insult (Fiorina, Ansari et al. 2006). CX3CL1, a leukocyte chemo-attractant and adhesion molecule, is expressed on T cells, NK cells and monocytes. Its expression is redistributed to the outer medulla in renal IRI and inhibition of its receptor, CX3CR1, attenuated fibrosis after IRI (Furuichi, Gao et al. 2006). Monocyte chemotactic protein 1 (MCP-1) is up-regulated in kidney IRI and deficiency of its receptor (CCR2) attenuated injury and macrophage infiltration (Furuichi, Wada et al. 2003).

2.2.3 Complement

The complement system has a pathogenic role early in renal IRI and all three pathways of activation (classical, alternative and mannose-binding lectin pathways) have been implicated (Farrar, Wang et al. 2004). Specific inhibition of, or deficiency in the alternative pathway protects kidneys in murine models of IRI (Thurman, Ljubanovic et al. 2003). Normally, epithelial cells lining the proximal tubules of the kidney express the complement inhibitor Crry on the basolateral membrane. After renal IRI, Crry is redistributed away from the basolateral surface of the cell, allowing deposition of C3 (the first component of the alternative pathway). Consistent with this finding, mice deficient in Crry are more susceptible to kidney IRI. C3a also has a role in the production of CXC chemokines by tubular epithelial cells observed after IRI (Thurman, Lenderink et al. 2007). C5a and the membrane attack complex (C5b-9) are implicated in kidney IRI and inhibition of C5a confers protection (Zhou, Farrar et al. 2000; Arumugam, Shiels et al. 2003; De Vries, Matthijsen et al. 2003). Mannose-binding lectin recognizes several endogenous ligands in post-ischaemic renal tissue. These include ligands expressed on apoptotic and necrotic cells and exposed cytokeratin on hypoxic endothelial cells (Moller-Kristensen, Ip et al. 2006). The role of complement is further strengthened by the observation that mice deficient in the complement regulators CD55 and CD59 were more sensitive to renal IRI (Yamada, Miwa et al. 2004).

2.2.4 Endothelial activation

The endothelium plays a central role in IRI with effects on inflammation, permeability, coagulation and vascular tone. The endothelial cell subjected to ischaemia undergoes several changes in enzymatic activity, mitochondrial function, cytoskeletal structure, membrane transport, and antioxidant defences. The intensity of endothelial injury may be particularly important in determining the degree of chronic damage that a kidney will develop following IRI. Compared to tubular cells, the regenerative capacity of the renal endothelium is limited which leads to vascular dropout (Horbelt, Lee et al. 2007). Vascular endothelial growth factor (VEGF) inhibitors are induced in ischaemia and, in a rat model of IRI, VEGF treatment attenuated vascular dropout (Basile, Fredrich et al. 2008; Leonard, Friedrich et al. 2008).

Ischaemia activates the endothelium and promotes the expression of various pro-inflammatory gene products such as cytokines (Pinsky, Yan et al. 1995) and adhesion molecules. More specifically, the expression of ICAM-1 (Kelly, Williams et al. 1996), P-selectin (Takada, Nadeau et al. 1997) and E-selectin (Singbartl and Ley 2000) is up-regulated and antibody blockade of ICAM-1 significantly attenuated IRI in rats.

Endothelium-dependent vasodilatation, mediated by nitric oxide (NO), is impaired in arterioles following IRI (Pang, Wu et al. 2000) and the disordered auto-regulation can persist for up to 1 week. In addition to vasodilatory effects, NO is both cytoprotective (antioxidant activity) and cytotoxic (by the production of peroxynitrite) and can inhibit neutrophil-mediated injury. These varying effects, which make the precise role of NO in IRI difficult to define, are in part due to differences between the isoforms of the NO synthase. In ischaemia, due to endothelial damage there is a reduction in endothelial nitric oxide synthase (eNOS) and a relative increase in inducible NOS (iNOS) and this imbalance is considered to contribute to injury, in part, by enhancing the thrombogenic tendancy of the endothelium (Goligorsky, Brodsky et al. 2004). Both deficiency and inhibition of iNOS protect in kidney IRI (Noiri, Peresleni et al. 1996; Ling, Edelstein et al. 1999). Furthermore, a NO inhibitor worsened, and treatment with the NOS substrate, L-arginine, attenuated kidney IRI in rats (Ogawa, Nussler et al. 2001; Chander and Chopra 2005).

The permeability of the endothelial barrier separating the capillary lumen from the interstitial space is increased in IRI. In vivo imaging studies suggest that this effect is maximal 24 hours after ischaemic injury and occurs within 2-4 hours (Sutton, Mang et al. 2003). A loss in the integrity of adeherens junctions as shown by the delocalisation of the adhesion molecule cadherin between endothelial cells was noted. Thus, the increased vascular permeability predominantly relates to para-cellular, rather than trans-cellular pathways. A role for the matrix metalloproteinases 2 and 9 has been postulated as their activation correlates with microvascular permeability. In murine IRI, an inhibitor of matrix metalloproteinase (minocycline) attenuated microvascular permeability (Sutton, Kelly et al. 2005).

2.2.5 Adenosine generation and signalling

Ischaemic injury results in the extrusion and transport of intra-cellular adenosine triphosphate (ATP) from injured or dying cells into the extra-cellular space. Here it undergoes serial hydrolysis by the ecto-enzyme CD39 (ectonucleoside-triphosphate-diphosphohydrolase-1) generating adenosine diphosphate (ADP) and adenosine monophosphate (AMP). AMP is further hydrolysed by the ecto-enzyme CD73 (ecto-5′-nucleotidase) generating adenosine (Zimmermann 1992; Kaczmarek, Koziak et al. 1996). The concentration of adenosine, which acts at 4 receptors, is therefore increased in ischaemia and is thought to provide adaptive responses to hypoxia and attenuate inflammation and apoptosis by several intra-cellular second messenger pathways. Conversely, signalling by ATP and ADP at P2 purinergic receptors have pro-inflammatory and pro-thrombotic effects. Although adenosine treatment has been shown to be protective in IRI models (Lee and Emala 2000), its extremely short half-life and systemic haemodynamic effects in vivo makes its clinical application difficult.

Manipulating the metabolic pathway of adenosine generation can influence kidney IRI. Transgenic over-expression of CD39 was protective in both warm and cold kidney IRI models. This finding is supported by the protection conferred by treatment with Apyrase (which provides CD39 enzymatic activity) and the severe injury noted in mice deficient in CD39 (Lu, Rajakumar et al. 2008; Crikis, Lu et al. 2010). CD73 is up-regulated in ischaemia by hypoxia-inducible factor 1 (Thompson, Eltzschig et al. 2004) and is thought to be part of an innate protective mechanism during hypoxia. Although soluble CD73 (5′ nucleotidase) treatment was protective in a murine kidney IRI model, this is inconsistent with other studies demonstrating protection with CD73 deficiency or inhibition. This may relate to differences in the IRI models (Van Waarde, Stromski et al. 1989; Grenz, Zhang et al. 2007; Rajakumar, Lu et al. 2010).

All four adenosine receptors are present in the kidney and expression is up-regulated by ischaemia. The precise localisation of each receptor has proven difficult but there is evidence that the A1 and A2B receptors are the dominant receptors in the pre-glomerular vasculature

(Jackson, Zhu et al. 2002) and that A2B receptor expression is more prominent on the renal vasculature than the tubular epithelial cells (Grenz, Osswald et al. 2008).

A1 receptor activation has generally been protective in kidney IRI. Mice deficient in the A1 receptor develop worse injury which is reversed by lentiviral reconstitution of the A1 receptor in the kidney (Kim, Chen et al. 2009). A1 receptor agonist treatment was protective in a mouse kidney IRI model. Treatment conferred both acute and delayed protection, interestingly, by different signalling mechanisms (Joo, Kim et al. 2007). A2A receptor signalling is also protective in kidney IRI. Adoptive transfer experiments using wild-type and A2A receptor deficient mice in a kidney IRI model demonstrated A2A expression on bone-marrow derived cells mediates the protective effect (Day, Huang et al. 2003). Furthermore, a specific protective role for the A2A receptor on CD4+ T lymphocytes has been demonstrated (Day, Huang et al. 2006). Regulatory T lymphocytes have a protective role in kidney IRI and A2A receptor signalling is known to promote their expansion (Zarek, Huang et al. 2008).

The A2B receptor has a lower affinity for adenosine than the other receptors and so may play a more prominent role in pathological states where there is increased adenosine generation. A2B receptor agonist treatment was protective in a mouse model of kidney IRI and a specific role in the protective phenomenon of ischaemic preconditioning was demonstrated. In contrast to the A2A receptor studies, adoptive transfer experiments localised the protective effect to A2B receptors on the renal parenchyma rather than infiltrating cells (Grenz, Osswald et al. 2008). The A3 receptor mediates injury in kidney IRI. Antagonist treatment protected, while agonist treatment worsened injury in a mouse model (Lee and Emala 2000).

2.2.6 Oxidative stress

In IRI, reperfusion is a trigger for the generation of reactive oxygen species (ROS) that mediate cell injury directly by lipid peroxidation of cellular membranes. ROS can increase activation, chemotaxis and endothelial adherence by stimulating adhesion molecules and cytokine gene expression through the activation of transcription factors such as NFκB (Toyokuni 1999).

Haemoxygenase (HO) is an enzyme that degrades haem to produce carbon monoxide, biliverdin and bilirubin. Free haem can mediate cellular toxicity whilst the metabolic products are generally cytoprotective (Sikorski, Hock et al. 2004). Specifically, bilirubin is protective in a rat model of kidney IRI; HO-up-regulation confers cytoprotection in the kidney and carbon monoxide induces HIF-α which up-regulates HO and over 100 other cytoprotective genes (Blydt-Hansen, Katori et al. 2003). Furthermore, carbon monoxide therapy was protective in a kidney transplant model (Neto, Nakao et al. 2006). Regulatory T cells have been shown to play a protective role in kidney IRI and HO expression on antigen-presenting cells has been shown to be necessary for their full suppressive ability (George, Braun et al. 2008; Kinsey, Huang et al. 2010).

The xanthine oxidase (XO) system is the major source of ROS production in mammals. During the ischaemic period, intracellular ATP is catabolised to hypoxanthine and hypoxic stress triggers the conversion of xanthine dehydrogenase (XDH) to the oxygen radical-producing XO (Younes, Schoenberg et al. 1984). During reperfusion, oxygen is reintroduced into the tissue, where it reacts with hypoxanthine and XO to produce a burst of oxygen free radicals; superoxide anion (O^{2-}) and hydrogen peroxide (H_2O_2) (Harrison 2002). Under physiological conditions, the damaging effects of O^{2-} are prevented in part by superoxide dismutase (SOD), which converts O^{2-} to H_2O_2. During reperfusion of ischaemic tissues, the capacity of these antioxidant pathways is exceeded leading to cellular injury and death. Mice deficient in SOD3 were shown to have increased oxidative stress and tubular cast formation in IRI (Schneider, Sullivan et al. 2010).

2.2.7 Peroxisome proliferator-activated receptors

The family of peroxisome proliferator-activated receptors (PPARs) nuclear hormone receptors play a regulatory role in inflammatory responses, lipid metabolism, cellular differentiation and cell survival and have attracted increasing attention in IRI. PPARα deficient mice have worse injury in kidney IRI (Portilla, Dai et al. 2000) while treatment with PPAR-α ligand or over-expression in the proximal tubules confers protection (Sivarajah, Chatterjee et al. 2002; Li, Nagothu et al. 2009). PPARγ agonist treatment protects in kidney IRI and PPARβ/δ activity is also protective (Sivarajah, Chatterjee et al. 2003; Letavernier, Perez et al. 2005).

2.3 Cellular mediators

2.3.1 Neutrophils, macrophages, dendritic cells and natural killer cells

Early infiltration of neutrophils into the post-ischaemic kidney has been demonstrated (Chiao, Kohda et al. 1997) and likely contributes to kidney IRI by the release of reactive oxygen species and proteases and by obstructing flow in the renal microvasculature. Inhibiting neutrophil infiltration is protective (Kelly, Williams et al. 1996) however only partial protection was observed with neutrophil blockade or depletion (Thornton, Winn et al. 1989).

The role of macrophages in renal IRI is via the production of pro-inflammatory cytokines (IL-1α, IL-6, IL-12p40/70, TNFα) and activation of other leucocytes. Macrophages infiltrate the kidney early in IRI (within 1 hour) and particularly target the outer medulla. The infiltration is mediated by CCR2 and CX3CR1 signalling (Li, Huang et al. 2008; Oh, Dursun et al. 2008). Depletion of macrophages prior to IRI prevents injury and reconstitution restores it (Day, Huang et al. 2005).

Dendritic cells (DC) form a link between the innate and adaptive arms of the immune system and are the most abundant resident leukocyte in the kidney interstitium. In particular, CD11c+MHC ClassII+ DC are abundant in the murine kidney suggesting an important role in regulating renal immunity and inflammation. Upon stimulation DCs becomes mature with phenotypic characteristics of increased expression of MHC Class II and co-stimulation molecules, the release pro-inflammatory factors and the ability to activate NKT cells (Dong, Swaminathan et al. 2005). Renal DC produce TNF-α, IL-6, C-C motif chemokine 2 and C-C motif chemokine 5 in kidney IRI and the amount of TNF-α produced after ischaemia is reduced after depletion of DCs (Dong, Swaminathan et al. 2007).

Natural killer cells (NK) are cytotoxic lymphocytes without B or T cell receptors. Infiltration by NK cells has been noted by 4 hours and depletion of NK cells protects in kidney IRI in a perforin-dependent manner (Zhang, Wang et al. 2008).

2.3.2 CD4+ effector T lymphocytes

Lymphocytes are the major mediators of adaptive immunity and so were initially not thought to contribute to IRI. Their significant role in IRI was, however, established with the demonstration that mice deficient in T cells are protected from IRI and the adoptive transfer of T cells restores injury (Burne-Taney, Yokota-Ikeda et al. 2005). Further confirmation of the importance of T cells in the pathogenesis of IRI is that the use of CTLA4-Ig to block the B7-CD28 co-stimulation of T cells significantly attenuates renal dysfunction (Ysebaert, De Greef et al. 2004) as does use of a monoclonal antibody specific to B7 (De Greef, Ysebaert et al. 2001). The Th1 subset of T lymphocytes that produce IFNγ are deleterious, while IL4 producing Th2 cells are protective in IRI (Yokota, Burne-Taney et al. 2003). Further confirmation of this is that adoptive transfer of CD4+ cells lacking CD28 are unable to restore this injury, as are CD4+ cells from IFNγ knock-out mice (Burne, Daniels et al. 2001).

In murine renal IRI the number of invariant NKT cells (cells that possess a conserved invariant T cell receptor together with the NK cell marker NK1.1) is significantly increased at 3 hours of reperfusion following 30 minutes of ischaemia and inhibition or depletion of this cell type prevents injury. NKT cell activation was reported to contribute to kidney injury by mediating neutrophil IFNγ production (Li, Huang et al. 2007).

The minor T cell subsets, the γ-δ T cell and the α-β T cell have a poorly understood role in kidney IRI. Deficiencies of these cell subsets have conferred protection (Savransky, Molls et al. 2006; Hochegger, Schatz et al. 2007).

2.3.3. Regulatory T cells

Regulatory T cells (Treg), known for their ability to suppress immune responsiveness, play a specific role in kidney IRI. Infiltration of Tregs was demonstrated 3 and 10 days after kidney IRI. Depletion of Tregs 24 hours after IRI resulted in increased tubular damage and cytokine production by infiltrating T effector cells. Infusion of Tregs resulted in early improvements in cytokine production and a late functional protective effect (Gandolfo, Jang et al. 2009). Correlating with this, Treg depletion was associated with an increased accumulation of neutrophils and macrophages, and increased inflammatory cytokine transcription, and Treg infusion prior to IRI attenuated inflammatory responses (Kinsey, Huang et al. 2010).

2.3.4 B lymphocytes

In kidney IRI the role of B lymphocytes remains unclear. They play a pathogenic role that relates to the production of natural antibodies, which develop without antigen stimulation. This is predominantly by B1 cells which are located in the pleural and peritoneal cavities. Depletion of peritoneal B1 cells reduced glomerular IgM deposition and protected mice from IRI. Conversely, the more abundant B2 cells likely play a protective role in kidney IRI mediated by IL-10 release (Renner, Strassheim et al. 2010).

2.4 Coagulation

Activation of the coagulation system has been noted in several IRI models. Ischaemia leads to a reduction in the expression of the anticoagulant thrombomodulin, the down-regulation of the endothelial protein C receptor (EPCR) and the up-regulation of tissue factor (Ogawa,

Shreeniwas et al. 1990). Thrombosis leads to further endothelial dysfunction and reduced tissue perfusion. Although anticoagulants such as heparin have been shown to be protective in IRI, the mechanism of protection relates to complement inhibition, the prevention of endothelial cell dysfunction and the release of vasoactive mediators from the endothelium, rather than direct anticoagulant effects (Kouretas, Kim et al. 1999). Kidney IRI was attenuated by soluble thrombomodulin treatment either before or after ischaemia. This was associated with reduced leukocyte adhesion and endothelial permeability and improved microvascular flow but was independent of its ability to generate activated protein C (APC) (Sharfuddin, Sandoval et al. 2009). Treatment with APC, which acts at the EPCR, is protective in a rat kidney IRI model. Again, the effect was considered to be independent of its anti-coagulant activity (Mizutani, Okajima et al. 2000).

3. Therapeutic implications

Based on recent advances in the understanding of the mechanistic basis of kidney IRI, several novel therapeutic approaches are being developed. Delineating the apoptotic cell death pathway has led to a pancaspase inhibitor and a p53 inhibitor that are currently in clinical trials for liver transplantation. The field of adenosine signalling is promising and an adenosine 2A receptor agonists is already available for myocardial diagnostic studies and selective adenosine 2B receptor agonists are being developed. The protective metabolic and anti-inflammatory effects of PPAR signalling have been demonstrated in murine kidney IRI models. Given thiazolidenediones (PPARγ ligand) and fibrates (PPARα ligand) are already available, this demonstrates the capacity for basic research in kidney IRI to identify potential new applications for existing treatments. Similarly, statin (HMG-CoA reductase inhibitor) therapy is widely used for dyslipidaemia and preclinical studies suggest it is protective in kidney IRI (Yokota, O'Donnell et al. 2003). The mechanism of protection is unrelated to cholesterol lowering and may relate to caspase-3 mediated anti-apoptotic effects (Haylor, Harris et al. 2011). Donor treatment with simvastatin is currently under investigation (NCT01160978).

Although erythropoietin treatment has a body of pre-clinical evidence suggesting protective effects (Sharples, Patel et al. 2004), clinical trials in both acute kidney injury and kidney transplantation have been disappointing to date (Endre, Walker et al. 2010; Martinez, Kamar et al. 2010). A greater understanding of the pathways of oxidative stress in kidney IRI have led to a focus on carbon monoxide. Given its systemic toxicity, donor compounds are being developed that may allow carbon monoxide release at the ischaemic tissue. Along a similar line, several anti-oxidant agents are currently being investigated. The significant role played by the complement system in several disease states has led to the development of treatments such as eculizumab (recombinant antibody targeting C5). This is being trialled in several clinical settings including kidney transplantation (Weitz, Amon et al. 2011).

Modulating cellular interactions, such us the endothelial-leukocyte adhesion, is promising based on pre-clinical studies in kidney IRI. Antibody blockade of ICAM1 showed disappointing results in an early trial (Salmela, Wramner et al. 1999). A recombinant blocking antibody to P-selectin has recently completed a phase 2 trial although an effect on delayed graft function has not yet been demonstrated (Osama Gaber, Mulgaonkar et al. 2011). The emerging role of T lymphocytes in kidney IRI has meant that inhibiting early T lymphocyte activation is a focus of investigation. Anti-thymocyte globulin induction for kidney transplantation has shown promising results and clinical trials are ongoing (NCT00733733/NCT01149993). Similarly, numerous agents that reduce T lymphocyte activation by blocking co-stimulation are under development. Belatacept, which prevents co-stimulation by binding to CD80 and CD86 on antigen-presenting cells was recently approved by the FDA for use in kidney transplant recipients (Vincenti, Dritselis et al. 2011).

Cell-based therapies show significant promise. On a background of positive pre-clinical studies (Togel, Hu et al. 2005), a clinical trial of autologous mesenchymal stem cell infusion in kidney transplantation is underway (NCT00752479). Haemopoietic stem cells, which may promote endothelial/microvascular repair also show promise (Becherucci, Mazzinghi et al. 2009). The recent pre-clinical finding that regulatory T cells protect in kidney IRI suggests ex-vivo expansion and infusion may also have therapeutic potential.

In addition to the recognized protective effects of hypothermia, insights into IRI mechanisms may improve reperfusion injury following cold ischaemia by modifying organ preservation methods. The University of Wisconsin (UW) solution widely used for preservation contains anti-oxidant ingredients such as allopurinol and glutathione. It also contains adenosine which may mediate cytoprotective effects. The addition of lecithinized SOD to the cold ischaemia preservation fluid improved early inflammation and later proteinuria and apoptosis in a rat kidney transplant model (Nakagawa, Koo et al. 2002). Similarly, carbon monoxide supplementation to UW preservation fluid led to improved histological damage and inflammatory responses in a pig transplant model (Yoshida, Ozaki et al. 2010). As an example of perfusion mediated protection, Yamauchi et al showed that flushing with the fibrinolytic agent streptokinase conferred protection in a non-heart beating donor rat kidney transplant model (Yamauchi, Schramm et al. 2003). A current clinical trial includes an experimental arm with infusion of the donor kidney with thymoglobulin which may attenuate T lymphocyte mediated injury with reperfusion (NCT01149993).

Brief periods of ischaemia can protect an organ from a subsequent ischaemic insult. This phenomenon is known as ischaemic preconditioning (IP) and was originally described in canine hearts (Murry, Jennings et al. 1986). Protection by IP in a murine model of renal IRI has been demonstrated using cycles of renal artery occlusion (Grenz, Eckle et al. 2007). Protection of an organ from an ischaemic insult is also observed when the cycles of short-term ischaemia are applied to a different anatomical site. This phenomenon is termed remote ischaemic preconditioning (RIP). Renal protection by RIP has been reported by cycles of ischaemia in the contra-lateral kidney in mice (Park, Chen et al. 2001). Several studies in humans have demonstrated the clinical applicability of RIP. A recent study demonstrated that cycles of lower limb ischaemia led to reduced ischaemic kidney injury in patients undergoing cardiac surgery (Zimmerman, Ezeanuna et al. 2011). While the phenomenon may be applied to transplantation, research into the mechanisms mediating RIP should also provide targets for future therapeutic strategies. Regulatory T cells play a dominant role in IP (Kinsey, Huang et al. 2010) as do CD39, CD73 and adenosine A2B receptor signalling (Grenz, Zhang et al. 2007; Grenz, Zhang et al. 2007; Grenz, Osswald et al. 2008). In various IRI models ATP-dependent potassium channels (Pell, Baxter et al. 1998), protein kinase C (Weinbrenner, Nelles et al. 2002), nitric oxide synthesis (Wang, Xu et al. 2001), bradykinin, heat shock proteins (Patel, van de Poll et al. 2004), haemoxygenase-1 (Amersi, Buelow et al. 1999) and TNFα (Teoh, Leclercq et al. 2003) have all been implicated. Clinical trials of remote preconditioning in kidney transplantation are currently underway (NCT01395719, NCT01289548).

4. Conclusion

Kidney ischaemia reperfusion injury is obligatory in transplantation. Given the significant impact of IRI on both short and long-term graft function, therapeutic strategies to minimise IRI are of considerable appeal. This is particularly relevant with the increasing utilisation of organs from extended-criteria/non-heart-beating donors. However, the pathophysiological mechanisms mediating kidney IRI are complex and involve the interaction of numerous biological systems. Novel insights regarding these interactions are leading to the development of applications to attenuate IRI in the fields of therapeutics, organ preservation and ischaemic preconditioning.

5. References

Amersi, F., R. Buelow, et al. (1999). "Upregulation of heme oxygenase-1 protects genetically fat Zucker rat livers from ischemia/reperfusion injury." *J Clin Invest* 104(11): 1631-1639.

Arumugam, T. V., I. A. Shiels, et al. (2003). "A small molecule C5a receptor antagonist protects kidneys from ischemia/reperfusion injury in rats." *Kidney Int* 63(1): 134-142.

Basile, D. P., K. Fredrich, et al. (2008). "Renal ischemia reperfusion inhibits VEGF expression and induces ADAMTS-1, a novel VEGF inhibitor." *Am J Physiol Renal Physiol* 294(4): F928-936.

Becherucci, F., B. Mazzinghi, et al. (2009). "The role of endothelial progenitor cells in acute kidney injury." *Blood Purif* 27(3): 261-270.

Blydt-Hansen, T. D., M. Katori, et al. (2003). "Gene transfer-induced local heme oxygenase-1 overexpression protects rat kidney transplants from ischemia/reperfusion injury." *J Am Soc Nephrol* 14(3): 745-754.

Burne-Taney, M. J., N. Yokota-Ikeda, et al. (2005). "Effects of combined T- and B-cell deficiency on murine ischemia reperfusion injury." *Am J Transplant* 5(6): 1186-1193.

Burne, M. J., F. Daniels, et al. (2001). "Identification of the CD4(+) T cell as a major pathogenic factor in ischemic acute renal failure." *J Clin Invest* 108(9): 1283-1290.

Chander, V. and K. Chopra (2005). "Renal protective effect of molsidomine and L-arginine in ischemia-reperfusion induced injury in rats." *J Surg Res* 128(1): 132-139.

Chiao, H., Y. Kohda, et al. (1997). "Alpha-melanocyte-stimulating hormone protects against renal injury after ischemia in mice and rats." *J Clin Invest* 99(6): 1165-1172.

Chien, C. T., S. K. Shyue, et al. (2007). "Bcl-xL augmentation potentially reduces ischemia/reperfusion induced proximal and distal tubular apoptosis and autophagy." *Transplantation* 84(9): 1183-1190.

Crikis, S., B. Lu, et al. (2010). "Transgenic overexpression of CD39 protects against renal ischemia-reperfusion and transplant vascular injury." *Am J Transplant* 10(12): 2586-2595.

Daemen, M. A., C. van 't Veer, et al. (1999). "Inhibition of apoptosis induced by ischemia-reperfusion prevents inflammation." *J Clin Invest* 104(5): 541-549.

Day, Y. J., L. Huang, et al. (2003). "Renal protection from ischemia mediated by A2A adenosine receptors on bone marrow-derived cells." *J Clin Invest* 112(6): 883-891.

Day, Y. J., L. Huang, et al. (2006). "Renal ischemia-reperfusion injury and adenosine 2A receptor-mediated tissue protection: the role of CD4+ T cells and IFN-gamma." *J Immunol* 176(5): 3108-3114.

Day, Y. J., L. Huang, et al. (2005). "Renal ischemia-reperfusion injury and adenosine 2A receptor-mediated tissue protection: role of macrophages." *Am J Physiol Renal Physiol* 288(4): F722-731.

De Greef, K. E., D. K. Ysebaert, et al. (2001). "Anti-B7-1 blocks mononuclear cell adherence in vasa recta after ischemia." *Kidney Int* 60(4): 1415-1427.

De Vries, B., R. A. Matthijsen, et al. (2003). "Inhibition of complement factor C5 protects against renal ischemia-reperfusion injury: inhibition of late apoptosis and inflammation." *Transplantation* 75(3): 375-382.

Del Rio, M., A. Imam, et al. (2004). "The death domain of kidney ankyrin interacts with Fas and promotes Fas-mediated cell death in renal epithelia." *J Am Soc Nephrol* 15(1): 41-51.

Deng, J., Y. Kohda, et al. (2001). "Interleukin-10 inhibits ischemic and cisplatin-induced acute renal injury." *Kidney Int* 60(6): 2118-2128.

Dong, X., S. Swaminathan, et al. (2005). "Antigen presentation by dendritic cells in renal lymph nodes is linked to systemic and local injury to the kidney." *Kidney Int* 68(3): 1096-1108.

Dong, X., S. Swaminathan, et al. (2007). "Resident dendritic cells are the predominant TNF-secreting cell in early renal ischemia-reperfusion injury." *Kidney Int* 71(7): 619-628.

Endre, Z. H., R. J. Walker, et al. (2010). "Early intervention with erythropoietin does not affect the outcome of acute kidney injury (the EARLYARF trial)." *Kidney Int* 77(11): 1020-1030.

Farrar, C. A., Y. Wang, et al. (2004). "Independent pathways of P-selectin and complement-mediated renal ischemia/reperfusion injury." *Am J Pathol* 164(1): 133-141.

Fiorina, P., M. J. Ansari, et al. (2006). "Role of CXC chemokine receptor 3 pathway in renal ischemic injury." *J Am Soc Nephrol* 17(3): 716-723.

Furuichi, K., J. L. Gao, et al. (2006). "Chemokine receptor CX3CR1 regulates renal interstitial fibrosis after ischemia-reperfusion injury." *Am J Pathol* 169(2): 372-387.

Furuichi, K., T. Wada, et al. (2003). "CCR2 signaling contributes to ischemia-reperfusion injury in kidney." *J Am Soc Nephrol* 14(10): 2503-2515.

Gandolfo, M. T., H. R. Jang, et al. (2009). "Foxp3+ regulatory T cells participate in repair of ischemic acute kidney injury." *Kidney Int* 76(7): 717-729.

George, J. F., A. Braun, et al. (2008). "Suppression by CD4+CD25+ regulatory T cells is dependent on expression of heme oxygenase-1 in antigen-presenting cells." *Am J Pathol* 173(1): 154-160.

Gogvadze, V., J. D. Robertson, et al. (2004). "Mitochondrial cytochrome c release may occur by volume-dependent mechanisms not involving permeability transition." *Biochem J* 378(Pt 1): 213-217.

Goligorsky, M. S., S. V. Brodsky, et al. (2004). "NO bioavailability, endothelial dysfunction, and acute renal failure: new insights into pathophysiology." *Semin Nephrol* 24(4): 316-323.

Grenz, A., T. Eckle, et al. (2007). "Use of a hanging-weight system for isolated renal artery occlusion during ischemic preconditioning in mice." *Am J Physiol Renal Physiol* 292(1): F475-485.

Grenz, A., H. Osswald, et al. (2008). "The reno-vascular A2B adenosine receptor protects the kidney from ischemia." *PLoS Med* 5(6): e137.

Grenz, A., H. Zhang, et al. (2007). "Protective role of ecto-5'-nucleotidase (CD73) in renal ischemia." *J Am Soc Nephrol* 18(3): 833-845.

Grenz, A., H. Zhang, et al. (2007). "Contribution of E-NTPDase1 (CD39) to renal protection from ischemia-reperfusion injury." *FASEB J* 21(11): 2863-2873.

Halloran, P. F., M. A. Aprile, et al. (1988). "Early function as the principal correlate of graft survival. A multivariate analysis of 200 cadaveric renal transplants treated with a protocol incorporating antilymphocyte globulin and cyclosporine." *Transplantation* 46(2): 223-228.

Harrison, R. (2002). "Structure and function of xanthine oxidoreductase: where are we now?" *Free Radic Biol Med* 33(6): 774-797.

Haylor, J. L., K. P. Harris, et al. (2011). "Atorvastatin improving renal ischemia reperfusion injury via direct inhibition of active caspase-3 in rats." *Exp Biol Med (Maywood)* 236(6): 755-763.

Hochegger, K., T. Schatz, et al. (2007). "Role of alpha/beta and gamma/delta T cells in renal ischemia-reperfusion injury." *Am J Physiol Renal Physiol* 293(3): F741-747.

Horbelt, M., S. Y. Lee, et al. (2007). "Acute and chronic microvascular alterations in a mouse model of ischemic acute kidney injury." *Am J Physiol Renal Physiol* 293(3): F688-695.

Jackson, E. K., C. Zhu, et al. (2002). "Expression of adenosine receptors in the preglomerular microcirculation." *Am J Physiol Renal Physiol* 283(1): F41-51.

Joo, J. D., M. Kim, et al. (2007). "Acute and delayed renal protection against renal ischemia and reperfusion injury with A1 adenosine receptors." *Am J Physiol Renal Physiol* 293(6): F1847-1857.

Kaczmarek, E., K. Koziak, et al. (1996). "Identification and characterization of CD39/vascular ATP diphosphohydrolase." *J Biol Chem* 271(51): 33116-33122.

Keizer, K. M., J. W. de Fijter, et al. (2005). "Non-heart-beating donor kidneys in the Netherlands: allocation and outcome of transplantation." *Transplantation* 79(9): 1195-1199.

Kelly, K. J., Z. Plotkin, et al. (2001). "Guanosine supplementation reduces apoptosis and protects renal function in the setting of ischemic injury." *J Clin Invest* 108(9): 1291-1298.

Kelly, K. J., Z. Plotkin, et al. (2003). "P53 mediates the apoptotic response to GTP depletion after renal ischemia-reperfusion: protective role of a p53 inhibitor." *J Am Soc Nephrol* 14(1): 128-138.

Kelly, K. J., W. W. Williams, Jr., et al. (1996). "Intercellular adhesion molecule-1-deficient mice are protected against ischemic renal injury." *J Clin Invest* 97(4): 1056-1063.

Kim, M., S. W. Chen, et al. (2009). "Kidney-specific reconstitution of the A1 adenosine receptor in A1 adenosine receptor knockout mice reduces renal ischemia-reperfusion injury." *Kidney Int* 75(8): 809-823.

Kinsey, G. R., L. Huang, et al. (2010). "Regulatory T cells contribute to the protective effect of ischemic preconditioning in the kidney." *Kidney Int* 77(9): 771-780.

Koesters, R., B. Kaissling, et al. (2010). "Tubular overexpression of transforming growth factor-beta1 induces autophagy and fibrosis but not mesenchymal transition of renal epithelial cells." *Am J Pathol* 177(2): 632-643.

Kouretas, P. C., Y. D. Kim, et al. (1999). "Nonanticoagulant heparin prevents coronary endothelial dysfunction after brief ischemia-reperfusion injury in the dog." *Circulation* 99(8): 1062-1068.

Lee, H. T. and C. W. Emala (2000). "Protective effects of renal ischemic preconditioning and adenosine pretreatment: role of A(1) and A(3) receptors." *Am J Physiol Renal Physiol* 278(3): F380-387.

Leemans, J. C., G. Stokman, et al. (2005). "Renal-associated TLR2 mediates ischemia/reperfusion injury in the kidney." *J Clin Invest* 115(10): 2894-2903.

Leonard, E. C., J. L. Friedrich, et al. (2008). "VEGF-121 preserves renal microvessel structure and ameliorates secondary renal disease following acute kidney injury." *Am J Physiol Renal Physiol* 295(6): F1648-1657.

Letavernier, E., J. Perez, et al. (2005). "Peroxisome proliferator-activated receptor beta/delta exerts a strong protection from ischemic acute renal failure." *J Am Soc Nephrol* 16(8): 2395-2402.

Li, L., L. Huang, et al. (2007). "NKT cell activation mediates neutrophil IFN-gamma production and renal ischemia-reperfusion injury." *J Immunol* 178(9): 5899-5911.

Li, L., L. Huang, et al. (2008). "The chemokine receptors CCR2 and CX3CR1 mediate monocyte/macrophage trafficking in kidney ischemia-reperfusion injury." *Kidney Int* 74(12): 1526-1537.

Li, S., K. K. Nagothu, et al. (2009). "Transgenic expression of proximal tubule peroxisome proliferator-activated receptor-alpha in mice confers protection during acute kidney injury." *Kidney Int* 76(10): 1049-1062.

Ling, H., C. Edelstein, et al. (1999). "Attenuation of renal ischemia-reperfusion injury in inducible nitric oxide synthase knockout mice." *Am J Physiol* 277(3 Pt 2): F383-390.

Lu, B., S. V. Rajakumar, et al. (2008). "The impact of purinergic signaling on renal ischemia-reperfusion injury." *Transplantation* 86(12): 1707-1712.

Martinez, F., N. Kamar, et al. (2010). "High dose epoetin beta in the first weeks following renal transplantation and delayed graft function: Results of the Neo-PDGF Study." *Am J Transplant* 10(7): 1695-1700.

Mizutani, A., K. Okajima, et al. (2000). "Activated protein C reduces ischemia/reperfusion-induced renal injury in rats by inhibiting leukocyte activation." *Blood* 95(12): 3781-3787.

Molitoris, B. A., P. C. Dagher, et al. (2009). "siRNA targeted to p53 attenuates ischemic and cisplatin-induced acute kidney injury." *J Am Soc Nephrol* 20(8): 1754-1764.

Moller-Kristensen, M., W. K. Ip, et al. (2006). "Deficiency of mannose-binding lectin greatly increases susceptibility to postburn infection with Pseudomonas aeruginosa." *J Immunol* 176(3): 1769-1775.

Murry, C. E., R. B. Jennings, et al. (1986). "Preconditioning with ischemia: a delay of lethal cell injury in ischemic myocardium." *Circulation* 74(5): 1124-1136.

Nakagawa, K., D. D. Koo, et al. (2002). "Lecithinized superoxide dismutase reduces cold ischemia-induced chronic allograft dysfunction." *Kidney Int* 61(3): 1160-1169.

Neto, J. S., A. Nakao, et al. (2006). "Low-dose carbon monoxide inhalation prevents development of chronic allograft nephropathy." *Am J Physiol Renal Physiol* 290(2): F324-334.

Nicholson, D. W. (2000). "From bench to clinic with apoptosis-based therapeutic agents." *Nature* 407(6805): 810-816.

Noiri, E., T. Peresleni, et al. (1996). "In vivo targeting of inducible NO synthase with oligodeoxynucleotides protects rat kidney against ischemia." *J Clin Invest* 97(10): 2377-2383.

Ogawa, S., R. Shreeniwas, et al. (1990). "The effect of hypoxia on capillary endothelial cell function: modulation of barrier and coagulant function." *Br J Haematol* 75(4): 517-524.

Ogawa, T., A. K. Nussler, et al. (2001). "Contribution of nitric oxide to the protective effects of ischemic preconditioning in ischemia-reperfused rat kidneys." *J Lab Clin Med* 138(1): 50-58.

Oh, D. J., B. Dursun, et al. (2008). "Fractalkine receptor (CX3CR1) inhibition is protective against ischemic acute renal failure in mice." *Am J Physiol Renal Physiol* 294(1): F264-271.

Osama Gaber, A., S. Mulgaonkar, et al. (2011). "YSPSL (rPSGL-Ig) for improvement of early renal allograft function: a double-blind, placebo-controlled, multi-center Phase IIa study(1,2,3)." *Clin Transplant* 25(4): 523-533.

Pang, S. T., M. S. Wu, et al. (2000). "University of Wisconsin preservation solution enhances intrarenal nitric oxide production." *Transplant Proc* 32(7): 1617-1618.

Park, K. M., A. Chen, et al. (2001). "Prevention of kidney ischemia/reperfusion-induced functional injury and JNK, p38, and MAPK kinase activation by remote ischemic pretreatment." *J Biol Chem* 276(15): 11870-11876.

Patel, A., M. C. van de Poll, et al. (2004). "Early stress protein gene expression in a human model of ischemic preconditioning." *Transplantation* 78(10): 1479-1487.

Pell, T. J., G. F. Baxter, et al. (1998). "Renal ischemia preconditions myocardium: role of adenosine receptors and ATP-sensitive potassium channels." *Am J Physiol* 275(5 Pt 2): H1542-1547.

Perico, N., D. Cattaneo, et al. (2004). "Delayed graft function in kidney transplantation." *Lancet* 364(9447): 1814-1827.

Pinsky, D. J., S. F. Yan, et al. (1995). "Hypoxia and modification of the endothelium: implications for regulation of vascular homeostatic properties." *Semin Cell Biol* 6(5): 283-294.

Portilla, D., G. Dai, et al. (2000). "Etomoxir-induced PPARalpha-modulated enzymes protect during acute renal failure." *Am J Physiol Renal Physiol* 278(4): F667-675.

Rajakumar, S. V., B. Lu, et al. (2010). "Deficiency or inhibition of CD73 protects in mild kidney ischemia-reperfusion injury." *Transplantation* 90(12): 1260-1264.

Renner, B., D. Strassheim, et al. (2010). "B cell subsets contribute to renal injury and renal protection after ischemia/reperfusion." *J Immunol* 185(7): 4393-4400.

Salmela, K., L. Wramner, et al. (1999). "A randomized multicenter trial of the anti-ICAM-1 monoclonal antibody (enlimomab) for the prevention of acute rejection and delayed onset of graft function in cadaveric renal transplantation: a report of the European Anti-ICAM-1 Renal Transplant Study Group." *Transplantation* 67(5): 729-736.

Savransky, V., R. R. Molls, et al. (2006). "Role of the T-cell receptor in kidney ischemia-reperfusion injury." *Kidney Int* 69(2): 233-238.

Schneider, M. P., J. C. Sullivan, et al. (2010). "Protective role of extracellular superoxide dismutase in renal ischemia/reperfusion injury." *Kidney Int* 78(4): 374-381.

Sharfuddin, A. A., R. M. Sandoval, et al. (2009). "Soluble thrombomodulin protects ischemic kidneys." *J Am Soc Nephrol* 20(3): 524-534.

Sharples, E. J., N. Patel, et al. (2004). "Erythropoietin protects the kidney against the injury and dysfunction caused by ischemia-reperfusion." *J Am Soc Nephrol* 15(8): 2115-2124.

Shi, Y., V. Y. Melnikov, et al. (2000). "Downregulation of the calpain inhibitor protein calpastatin by caspases during renal ischemia-reperfusion." *Am J Physiol Renal Physiol* 279(3): F509-517.

Shigeoka, A. A., T. D. Holscher, et al. (2007). "TLR2 is constitutively expressed within the kidney and participates in ischemic renal injury through both MyD88-dependent and -independent pathways." *J Immunol* 178(10): 6252-6258.

Shoskes, D. A. and J. M. Cecka (1998). "Deleterious effects of delayed graft function in cadaveric renal transplant recipients independent of acute rejection." *Transplantation* 66(12): 1697-1701.

Sikorski, E. M., T. Hock, et al. (2004). "The story so far: Molecular regulation of the heme oxygenase-1 gene in renal injury." *Am J Physiol Renal Physiol* 286(3): F425-441.

Singbartl, K. and K. Ley (2000). "Protection from ischemia-reperfusion induced severe acute renal failure by blocking E-selectin." *Crit Care Med* 28(7): 2507-2514.

Sivarajah, A., P. K. Chatterjee, et al. (2002). "Agonists of peroxisome-proliferator activated receptor-alpha (clofibrate and WY14643) reduce renal ischemia/reperfusion injury in the rat." *Med Sci Monit* 8(12): BR532-539.

Sivarajah, A., P. K. Chatterjee, et al. (2003). "Agonists of peroxisome-proliferator activated receptor-gamma reduce renal ischemia/reperfusion injury." *Am J Nephrol* 23(4): 267-276.

Sutton, T. A., K. J. Kelly, et al. (2005). "Minocycline reduces renal microvascular leakage in a rat model of ischemic renal injury." *Am J Physiol Renal Physiol* 288(1): F91-97.

Sutton, T. A., H. E. Mang, et al. (2003). "Injury of the renal microvascular endothelium alters barrier function after ischemia." *Am J Physiol Renal Physiol* 285(2): F191-198.

Takada, M., K. C. Nadeau, et al. (1997). "The cytokine-adhesion molecule cascade in ischemia/reperfusion injury of the rat kidney. Inhibition by a soluble P-selectin ligand." *J Clin Invest* 99(11): 2682-2690.

Teoh, N., I. Leclercq, et al. (2003). "Low-dose TNF-alpha protects against hepatic ischemia-reperfusion injury in mice: implications for preconditioning." *Hepatology* 37(1): 118-128.

Thompson, L. F., H. K. Eltzschig, et al. (2004). "Crucial role for ecto-5'-nucleotidase (CD73) in vascular leakage during hypoxia." *J Exp Med* 200(11): 1395-1405.

Thornton, M. A., R. Winn, et al. (1989). "An evaluation of the neutrophil as a mediator of in vivo renal ischemic-reperfusion injury." *Am J Pathol* 135(3): 509-515.

Thurman, J. M., A. M. Lenderink, et al. (2007). "C3a is required for the production of CXC chemokines by tubular epithelial cells after renal ishemia/reperfusion." *J Immunol* 178(3): 1819-1828.

Thurman, J. M., D. Ljubanovic, et al. (2003). "Lack of a functional alternative complement pathway ameliorates ischemic acute renal failure in mice." *J Immunol* 170(3): 1517-1523.

Togel, F., Z. Hu, et al. (2005). "Administered mesenchymal stem cells protect against ischemic acute renal failure through differentiation-independent mechanisms." *Am J Physiol Renal Physiol* 289(1): F31-42.

Toyokuni, S. (1999). "Reactive oxygen species-induced molecular damage and its application in pathology." *Pathol Int* 49(2): 91-102.

Van Waarde, A., M. E. Stromski, et al. (1989). "Protection of the kidney against ischemic injury by inhibition of 5'-nucleotidase." *Am J Physiol* 256(2 Pt 2): F298-305.

Vincenti, F., A. Dritselis, et al. (2011). "Belatacept." *Nat Rev Drug Discov* 10(9): 655-656.

Wang, Y., H. Xu, et al. (2001). "Intestinal ischemia induces late preconditioning against myocardial infarction: a role for inducible nitric oxide synthase." *Cardiovasc Res* 49(2): 391-398.

Weinbrenner, C., M. Nelles, et al. (2002). "Remote preconditioning by infrarenal occlusion of the aorta protects the heart from infarction: a newly identified non-neuronal but PKC-dependent pathway." *Cardiovasc Res* 55(3): 590-601.

Weitz, M., O. Amon, et al. (2011). "Prophylactic eculizumab prior to kidney transplantation for atypical hemolytic uremic syndrome." *Pediatr Nephrol* 26(8): 1325-1329.

Wolfs, T. G., W. A. Buurman, et al. (2002). "In vivo expression of Toll-like receptor 2 and 4 by renal epithelial cells: IFN-gamma and TNF-alpha mediated up-regulation during inflammation." *J Immunol* 168(3): 1286-1293.

Wu, H., G. Chen, et al. (2007). "TLR4 activation mediates kidney ischemia/reperfusion injury." *J Clin Invest* 117(10): 2847-2859.

Yamada, K., T. Miwa, et al. (2004). "Critical protection from renal ischemia reperfusion injury by CD55 and CD59." *J Immunol* 172(6): 3869-3875.

Yamauchi, J., R. Schramm, et al. (2003). "Improvement of microvascular graft equilibration and preservation in non-heart-beating donors by warm preflush with streptokinase." *Transplantation* 75(4): 449-453.

Yang, C., V. Kaushal, et al. (2008). "Transcriptional activation of caspase-6 and -7 genes by cisplatin-induced p53 and its functional significance in cisplatin nephrotoxicity." *Cell Death Differ* 15(3): 530-544.

Yokota, N., M. Burne-Taney, et al. (2003). "Contrasting roles for STAT4 and STAT6 signal transduction pathways in murine renal ischemia-reperfusion injury." *Am J Physiol Renal Physiol* 285(2): F319-325.

Yokota, N., M. O'Donnell, et al. (2003). "Protective effect of HMG-CoA reductase inhibitor on experimental renal ischemia-reperfusion injury." *Am J Nephrol* 23(1): 13-17.

Yoshida, J., K. S. Ozaki, et al. (2010). "Ex vivo application of carbon monoxide in UW solution prevents transplant-induced renal ischemia/reperfusion injury in pigs." *Am J Transplant* 10(4): 763-772.

Younes, M., M. H. Schoenberg, et al. (1984). "Oxidative tissue damage following regional intestinal ischemia and reperfusion in the cat." *Res Exp Med (Berl)* 184(4): 259-264.

Ysebaert, D. K., K. E. De Greef, et al. (2004). "T cells as mediators in renal ischemia/reperfusion injury." *Kidney Int* 66(2): 491-496.

Zarek, P. E., C. T. Huang, et al. (2008). "A2A receptor signaling promotes peripheral tolerance by inducing T-cell anergy and the generation of adaptive regulatory T cells." *Blood* 111(1): 251-259.

Zhang, Z. X., S. Wang, et al. (2008). "NK cells induce apoptosis in tubular epithelial cells and contribute to renal ischemia-reperfusion injury." *J Immunol* 181(11): 7489-7498.

Zhou, W., C. A. Farrar, et al. (2000). "Predominant role for C5b-9 in renal ischemia/reperfusion injury." *J Clin Invest* 105(10): 1363-1371.

Zimmerman, R. F., P. U. Ezeanuna, et al. (2011). "Ischemic preconditioning at a remote site prevents acute kidney injury in patients following cardiac surgery." *Kidney Int.*

Zimmermann, H. (1992). "5'-Nucleotidase: molecular structure and functional aspects." *Biochem J* 285 (Pt 2): 345-365.

12

Ischemia-Reperfusion Injury in the Transplanted Kidney Based on Purine Metabolism Markers and Activity of the Antioxidant System

Leszek Domański, Karolina Kłoda and Kazimierz Ciechanowski
Clinical Department of Nephrology, Transplantology and Internal Medicine of the Pomeranian Medical University in Szczecin
Poland

1. Introduction

The pathophysiology of ischemia and reperfusion stress linked with the generation of reactive oxygen species (ROS), as well as the activation of antioxidant defense mechanisms are an integral part of non-immune factors implicated in the early and delayed graft function (DGF). Oxygen free radicals are central mediators of cellular injury that occurs upon postischaemic reperfusion. Studies on the mechanisms of reperfusion injury in the cold-preserved kidney transplant model have suggested an important role for free radicals generated at reperfusion from oxygen by activated xanthine oxidase. Generation of ROS is the main mechanism inducing ischemic/reperfusion damage of the organ. Oxygen burst is a trigger for complex biochemical reactions leading to generation of oxygenated lipids and changes in microcirculation with recruitment of neutrophils to the graft. Recently, radical generation has been measured in postischaemic tissues using electron paramagnetic resonance spectroscopy. Electron paramagnetic resonance techniques have demonstrated that presence of oxygen burst after postischaemic reperfusion of the graft (Hirayama et al.,2004). Moreover, it has been shown that free radical generation is correlated with the activity of the anti-oxidative system. Many markers have been researched to prove the presence of ROS in the transplanted tissue including malondialdehyde (MDA), glutathione (GSH), superoxide dismutase (SOD) and catalase (CAT). They are involved in protection against free radicals. Elucidation of inter-relations between these factors is important for our understanding of the phenomena and for implementation of perioperative procedures aimed at prolonging graft survival. Organ preservation seeks to ensure the functional viability of transplanted organs. Preservation during ischemia includes steps against acidosis, steps to maintain cell volume and for optimal utilization of anaerobic energy reserves. Previous studies have demonstrated that apart from ischemic damage, additional tissue injury evolves as a result of reperfusion and reoxygenation (Tilney et al., 2001). Energy-dependent processes occurring during cold ischemia of the graft require adequate levels of ATP and other high-energy compounds generated in the majority during oxidative catabolism of various substrates. Because oxygen is required for such reactions, the ability to maintain adequate levels of high-energy phosphates would appear to depend on oxygen delivery to graft cells (Chien et al., 2001a). Oxygen delivery during reperfusion is insufficient to maintain an aerobic environment in graft tissue. It is plausible that such tissue hypoxia may be associated with alterations in concentrations of high-energy phosphates and their metabolites (Grinyo et al., 2001). Various molecular mechanisms of ischemic changes in the graft tissue have been demonstrated. The graft's adenine nucleotide metabolism is directly linked to high-energy phosphate turnover and graft functioning. Some studies have shown that prolonged graft ischemia is accompanied by nucleotide degradation, but clinical data concerning nucleotide pool changes in renal and peripheral veins is lacking (Harris et al., 1996; Rabb et al., 1997). ATP is catabolized to adenosine and then to hypoxanthine. Nucleosides and oxypurines are released to plasma, but part of them are transported to erythrocytes where they are metabolized to other nucleosides and nucleotides. Ischemia-reperfusion injury is a not only a major cause of acute renal damage but also affects its clinical expression, mentioned earlier: delayed graft function. DGF has a significant impact on short- and long-term graft survival (Chien et al., 2001b). DGF is defined as a requirement for dialysis in the first week post-transplantation and includes a spectrum of clinical manifestations, ranging from borderline function to a complete absence of graft function. According to recent studies (Azevedo et al., 2005; Carter et al., 2005; Woodle et al., 2005), the rate of DGF varies between 20% and 50% in patients receiving a first cadaver graft. Consequently, estimation of the ischemic damage is important and it is essential to define reliable markers in order to properly assess renal ischemic damage and predict DGF. Determination of such parameters should improve the early follow-up of renal transplantation and the management of patients who receive nephrotoxic immunosuppressive compounds such as cyclosporine, which may enhance acute tubular injury and reduce the long-term prognosis of the graft functions. The pathophysiology of acute ischemia and the pathophysiology of reperfusion of the kidney graft require further studies and more focus on clinical parameters.

2. Objectives of ischemia-reperfusion injury analysis in the transplanted kidney

The impairment of organ function derived from ischemia–reperfusion injury is still an important problem in solid organ transplantation. Cell alterations induced by ischemia prime the tissue for the subsequent damage that occurs during the reperfusion phase. Ischemia–reperfusion injury affects early graft function and influences the development of chronic graft dysfunction.

Therefore the objective of the study was to determine:

- The concentration profile of oxypurines and purine nucleosides in the renal vein of the kidney graft in humans during reperfusion as a marker of the energy status of kidney tissue and as a prognostic factor for graft function;
- The activity of superoxide dismutase, catalase, and glutathione peroxidase in erythrocytes during reperfusion of the kidney graft in humans and their effect on graft function;
- The relationship between purine concentrations in blood and the activity of anti-oxidative enzymes in erythrocytes during reperfusion of the renal graft in humans;
- The effect of trimetazidine on the concentration of purine nucleotides as markers of ischemia in rat kidney with ischemia-reperfusion injury.

2.1 Oxypurine and purine nucleoside concentrations in renal vein of allograft as potential markers of energy status of renal tissue

Purine nucleosides and oxypurines are products of adenine nucleotides degradation. Reperfusion and reoxygenation are accompanied by production of reactive oxygen species and free radicals, which lead to damage of graft tissue. The aim of our study was to measure concentrations of adenine nucleotides and their metabolites in renal allograft vein as well as in recipient's peripheral veins during the reperfusion period and to evaluate their usefulness as markers of tissue metabolism in kidney allografts.

The study included 20 deceased donor kidney transplant recipients (11 males, 9 females, mean age 52 ± 8 years, cold ischemia time 19.9 ± 8.8 h, warm ischemia time 19.3 ± 5.7 min). The harvested grafts were perfused with EuroCollins preservation solution. All patients received standard immunosuppressive protocol with triple drug therapy including cyclosporine A, azathioprine, and steroids. The first blood sample (UV0) was taken from the recipient's ulnar vein before anastomosing of the kidney allograft vessels with recipient's iliac vessels. Next, samples were taken from the graft's renal vein (RV1) and recipient's ulnar (UV1) vein at 5 min of graft reperfusion. Five ml of blood was aliquoted into heparin-containing tubes kept on ice. Reperfusion of the transplanted kidney was followed precisely with ThermaCAM SC500 thermovision camera (FLIR Systems), which detects infrared radiation and records digital images presenting surface temperature distribution of the object. We assumed that the process of total reperfusion was completed when thermal scans showed the homogeneous distribution of graft's temperature. Samples RV1 and UV1 were taken from plastic microcatheters inserted into the renal allograft and ulnar veins after total tissue reperfusion when the temperature of the graft reached 35.0°C. Two mL of blood was mixed with the same volume of 1.3 mol/L HClO4 and stored at -80°C until assayed. The remaining blood was centrifuged within 15 min from collection at 4°C for 10 min. Three hundred mL of plasma was supplemented with 300 mL of 1.3 mol/L perchloric acid and vortexed. Subsequently, plasma and blood samples were centrifuged at 20,000 x g and 4°C for 5 min. Four hundred mL of the acid supernatant was removed and neutralized with 130-160 mL of 1 mol/L potassium phosphate to pH 5-7. Centrifugation was repeated and the supernatant was withdrawn for chromatography. High-performance liquid chromatography (HPLC) was done to measure blood and plasma concentrations of adenosine triphosphate (ATP), adenosine monophosphate (AMP), guanosine (Guo), inosine (Ino), hypoxanthine (Hyp), xanthine (Xan), uric acid (UA), and uridine (Urd). Analyses were performed with Hewlett-Packard 1050 series chromatography system consisting of a quaternary gradient pump with vacuum degassing and piston desalting modules, Rheodyne 7125 manual injection valve with 20 uL loop, UV-VIS detector, and series 1100 thermostatted column compartment. Separations were achieved on Hypersil BDS 125 x 3 mm, 3-mm particle size column (Agilent Technologies). Modifications were introduced into the original method (Smolenski et al., 1990). The mobile phase flowed at a rate of 0.5 mL/min and column temperature was 20.5°C. Buffer composition remained unchanged (A: 150 mmol/L, phosphate buffer, pH 6.0, containing 150 mmol/L potassium chloride; B: 15% acetonitrile in buffer A). The gradient profile was modified to the following content of buffer B in the mobile phase: 0% at 0.00 min, 2% at 0.05 min, 7% at 2.45 min, 50% at 5.05 min, 100% at 5.35 min, 100% at 7.00 min, 0% at 7.10 min. Samples of 100 mL were injected every 12 min into the injection valve loop. Absorbance was read at 254 nm. Concentrations were expressed as mmol/liter of blood or plasma. Adenylate energy charge (AEC) was calculated using the following formula: AEC = (ATP + ADP/2)/(ATP + ADP + AMP).

Hyp concentrations in whole blood were significantly increased in renal allograft vein after reperfusion as compared with peripheral (ulnar) vein before (1.82 times higher) as well as after reperfusion (1.61 times higher). Moreover, there was no statistically significant difference in Hyp peripheral vein concentrations before and after reperfusion. Similar differences were observed for Hyp concentrations in plasma. Plasma Hyp concentrations in renal vein after reperfusion were 155% and 162% higher than in peripheral vein before and after reperfusion, respectively. Xan concentrations in whole blood and plasma were significantly higher in renal vein in comparison with peripheral vein. Xan concentrations in plasma and whole blood from the renal vein were 155% and 163% higher before reperfusion and 162% and 129% after reperfusion, respectively. Ino concentrations in plasma and whole blood were significantly higher in renal allograft vein compared with peripheral vein in the post-reperfusion period. Moreover, peripheral vein Ino concentrations were significantly decreased after reperfusion. Guo concentrations in plasma and whole blood were higher in peripheral vein than in renal allograft vein after reperfusion. There was no significant difference in Guo peripheral vein concentrations before and after reperfusion. There was no significant difference between concentrations of uric acid and uridine in renal and peripheral veins before and after reperfusion. There was no significant difference in whole blood concentrations of ATP in renal and peripheral veins before and after reperfusion. AMP concentration in peripheral vein was decreased by 24% after reperfusion, which was associated with a slight increase in AEC. There was found many strong positive correlations between concentrations of purines in plasma and whole blood. Positive correlations between concentrations of most purines in plasma from the renal allograft vein and cold ischemia time, as well as warm ischemia time were showed. Correlations were most significant for Xan (with cold and warm ischemia time) and Ino and Guo (warm ischemia time only).

Long ischemia time can alter electron transport in the respiratory chain. All complexes involved in the process show a reduction in their activity associated with structural damage. ATP hydrolysis during ischemia causes a rise in free inorganic phosphate, which increases membrane permeability. ATP hydrolysis and anaerobic glycolysis decrease the intracellular pH which is a factor that may protect cells from death during ischemia (Smoleński et al., 1989). Extended ischemia causes progressive reduction of the iron-sulfur proteins associated with NADH dehydrogenase. During renal ischemia, ATP is degraded via ADP, AMP, adenosine and inosine to hypoxanthine, which is next oxidized to xanthine and uric acid. Catabolism of adenine nucleotides results in accumulation of hypoxanthine in ischemic cells. Ischemia also promotes the proteolytic conversion of xanthine dehydrogenase to xanthine oxidase (Arduini et al., 1988). Xanthine acts as a substrate for xanthine oxidase and enhances superoxide generation (Li et al., 1995). When xanthine oxidase converts hypoxanthine to xanthine in the presence of molecular oxygen, superoxide radicals are released. Reactive oxygen species generated during ischemia-reperfusion play a major role in microvascular dysfunction and exert direct tissue damage, leading to lipid peroxidation, denaturation of proteins, and oxidation of DNA (Dowell et al., 1993). During ischemia, elevated concentrations of inosine, hypoxanthine and xanthine may occur due to the breakdown of ATP (Kurokawa et al., 1996). Administration of cyclosporine, which inhibits adenosine uptake by erythrocytes but not adenosine catabolism to inosine mediated by adenosine deaminase, is an additional factor for increasing concentrations of these nucleotides in recipient's plasma (Guieu et al., 1998). However, we were not able to verify this hypothesis because all our patients were treated with cyclosporine. Previous studies on the effect of xanthine or xanthine oxidase as inducers of renal injury have produced inconsistent results. It was found that infusion of xanthine into isolated perfused kidneys increases the generation of oxygen free radicals and impairs renal function (Galat et al., 1989). Another study showed that xanthine oxidase depletion improved renal function after reperfusion (Linas et al., 1990). However, some authors have revealed a lack of effect of inhibitors of xanthine oxidase or of xanthine itself (Zager & Gmur, 1989). Purine metabolism during kidney transplantation in humans were assessed (Vigues et al., 1993). ATP levels in renal bioptates were decreased, whereas degradation products (IMP, inosine, adenosine, hypoxanthine) increased during cold storage. Moreover, adenylate energy charge was reduced by half. Kidneys with subsequent acute tubular necrosis (ATN) had significantly lower levels of the total pool of adenine nucleotides at reperfusion, but there was no correlation between incidence of ATN and concentrations of ATP and other metabolites in the kidneys before and during cold preservation. Lipid peroxidation during ischemia-reperfusion of rat kidney (Akcetin et al., 1999, 2000) was observed with decreased ATP levels and consecutive accumulation of hypoxanthine at the end of the ischemic period as well as a subsequent decline of hypoxanthine during reperfusion. In our study we measured levels of hypoxanthine, xanthine, inosine, guanosine, uric acid, uridine, ATP, and AMP in renal allograft and ulnar veins during reperfusion of kidney allografts. All these purines are present physiologically in the blood (Chouker et al., 2005). After reperfusion, Hyp and Xan concentrations in whole blood and plasma increased to the greatest extent. The catabolism of adenine nucleotides leads to generation of Hyp, which is metabolized to Xan. Xanthine is metabolized to uric acid, the final product of purine degradation in humans (Colpaert & Lefebvre, 2000). In our study we did not observe differences in the concentrations of uric acid between peripheral and renal veins. This finding can be explained by high basal concentrations of uric acid in blood and relatively low xanthine oxidoreductase activity in renal grafts (Sun et al., 2004). The relatively higher Hyp concentrations (which is a substrate for xanthine oxidoreductase) in renal vein than Xan concentrations (product of xanthine oxidoreductase) seem to confirm this hypothesis. Under conditions of low xanthine oxidoreductase activity, hypoxanthine is phosphoribosylated by hypoxanthine-guanine phosphoribosyltransferase to IMP (salvage pathway). We have shown that guanosine and uridine are not synthesized during ischemia and reperfusion and therefore are not useful for monitoring of kidney graft metabolism during reperfusion. A relatively stable erythrocyte adenine nucleotide concentration in the pre- and post-reperfusion period suggests that the process does not lead to disturbances of purine metabolism in erythrocytes. We found increased concentrations of oxypurines and nucleosides in plasma as well as in whole blood. Therefore, plasma or whole blood may be used to determine the release of these metabolites by the graft. However, when quick centrifugation of blood after collection is not possible, the only way to measure purine content is precipitation of whole blood with perchloric acid, which can be done immediately at the collection site. In the present study we also examined differences in concentrations of purine metabolites in renal allograft and peripheral veins. Concentrations of Hyp and Xan were significantly higher in the renal vein compared with peripheral vein. Higher Hyp and Xan concentrations in the renal vein were associated with increased ischemic duration and can represent accelerated high-energy product breakdown. Therefore, we suggest that the differences in Hyp and Xan concentrations between renal and peripheral veins reflect changes and damage to renal tissue during reperfusion and might be useful for monitoring graft function during reperfusion.

2.2 Oxypurine and nucleoside concentrations in renal veins during reperfusion as predictors of early graft function

Perfusion is a process which creates the possibility of graft injury. A high perfusion pressure or an improper fluid composition may cause diffuse endothelial damage, creation of thrombi in small vessels and neutrophil infiltration (Gulec et al., 2006). Hypothermia downregulates the metabolism and prevents protease-dependent cell degranulation. Negative consequences of hypothermia and ischemia include cessation of ATP synthesis and Na-K-ATP synthase inhibition (Giligan et al., 2004). ATP is catabolized intracellularly to adenosine and then to hypoxanthine (Princemail et al., 1993; Hower et al., 1996). Both products migrate from the cell by means of a sophisticated membrane transport system. Under such conditions, xanthine oxidoreductase oxidizes hypoxanthine to xanthine and xanthine to uric acid. Hypoxanthine, xanthine and uric acid have only oxo substituents in their purine rings and are therefore called oxypurines. Uric acid is the final product of purine catabolism in humans. Superoxide radical is another product of reactions catalysed by xanthine oxidoreductase. It is toxic to the cell membrane, may cause structural damage to proteins and enzymes and finally may activate the arachidonic acid cascade, leading to production of inflammatory mediators (Grinyo et al., 2001; Skrzycki & Czeczot, 2004). The aim of this study was to examine whether purine and pyrimidine nucleoside concentrations as well as oxypurine concentrations in renal allograft and peripheral veins correlate with graft function.

The study population comprised 25 recipients of cadaver kidney transplant. A first blood sample was taken from the recipient's peripheral vein before anastomosing the kidney allograft vessels with the recipient's iliac vessels. Subsequent samples were taken from the allograft renal vein and the recipient's peripheral vein 5 min after beginning reperfusion. High-performance liquid chromatography was done to measure plasma concentrations of the oxypurines: hypoxanthine, xanthine and uric acid and the nucleosides: guanosine, inosine and uridine. Concentrations of Hyp, Xan and Ino were significantly higher in the renal than the peripheral vein. The differences between the Xan, Hyp, Ino and Urd plasma concentrations in the renal and peripheral veins before and 5 min after reperfusion correlated positively and significantly with serum creatinine concentrations 24 and 72 h after graft transplantation. Moreover, the concentrations of Hyp were significantly increased in renal transplant recipients with delayed graft function.

Preservation of the harvested organ constitutes a prerequisite for organ transplantation. For kidney preservation, hypothermic storage remains the commonest technique in use. However, hypothermic organ preservation is associated with oxygen deprivation, which inevitably leads to some degree of ischemia-reperfusion injury upon transplantation (Smolenski et al., 1989). During renal storage before transplantation, hypothermic swelling of the medullary thick ascending tubules results in mechanical constriction of the peritubular capillaries and vasa recta (Corner et al., 2003). During reperfusion, a large amount of reactive oxygen species (superoxide anions, hydroxyl radicals and hydrogen peroxides) is produced by the re-entry of oxygenated blood into the ischemic tissue. A long period of ischemia can alter the electron transport complexes. All of the complexes show a reduction in their activity associated with structural damage. ATP hydrolysis during ischemia causes a rise in free inorganic phosphate, which increases membrane permeability. ATP hydrolysis and anaerobic glycolysis decrease the intracellular pH, a factor that may protect cells from death during ischemia (Arduini et al., 1988). During renal ischemia ATP, as mentioned earlier, is degraded via adenosine diphosphate, adenosine monophosphate, adenosine and Ino to Hyp, which is oxidized to Xan and UA. The catabolism of adenine nucleotides results in an accumulation of Hyp in ischemic cells. Also, ischemia is associated with the proteolytic conversion of xanthine dehydrogenase to xanthine oxidase (Dowell et al., 1993). When xanthine oxidase converts Hyp to Xan in the presence of molecular oxygen, superoxide radical is generated. Reperfusion and reactive oxygen species which are generated during ischemia play a major role in microvascular dysfunction and cause direct tissue damage, leading to lipid peroxidation, denaturation of protein and oxidation of DNA (Chouker et al., 2005). During ischemia, elevated concentrations of Ino, Hyp and Xan may occur due to the breakdown of ATP (Colpaert & Lefebvre, 2000). Xan acts as a substrate for xanthine oxidase and enhances superoxide generation (Li et al., 1995). These two events may influence renal injury, but previous studies on the effect of Xan or xanthine oxidase as inducers of renal injury are inconsistent. It was shown in some studies (Galat et al., 1989) that infusion of Xan into isolated perfused kidneys increases the generation of oxygen free radicals and impairs renal function. It was found that xanthine oxidase depletion improved renal function after reperfusion (Linas et al., 1990), while other authors (Zager et al., 1989) revealed a lack of effect of inhibitors of xanthine oxidase. Assessement of purine metabolism during kidney transplantation in humans showed (Vigues et al., 1993), that ATP levels in renal bioptates were decreased whereas levels of the degradation products (inosine monophosphate, Ino, adenosine, Hyp) increased during cold storage. Moreover, the adenylate energy charge was reduced by half. Kidneys with acute tubular necrosis (ATN) had significantly lower levels of the total pool of adenine nucleotides at reperfusion, but there was no correlation between the incidence of ATN and concentrations of ATP and other metabolites in the kidneys before and during cold preservation. In another study (Lopez-Marti et al., 2003), tissue levels of adenosine in rats decreased significantly 30 min following ischemia, whereas Xan/Hyp levels increased concomitantly with renal dysfunction and histological damage. In our study, which to our knowledge is the first to evaluate the purine and pyrimidine nucleoside as well as oxypurine concentrations in renal and peripheral veins during reperfusion of kidney allografts in humans, we examined plasma levels of Hyp, Xan, Ino, Guo, UA and Urd. After reperfusion we observed increased concentrations of all metabolites, with the greatest increase occurring in the concentrations of Hyp and Xan in renal allograft veins. This finding is in concordance with those of previous studies carried out in animal models and may result from disturbances in purine metabolism during kidney allograft reperfusion. The catabolism of adenine nucleotides leads to the generation of Hyp, which is metabolized to Xan. Xan is metabolized to UA, the final product of purine degradation in humans (Sun et al., 2004). A lack of significant differences in UA concentrations between the studied blood samples may have been due to high basal plasma concentrations of UA in the systemic circulation. Hyp and Xan are the factors that may be modified depending on the duration and severity of ischemia. The renal content of Hyp and Xan changes after renal ischemia as a consequence of ATP breakdown (Li et al., 1995).

Increased Hyp and Xan concentrations in the renal compared with the peripheral vein are manifestations of ATP breakdown in renal tissue, which occurs during reperfusion. Therefore, the differences between metabolite concentrations in the renal and peripheral veins may most precisely reflect the degree of metabolic changes in renal tissues during reperfusion. Moreover, we correlated the differences between metabolite concentrations in renal and peripheral veins with graft function and creatinine concentrations at follow-up. The Hyp concentrations correlated with creatinine concentrations during the first 3 days after transplantation, whereas there was no correlation with long-term graft function. The differences in Guo concentration correlated negatively with the recipients' serum creatinine concentration 6 and 12 months after transplantation. Guo is metabolized to Xan by the kidney. Therefore, decreased metabolism of Guo to Xan may correlate with improved late graft function. Moreover, Hyp concentrations correlated with DGF in graft recipients. These results suggest that Hyp may be a useful predictor of early graft function. Another aim of the study was to determine whether disturbances of purine metabolism in the graft are associated with graft function. At transplantation it is not known when the graft will be fully functional, but a high concentration of Hyp in the graft's renal vein may indicate an increased risk of DGF. We conclude that disturbances in purine metabolism may be involved in the pathomechanisms of DGF.

2.3 Early phase of reperfusion of human kidney allograft and the erythrocyte anti-oxidative system

Although the problem of anti-oxidant defence is often brought up in the literature, authors are not precise in describing the activity of the enzymes during the first minutes after reperfusion. Previous studies on the animal model have shown increased free radicals generation during the first minutes of kidney allograft reperfusion with simultaneous activation of protecting mechanisms (Singh et al., 1993; Davies et al., 1995). The erythrocyte anti-oxidative system plays an important role in the protection against free radicals generated during the first minutes of reperfusion. The majority of reports regarding the erythrocyte anti-oxidative system derive from animal studies. Studies in humans are inconsistent. Therefore, the aim of our study was to examine the activity of the erythrocyte anti-oxidative system: superoxide dismutase (SOD), catalase (CAT), glutathione peroxidase (GPx) and glutathione (GSH) during reperfusion of the transplanted kidney.

The study included 40 renal transplant recipients (22 men, 18 women, mean age 51 ± 7 years, cold ischaemia time 25 ± 5 h). The grafts were perfused with EuroCollins preservation solutions. All patients received standard immunosuppressive protocol with triple drug therapy including cyclosporine A, azathioprine and steroids. The '0' blood sample was taken from the iliac vein before anastomosing of the kidney vessels with recipient's iliac vessels. Then, the renal vein of the graft was cannulated and blood samples I, II and III were taken. The reperfusion of the transplanted kidney was measured precisely with ThermaCAM SC500 (AGEMA, Infrared System AB, Danderyd, Sweden) thermovision camera, which detects infrared radiation and records digital images presenting surface temperature distribution of tested objects. The process of total reperfusion was completed when the scans from thermovision camera showed the whole organ filled with recipient's blood. Sample I was taken from the inserted catheter after total tissue reperfusion had been demonstrated on the scan monitor and after the temperature of the graft had reached 34 °C.

Blood samples II and III were taken 2 and 4 min after blood sample I. The erythrocytes were separated by centrifugation (300 *g*, 10 min), washed three times with buffered 0.9% NaCl solution (PBS: 0.01 mol phosphate buffer; 0.14 mol NaCl, pH 7.4) chilled to 4 °C and finally frozen at −70 °C. Before the analysis, erythrocytes were thawed and the haemolysate of washed red blood cells was diluted with distilled water and chilled to 4 °C. SOD, CAT, GPx activity and GSH concentrations were measured with Bioxytech (Oxis Research, Portland, OR, USA) kit using UV/ VIS Lambda 40 (Perkin Elmer, Wellesley, MA, USA) spectrophotometer. Friedmann ANOVA was used to assess statistical significance of changes of studied parameters. Spearman's rank correlation coefficient was used to measure correlations between measured parameters. There were no statistically significant differences in the activity of superoxide dismutase, catalase, glutathione peroxidase as well as glutathione concentrations during the first 4 min after total graft reperfusion and after having reached the temperature of 34.0 °C by the graft. Nevertheless, there was a positive correlation between the activity of superoxide dismutase and glutathione peroxidase ($P < 0.005$). The activity of glutathione peroxidase correlated positively with the concentration of glutathione in the fourth minute after total reperfusion ($P < 0.005$). Moreover, there was negative correlation between superoxide dismutase activity and glutathione concentration. This correlation was statistically significant before and 2 min after reperfusion ($P < 0.05$).

Oxidative reperfusion injury is thought to be a central mechanism of cellular damage affecting all organs and tissues after ischaemia. The mechanisms of this damage, however, are still not fully understood. Ischaemia results in the impairment of mitochondrial anti-oxidant defences and thereby renders cells more susceptible to oxidative stress (Arduini et al., 1988). The activity of anti-oxidative enzymes seems to be relatively stable during ischaemia (Kurokawa et al., 1996). However, glutathione peroxidase levels may decrease during both warm ischaemia and cold storage (Jassem et al., 1996). It has been demonstrated in isolated perfused kidney that oxygen free radicals are generated on postischaemic reperfusion (Paller et al., 1984). Several sources may be responsible for oxygen free radical production during ischaemia-reperfusion. These include alterations in mitochondrial electron transport, arachidonic acid metabolism, activation of xanthine oxidase, catecholamines or haemoglobin oxidation, as well as massive release of iron (Jassem et al., 2002). The results from previous studies indicate that leucocytes play a key role in ischaemia-reperfusion injury (Harris et al., 1996). The phenomenon also involves components of a typical inflammatory reaction. Oxygen free radicals can directly trigger the activation of leucocytes and adhesion molecules. Leucocyte activation is significantly enhanced within minutes after the onset of reperfusion and remains elevated for hours (Rabb et al., 1997). The measurement of the activity of enzymes involved in the anti-oxidative system is considered to be one of the reliable and sensitive assays of ischaemia-reperfusion period. Nevertheless, only a few studies have been conducted in humans to investigate the activity of the anti-oxidative system in erythrocytes during ischaemia and reperfusion. In the present study changes in activities of superoxide dismutase, catalase, glutathione peroxidase and glutathione concentrations in erythrocytes during the first 4 min after total kidney graft reperfusion were examined. The authors did not find statistically significant changes in the activities of enzymes involved in the anti-oxidative system. However, there was significant positive correlation between the activities of superoxide dismutase and glutathione peroxidase. This correlation may indicate the presence of mechanisms coordinating the activity of these enzymes. This mechanism might be of clinical importance increasing the effectiveness of superoxide radical inactivation, because H2O2, which is the product of superoxide dismutase, is at the same time the substrate for glutathione peroxidase. Moreover, there was no significant association between the erythrocyte anti-oxidative system and transplant outcome such as delayed graft function and acute rejection. In the present we analysed the enzymatic anti-oxidative system in the renal vein only and have not detected any changes in their activity in first 4 min of graft reperfusion. We have not analysed the enzymatic and non-enzymatic anti-oxidative systems in serum, as well as markers of biological membranes oxidative damage such as lipid peroxidation products. The lack of unfavourable changes during the early period of reperfusion such as decreased glutathione concentration, decreased glutathione peroxidase or SOD activity may indicate the very high capacity of anti-oxidative systems. It is possible that besides the erythrocyte anti-oxidative system other anti-oxidative systems such as plasmatic (Muzakova et al., 2000; Pechan et al., 2003;) or tissue antioxidative system (Dobashi et al., 2000) are involved in the defence against free radicals during allograft reperfusion. Nevertheless, a better understanding of changes in the anti-oxidative systems protecting against free radicals generation during allograft reperfusion requires further investigations.

2.4 Activity of CuZn-superoxide dismutase, catalase and glutathione peroxidase in erythrocytes in kidney allografts during reperfusion and delayed graft function

Many markers have been researched to prove the presence of ROS in the transplanted tissue. Some of them, like superoxide dismutase, catalase, and glutathione peroxidase are considered to play a major role in graft protection against oxygen stress during reperfusion. The SODs appear to be the most important enzymes involved in the defense system against ROS, particularly against superoxide anion radicals. Three distinct isoforms of SOD have been identified in mammals and their genomic structure, c-DNA, and protein structure have been described (Skrzycki & Czeczot, 2004). Two isoforms of SOD have Cu and Zn in their catalytic center and are localized in either intracellular cytoplasmatic compartments (CuZn-SOD or SOD1) or in extracellular elements (EC-SOD or SOD3). SOD1 is a homodimer with a molecular mass of about 32 kDa (Fattman et al., 2003; Zelko et al., 2002). It has been found in the cytoplasm, nuclear compartments and lysosomes of mammalian cells. SOD3 is a homotetramer of 135 kDa with a high affinity to heparin (Lookene et al, 2000; Oury et al., 1996). Manganese (Mn) is the cofactor of the third SOD isoform (Mn-SOD or SOD2) which is localized in aerobic cells' mitochondria (Petersen et al., 2003; Tibell et al., 1997). Early reperfusion is definitely associated with upregulating of SODs activity, but is also a factor that may lead to their rapid depletion (Davies et al., 1995; Singh et al., 1993) as huge amounts of ROS are released during that process. The aim of the study was to examine the activity of erythrocyte antioxidative system (SOD1, GPx, and CAT activity as well as GSH concentration) among patients with or without DGF.

Forty patients undergoing kidney transplantation at our center were assigned to two groups: with or without delayed graft function. Before anastomosing kidney vessels with recipient's iliac vessels, the '0' blood sample was taken from the iliac vein. Next blood samples I, II and III were taken from the graft's renal vein. The reperfusion of the transplanted kidney was evaluated precisely with the thermovision camera. Erythrocyte SOD1, CAT and GPx activity was measured with a spectrophotometric method. We did not observe statistically significant changes in SOD1, CAT and GPx activity in erythrocytes during the early phase of reperfusion in patients with and without DGF.

In humans, only a few studies have been conducted to investigate the activity of antioxidative system in erythrocytes during ischemia reperfusion. The excess of ROS, particularly of superoxide anion radicals is the main factor, which activates SODs. These enzymes are essential for cell protection against oxygen toxicity. As a result of the reaction catalyzed by SODs, hydrogen superoxide is generated and becomes a substrate for further reactions involving GPx and CAT. In our study the activity of erythrocyte antioxidative system, after total graft reperfusion in patients with and without DGF was assessed. SOD, CAT and GPx are the most important enzymes involved in antioxidative system during reperfusion. The SOD1 gene has been mapped to chromosome 21 (region 21q22) in humans (Levanon et al., 1985). Despite the fact that SOD1 is considered to be constitutively expressed, transcriptional regulation of SOD1 is highly controlled depending on extra- and intracellular conditions (Crapo et al., 1992). SOD1 mRNA level elevates in response to a wide array of mechanical, chemical and biological messengers such as heat shock, shear stress or hydrogen peroxide (Dimmerel et al., 1999; Hass & Massaro, 1988; Inoue et al., 1996; Yoo et al., 1988). SOD1 was fund to have a widespread distribution in a variety of tissues (Crapo et al., 1992). Early reperfusion is definitely associated with upregulating of SODs activity, but is also a factor that may lead to their rapid depletion (Davies et al., 1995; Singh et al., 1993) as huge amounts of ROS are released during that process. It was shown that MDA concentration as a marker of lipid peroxidation in the renal vein after 2 min of reperfusion increased by 30% compared with the systemic baseline value (Hower et al., 1996). In rats, the endogenous scavenger SOD, especially the cytoplasm copper-zinc (CuZn) form, is rapidly depleted during ischemia and reperfusion (Davies et al., 1995; Singh et al., 1993). Numerous studies have assessed the potential benefits of exogenous SOD administration in preventing reperfusion injury, but conclusions are ambiguous. In one study (Land et al., 1994) intraoperative human recombinant CuZn-SOD administration led to a significant reduction of early and late immunological complications. The effect, according to the authors, could be related to the enzyme's antioxidant action on ischemia-reperfusion injury of the renal allograft, which is a potential factor that reduces the immunogenicity of the graft. In another experimental study protective effect of exogenous Cu/Zn SOD proved to be minimal, probably because of very short half-period of SOD counted in minutes (Bayati et al., 1988; Johnson & Weinberg, 1993). In those studies, however, the authors did not specify which form of Cu/ Zn SOD was administered. An experimental study observed (Yin et al., 2001), that increased levels of intracellular SOD in kidney induced by its transfection with an adenoviral vector minimized ischemia-reperfusion induced tubular injury and improved post-ischemic renal function. Results of the studies suggest that some changes in SOD activity occur in graft's vein during the first few minutes after reperfusion. In our experiment no significant changes in graft's vein SOD1 activity were observed either in the group of patients with DGF or in the group without DGF, as the enzyme activity in sample III was comparable with its activity in sample 0. Early period of reperfusion from clamp removal till the whole graft is filled with recipient's blood and reaches the temperature of 36.6°C is essential for further graft function. Therefore appropriate assessment of the process is very important. The use of thermovision camera was the important point of our research. In most cases the assessment of graft reperfusion is performed by the surgeon without any objective method during the operation. However, proper evaluation of the process seems to be crucial in everyday practice as well as in experimental studies. Thermovision camera helped us to determine the moment when the whole graft was perfused with recipient's blood (Gnaiger et al., 1999; Jassem et al., 2002; Ostrowski et al., 2004). We suggest that this method is an important step to objective assessment of early reperfusion. In our study the erythrocyte antioxidative system remained stable after total reperfusion. The activity of SOD, CAT, GPx as well as GSH concentrations did not change statistically significantly during the reperfusion. Taking into consideration the results of our and previous studies which proved the beneficial effect of Cu/Zn SOD on the graft in the early stages after transplantation, we suggest that extracellular antioxidative system proves to be essential for protection against ROS during early stages after reperfusion. Extracellular matrix and the cell surface is the main EC SOD (SOD3) localization (Marklund, 1984, 1994) and structural differences between SOD1 and SOD3 seem to be the main factor that influences their activity and the place of action. In experiments with fluorescently labeled SOD (Emerit et al., 2002) clearly, it was showed that the enzyme binds to cellular membranes and the intensity of binding varies according to cell type. The differences observed for binding were concomitant with decreased inhibition of stimulated superoxide production. Taking into account the results of present study we suggest that the erythrocyte antioxidative system during the reperfusion is stable, and the main protective role against free radicals plays the extracellular antioxidative system, nevertheless this hypothesis requires further investigations.

2.5 Hypoxanthine as a graft ischemia marker and catalase activity during reperfusion

It has been proposed that xanthine oxidase may be a central mechanism of postischemic free radical generation in a variety of cells. Superoxide dismutase, catalase, glutathione and glutathione peroxidase are involved in protection against free radicals (Colpaert &Lefebrve, 2000; Komada et al., 1999; Radi et al., 1997). The aim of the study was to examine the correlation between the concentrations of ischemia markers: hypoxanthine or inosine and the activity of erythrocyte SOD, CAT as well as GPx.

The study included 40 renal transplant recipients. Before anastomosis of the kidney vessels with the recipient's iliac vessels, a "0" blood sample was taken from the iliac vein. Then, after anastomosis, the renal vein of the graft was cannulated and blood samples I, II, and III were obtained. The reperfusion of the transplanted kidney was measured with a thermovision camera ThermaCAM SC500. The study included 40 renal transplant recipients (21 men, 19 women), of mean age 52 ± 8 years with mean cold ischemia time of 26 ± 3 hours. The grafts were perfused with EuroCollins preservation solution. All patients received cyclosporine, azathioprine, and steroids. The "0" blood sample was taken from the iliac vein before anastomosing the kidney vessels with recipient iliac vessels. Then, the graft renal vein was cannulated to obtain blood samples I, II, and III. The reperfusion of the transplanted kidney was measured with thermovision camera (ThermaCAM SC500), which detects infrared radiation, recording digital image presenting the surface temperature distribution of the organ. The process of total reperfusion was completed when the scans from thermovision camera showed the whole organ filled with recipient blood. The sample I was taken from the inserted catheter after total tissue reperfusion had been shown by the scan monitor and after the temperature of the graft had reached 34°C. Blood samples II and III were taken 2 and 4 minutes after blood sample I, respectively. Blood was aliquoted into heparin containing tubes kept in ice. One tube was centrifuged within 15 minutes from collection. Plasma (300 μL) was supplemented with 300 μL of 1.3 mol/L perchloric acid, vortexed, and centrifuged (5 min/20000 *g*/4°C). The acid supernatant (400 μL) was removed and neutralized with 130 to 160 μL of 1 mol/L potassium phosphate to pH 5 to 7.7 Centrifugation was repeated and the supernatant withdrawn for high-performance liquid chromatography (HPLC) to measure plasma concentrations of Hyp and Ino. Analyses were performed with a Hewlett-Packard (now Agilent) Series 1050 chromatography System. SOD, CAT, and GPx activities were measured with spectrophotometric methods using an UV/VIS Lambda 40 (Perkin Elmer) spectrophotometer. We used Bioxytech (Oxis Research, USA) kits. The results are presented per gram of hemoglobin, measured using Drabkin's method. Friedmann ANOVA was used to assess the significance of changes in the studied parameters. Spearman's rank correlation coefficient was used to measure correlations between analysed parameters.

The plasma concentrations of Hyp and Ino increased in statistically significant fashion immediately after total tissue reperfusion ($P < .0001$) then gradually decreasing. There were no statistically significant differences in the activities of CAT, SOD, and GPx. The activity of catalase at 4 minutes after total tissue reperfusion (sample III) correlated positively with hypoxanthine concentrations immediately after total tissue reperfusion (sample I; Rs = +0.49), 2 minutes after total tissue reperfusion (sample II; Rs = +0.47), and 4 minutes after total tissue reperfusion (sample III; Rs = +0.46). There were no statistically significant correlations between CAT activity and Hyp concentrations in the iliac vein before transplantation. Similar correlations were observed between CAT activity and Ino concentrations; those values, however, did not reach statistical significance ($P < .07$). Moreover, there were no statistically significant correlations between Hyp and Ino concentrations and SOD and GPx activities.

For kidney preservation, hypothermic storage remains the most common technique. However, hypothermic organ preservation is associated with oxygen deprivation, which inevitably leads to some degree of ischemia-reperfusion injury upon transplantation (Hower et al., 1996). During reperfusion, a large amount of reactive oxygen species (superoxide anions, hydroxyl radicals, and hydrogen peroxides) are produced by the reentry of oxygenated blood into the ischemic tissue (Grinyo, 2001). The catabolism of adenine nucleotides results in an accumulation of Hyp in ischemic cells. Ischemia is also associated with the proteolytic conversion of xanthine dehydrogenase to xanthine oxidase (Sermet et al. 2000). When xanthine oxidase converts Hyp to xanthine in the presence of molecular oxygen, superoxide radical is generated. SOD, CAT, GSH, and GPx are involved in defense against these processes (Dowell et al., 1993). In the present study we evaluated the correlation between the concentration of ischemia markers (Hyp or Ino) and the activity of erythrocyte SOD, CAT, as well as GPx. Immediately after total reperfusion we observed a statistically significant increase in Hyp and Ino plasma concentrations, changes which retreated after reperfusion. Elevated concentrations of Hyp and Ino during ischemia may occur due to ATP breakdown. The elevated concentrations of Hyp and Ino correlated with increased activity of catalase in erythrocytes. We did not, however, observe a correlation with SOD activity. Characterization of the human SOD gene has revealed several potential transcriptional regulatory sites, none of which have been demonstrated to be active in the human SOD gene (Foltz & Carpo, 1994). The presence of those possible regulatory sequences suggests that SOD expression may be regulated by multiple stimuli. Recently SOD expression has been shown to be regulated by several cytokines. Interferon-γ results in an increased expression of SOD, whereas tumor necrosis factor-α and transforming growth factor- β decrease enzyme expression (Marklund 1992). Various forms of direct oxidative stress do not, however, seem to affect SOD expression (Stralin & Marklund, 1994). The results of the present study suggested that CAT activity may correlate with the concentration of Hyp and other mediators of oxidative stress in the graft renal vein. We hypothesize that catalase activity is regulated by factors that protect against a burst of free radicals upon postischemic reperfusion. The hypothesis requires further investigation.

2.6 Effect of trimetazidine on the nucleotide profile in rat kidney with ischemia–reperfusion injury

Total adenine nucleotide concentration (TAN) is a measure of pool of all (high- and low-energy) nucleotides containing adenine moiety (ATP + ADP + AMP). The balance between these three nucleotides is maintained by the action of adenylate kinase which catalyzes the reversible transphosphorylation of two molecules of ADP to one ATP and one AMP (Saiki et al., 1997). Adenylate energy charge is a measure of the balance between adenine nucleotides. Its value (Atkinson & Walton, 1967) is between 0 (when only low-energy AMP is present in the cell) and 1 (when only high-energy ATP is present). Dephosphorylation of AMP to adenosine catalyzed by 5′-nucleotidases is responsible for loss of AMP and decrease in TAN concentration (Welsh & Lindinger, 1997). Preservation of TAN pool is crucial to maintenance of normal purine metabolism in the cell since the replenishment of the lost adenine nucleotide molecules (via synthesis "de novo" or salvage reactions) would require additional energy, which is lacking during ischemia. Therefore considerable loss of adenine nucleotides during ischemia results in vicious circle leading to irreversible deficit of energy which cannot be recovered during reperfusion (Hiraoka et al.,1993). The catabolism of adenine nucleotides results in an accumulation of hypoxanthine in ischemic cells. Ischemia is also associated with proteolytic conversion of xanthine/hypoxanthine dehydrogenase to xanthine/hypoxanthine oxidase (Colpaert & Lefebvre, 2000; Komada et al., 1999; Sun et al., 2004). With the supply of molecular oxygen upon reperfusion of ischemic tissues, xanthine oxidase metabolizes xanthine and hypoxanthine to uric acid and free radicals are generated. The generation of oxygen free radicals during reperfusion may overcome the capacity of physiologic scavengers. The excess of these highly reactive species results in cytotoxicity and induces peroxidation of the lipid cell membrane (Akcetin et al., 2000; Pincemail et al., 1993). It has been shown that the free radicals generation correlates with the activity of antioxidative system (Singh et al., 1993). The excess of ROS, particularly of superoxide anion radicals is the main factor which activates superoxide dismutases. These enzymes are essential for cell protection against oxygen toxicity. As a result of the reaction catalyzed by SODs, hydrogen superoxide is generated and becomes a substrate for further reactions involving glutathione peroxidase and catalase (Gulati et al., 1993; Yoo et al., 1999). In experimental systems of ischemia-reperfusion injury, it has been shown that mitochondria may play a key role in oxidative injury (Vlessis & Mela-Riker, 1989). Mitochondria are the powerhouse of the cell and provide ATP through the oxidative phosphorylation process.

Moreover, mitochondria were identified as an important source of hydrogen peroxide (Jassem et al., 2002). Ischemia causes also extensive cytoskeletal and mitochondrial damage and uncoupling of oxidative phosphorylation (Akcetin et al., 1999; Caraceni et al., 2005). The effect of trimetazidine on the mitochondrial function of ischemic Wistar rat was studied (Monteiro et al., 2004). In this model, trimetazidine had a preferential action on the oxidative system, increasing its enzyme activity and decreasing O2 consumption after phosphorylation; this could decrease oxygen free radical production and increase mitochondrial integrity, thus allowing the maintenance of the electrical potential. Trimetazidine (TMZ) is an anti-ischemic agent. Its anti-ischemic effects have been experimentally assessed in various models including cell cultures, isolated and perfused organs, and also in vivo (Baumert et al., 1999; Hauet et al., 2000). TMZ mostly acts on mitochondria by restoring ATP synthesis, which was blocked by the Ca overload, by releasing Ca accumulation in the matrix, and by restoring the mitochondrial membrane impermeability and its affinity for protons. Moreover, TMZ inhibits the excessive release of oxygen free radicals, increases glucose metabolism, limits intracellular acidosis, protects ATP stores, reduces membrane lipid peroxydation and inhibits neutrophils infiltration after ischemia and reperfusion (Catroux et al., 1990; Hauet et al., 1998a). The aim of the study was to examine the effect of TMZ on nucleotide profile in rat kidney with ischemia–reperfusion injury.

Male Wistar rats weighing 300–350 g were used in this experiment. They were allowed to acclimatize for a minimum of 10 days prior to the study. The rats were housed in the room maintained at 21 ± 1 °C with 12 h light–dark cycle with the light cycle beginning at 6:00 a.m. All animals were fed standard rat chow and water ad libitum. Food was withheld overnight before surgery. Animals were divided into two groups: animals treated with TMZ (n = 14) and control group receiving placebo (n = 13). The aqueous solution of trimetazidine 10 mg/kg/day was administrated by gavages vehicle twice a day at 8.00 a.m. and 18.00 p.m. for 30 days. In this study, the effect of trimetazidine on adenine nucleotide profile was examined after ischemia-reperfusion as well as by normal renal blood flow. Therefore the left kidney artery was clamped to induce the ischemia-reperfusion injury, whereas the blood flow in right kidney artery remained unchanged. The rats were anesthetized with ketamine (Ketolar). The abdominal cavity was opened via middle incision. The aorta, vena cava inferior, and finally left and right renal vessels were atraumatically isolated. An atraumatic microvascular clamp was placed on the left renal artery for 15 min to induce the ischemia of renal tissue. The catheter (Becton Dickinson Vascular Access Inc., Sandy, Utah, USA) was inserted in aorta. After clamp removal from the left renal artery, the aorta and vena cava superior were clamped over the right and left renal artery, and then vena cava inferior was catheterized to enable the outflow of perfusion solution. The EuroCollins solution was perfused continuously at 100 ml/h during 12 min (temperature of the solution, +4 ◦C; volume of injected solution, 20 ml). Finally, bilateral nephrectomy was performed. After obtaining tissue samples from both kidneys for histological analysis the right and left kidneys were immediately frozen in liquid nitrogen within a few seconds from collection and transferred to 1.5 mL airtight tubes immersed in liquid nitrogen. Subsequently, they were minced with a metal homogenizer pre-cooled in liquid nitrogen, transferred to capped 1.5 mL tubes containing 500 μL of 0.4 mol/L cold perchloric acid, and homogenized for 15 s with a knife microhomogenizer (Dispergierstation T8.10, IKA). Centrifugation followed at 4 ◦C (16,000 × g, 5 min), 400 μL of the supernatant was transferred to a test tube and neutralized with 115 μL of 1 mol/L potassium phosphate. Centrifugation was repeated and the supernatant was taken for high performance liquid chromatography. HPLC was done to measure tissue and whole blood concentrations of the following 17 nucleotides, nucleosides, and oxypurines: adenosine triphosphate (ATP), adenosine diphosphate (ADP), adenosine monophosphate (AMP), adenosine (Ado), guanosine triphosphate (GTP), guanosine diphosphate (GDP), guanosine monophosphate (GMP), guanosine (Guo), inosine monophosphate (IMP), inosine (Ino), hypoxanthine (Hyp), xanthine (Xan), uric acid (UA), uridine (Urd), nicotinamide adenine dinucleotide (NAD) and nicotinamide adenine dinucleotide phosphate (NADP). Analyses were performed with Hewlett–Packard Series 1050 chromatography system consisting of a quaternary gradient pump with vacuum degassing and piston desalting modules, Rheodyne 7125 manual injection valve with 20 μL loop, UV–vis detector, and series 1100 thermostatted column compartment. Separations were achieved on Hypersil BDS 125 mm × 3 mm, 3 μm particle size column (Agilent). The mobile phase flowed at a rate of 0.5 mL/min and column temperature was 20.5 °C. Buffer composition remained unchanged (A: 150 mmol/L phosphate buffer, pH 6.0, containing 150 mmol/L potassium chloride; B: 15% acetonitrile in buffer A). The gradient profile was modified to the following content of buffer B in the mobile phase: 0% at 0.00 min, 2% at 0.05 min, 7% at 2.45 min, 50% at 5.05 min, 100% at 5.35 min, 100% at 7.00 min, 0% at 7.10 min. Samples of 100 μL were injected every 12 min into the injection valve loop. Absorbance was read at 254 nm. Concentrations were expressed as median in nmol/mg protein. For histology, kidneys were fixed in buffered formalin and 2 μm paraffin-embedded sections were stained using hematoxylin–eosin and periodic acid-Schiff (PAS). Twenty randomly selected areas in a renal cortex were examined under light microscopy at 400×. Severity of acute tubular damage was semi-quantitatively scored by estimating the percentage of tubules that showed epithelial necrosis or had necrotic debris as follows: 0, none; 1+ (mild), <10%; 2+ (moderate), 10–50%; 3+ (severe), >50%. Mann–Whitney test was performed to compare each parameter between two groups. The significance of the differences between the parameters in the left (clamped, with ischemia) and the right (non-clamped, without ischemia) kidney was assessed using Wilcoxon test. Severity of acute tubular damage was compared between groups with x2-test.

Tissue concentrations of ATP, ADP, AMP, TAN and AEC were significantly increased in kidneys from rats treated with TMZ in comparison with rats receiving placebo. Concentrations of products of nucleotide degradation: inosine, guanosine and uridine, as well as oxypurines: Hyp and Xan, were significantly decreased in rats treated with trimetazidine. Moreover, significantly less pronounced acute tubular necrosis was observed in kidneys of rats treated with TMZ. Tissue concentrations of ATP, ADP, AMP, TAN and AEC values were significantly increased in kidneys with or without ischemia in rats treated with trimetazidine in comparison with rats receiving placebo. Moreover, the concentrations of GTP and GDP were increased, although the concentrations of GMP were decreased in kidney from rats treated with trimetazidine. The concentrations of products of nucleotide degradation: Ino, Guo and Urd, as well as oxypurines: Hyp and Xan, were significantly decreased in rats treated with trimetazidine. These results suggest the protecting activity of trimetazidine against the dephosphorylation of nucleotides. Nevertheless, the concentration of Ado was significantly increased in rats treated with trimetazidine. The increased Ado concentrations may be the result of increased adenine nucleotide synthesis or inhibition of adenosine to inosine degradation. The increased tissue adenosine concentrations may be the important kidney preconditioning factor improving the tissue metabolism during ischemia. Concentrations of NAD were significantly increased in kidneys from rats treated with trimetazidine. It might be associated with enhanced ATP availability, essential for NAD synthesis. NADP concentrations were decreased in rats treated with trimetazidine. Decreased NADP concentrations may suggest the increase in NADPH/NADP ratio. NADPH is involved in the antioxidative system; therefore the increased NADPH concentration may have beneficial effects in ischemic tissues. Analyzing tissue concentrations of ATP, ADP, AMP, GDP, GMP and TAN between kidneys with and without ischemia we observed the decrease of these nucleotide concentrations associated with ischemia in rats treated with TMZ, although the concentrations in rats receiving TMZ remained significantly higher as compared to values in rats from control group. There were no statistically significant differences in NAD concentration between kidney with and without ischemia, the NADP concentrations were significantly decreased in kidney with ischemia in rats treated with trimetazidine as well as placebo. Tissue concentrations of Guo were significantly decreased in kidneys after ischemia in rats treated with trimetazidine. It may be the result of decreased guanylate degradation in kidneys treated with trimetazidine during ischemia. Hyp concentrations were significantly decreased in kidneys after ischemia in rats treated with trimetazidine, but in rats receiving placebo these values were increased. Decreased tissue concentrations of Hyp may be associated with diminished degradation of adenine nucleotides during ischemia in rats treated with trimetazidine. The histological changes of ischemic acute tubular necrosis depends on the intensity of ischemic trigger and varies with the evolution of the lesion in relationship to the onset of initial injury. Among many histologic features of ATN individual, cell necrosis with denudation of the basement membrane, shedding of epithelial cells and necrotic debris into the lumen are most characteristic whereas glomerular morphology typically remains unchanged. The commonest finding in kidneys from control group was moderate ATN followed by complete necrosis of epithelial tubular cells and denudation of basement membranes seen in many tubules. Mild ATN characterized by the presence of fragments of cells within the tubular lamina of single tubules was significantly more frequent in kidneys from rats treated with trimetazidine than in control groups ($p < 0.001$ and <0.05, respectively). Severe ATN in kidneys from the trimetazidine treated rats was not detected. The intensity of ATN did not differ significantly between kidneys with and without ischemia. The significantly less pronounced ATN observed in kidneys of rats treated with TMZ suggests that TMZ protects the tubules from ischemic damage.

Ischemia-reperfusion injury affects early graft function and influences the development of chronic graft dysfunction. Ischemia favors the depletion of cellular adenosine nucleotides, alterations in membrane ATP-dependent ionic transporters, and the intracellular accumulation of Ca, Na and water. The great swelling of endothelial and tubular epithelial cells due to ischemia not only increases the acidosis caused by anaerobic metabolism, but also alters cell permeability and favors the obstruction of capillary flow (Facundo et al., 2005). The reperfusion of ischemic tissues also increases the release of intracellular enzymes. In anaerobic metabolism the energy production for essential processes is greatly reduced. Failure of ion pumping with rapid loss of electrochemical gradients results in translocation of ions. The production of oxygen-derived free radicals is considerably increased during tissue ischemia caused by dissociation of oxidative phosphorylation, which results in univalent reduction of oxygen, catabolism of ATP into hypoxanthine and uric acid (Elsner et al., 1998). In particular, the reduced form of NADH, the essential coenzyme for all the oxidative enzymatic reactions, accumulates and is only utilized in reactions such as lactate formation from pyruvate, which under ischemia cannot be used in Krebs cycle. A general assumption is that NADP - the cofactor of anabolic enzymatic reactions - accumulates in the reduced form (NADPH), following the same pattern of the NADH/NAD redox couple. Under conditions of impaired NADPH production, the possible utilization of cofactor can remain unbalanced. There is clear evidence that a highly-reduced state of NADP and of glutathione redox couples exerts a major protective function (Hai et al., 2005). In particular glutathione is involved in the protection against free radical induced damage through glutathione peroxidase. Interruption of blood supply and lack of oxygen during ischemia lead to anaerobic metabolism that entails a depletion of ATP (Cruthirds et al., 2005). In this study we examined the effect of TMZ on nucleotide concentrations in renal tissue after ischemia–reperfusion. The animals received TMZ 4 weeks before the experiment. Tissue concentrations of the majority of nucleotides involved in energetic processes in cells were significantly increased in renal tissues from animals receiving TMZ as compared to rats receiving placebo. Although the concentrations of purine nucleotides decreased during ischemia in rats treated with TMZ, they remained still significantly increased as compared to control group. Our results suggest that TMZ increases the synthesis of purine and pyridine nucleotides leading to improvement of energy status of cells. Moreover in histological pictures the severe tubular necrosis in kidneys from animals treated with TMZ was not detected. In kidneys from animals receiving TMZ the prevalence of mild ATN was observed. Various experimental studies have shown that TMZ has preserved the intracellular concentration of ATP and inhibited the extracellular leakage of K+ during cellular ischemia (Hauet et al., 1998b). Additionally it prevents excessive release of free radicals, which are particularly toxic to phospholipid membranes and are responsible for both the fall in intracellular ATP concentration and the extracellular leakage of K+ (Catroux et al., 1990; Maupoil et al., 1990). The protective effect of TMZ on the decreased levels of NADPH caused by ischemia-reperfusion suggests that this agent has some beneficial effects against the activation of NADPH-dependent oxidases. They represent the most significant O2 source in tissues. TMZ is also efficient in preventing inflammatory cell infiltration (Baumert et al., 2004). Current immunosuppressive protocols use treatments that might worsen nonimmunological mechanisms such as ischemia, hypertension and direct drug nephrotoxicity. TMZ has been shown to restore ATP synthesis from cyclosporine-treated isolated mitochondria suspensions (Simon et al., 1997). Moreover, it has been shown that TMZ significantly reduced lipid peroxidation after 60 min warm renal ischemia followed by 15 min reperfusion (Hauet et al., 1998c). TMZ decreased also the concentrations of malondialdehyde and increased the activity of glutathione peroxidase in rat's kidney after warm ischemia (Ozden et al., 1998). Recipient treatment with trimetazidine improved graft function and protected energy status after lung transplantation (Inci et al., 2001). The effects of trimetazidine in a rat model of renal ischemia–reperfusion injury were investigated (Kaur et al., 2003). The ischemic kidneys of rats showed severe hyaline casts, epithelial swelling, proteinaceous debris, tubular necrosis, medullary congestion and hemorrhage. Trimetazidine markedly reduced elevated levels of tissue lipid peroxidation and significantly attenuated renal dysfunction and morphological changes in rats subjected to renal ischemia–reperfusion. Singh et al. studied the effect of trimetazidine on ischemia–reperfusion induced renal failure in rats as well as the protective effect of trimetazidine against the damage inflicted by reactive oxygen species. Pretreatment of animals with trimetazidine markedly attenuated renal dysfunction, morphological alterations and restored the depleted renal antioxidant enzymes (Singh & Chopra, 2004). The results of present study have shown that trimetazidine reduced the dephosphorylation of nucleotides caused by renal ischemia-reperfusion and this correlated with a reduction of histological evidence of renal injury. Because the rejection is initiated by the response to injury sustained during the transplant process and because TMZ may diminish the reperfusion injury, it seems that this drug could be useful in limiting the complications after cadaver organ transplantation and preventing the initiation of rejection.

3. Conclusion

1. The profile of oxypurines and purine nucleosides in the renal vein of the reperfused graft in humans appears to be a reliable marker of the energy status of kidney tissue and a prognostic factor for early graft function.
2. Concentrations of hypoxanthine and xanthine in the renal and peripheral vein are useful for monitoring the energy status of the graft during reperfusion.
3. The early phase of reperfusion in humans is without significant effect on the activity of superoxide dismutase, catalase, or glutathione peroxidase in erythrocytes from the graft vein. The activity of anti-oxidative enzymes in erythrocytes from the graft vein does not correlate with early graft function and as such is without value as a prognostic factor for graft function.
4. Hypoxanthine appears to stimulate catalase activity which is an important element of the antioxidant system.
5. Trimetazidine inhibits dephosphorylation of purine nucleotides and histological changes in tubules of the ischemic rat kidney, thereby limiting the extent of ischemia-reperfusion injury.

4. Acknowledgment

The present study was financed by the State Committee for Scientific Research of Poland (grant number - 3P05C07324p05).

5. References

Akcetin, Z.; Busch, A.; Kessler, G.; Heynemann, H.; Holtz, J. & Bromme, H.J. (1999). Evidence for only a moderatelipid peroxidation during ischemia-reperfusion of rat kidney due to its high antioxidative capacity. *Urol Res* Vol.27, pp. 280-284

Akcetin, Z.; Pregla, R.; Busch, A.; Kessler, G.; Heynemann, H.; Holtz, J. & Bromme, H.J. (2000). Lipid peroxidationand the expressional regulation of the heatshock response during ischemia-reperfusion of rat kidney. *Urol Int* Vol.65, pp. 32-39

Arduini, A.; Mezzetti, A.; Porreca, E.; Lapenna, D.; DeJulia, J.; Marzio, L.; Polidoro, G. & Cuccurullo, F. (1988). Effect of ischemia and reperfusion on antioxidant enzymes and mitochondrial inner membrane proteins in perfused rat heart. *Biochim Biophys Acta* Vol.970, No.2, pp. 113-21

Atkinson, D.E. & Walton, G.M. (1967). Adenosine triphosphate conservation in metabolic regulation. Rat livercitrate cleavage enzyme. *J. Biol. Chem.* Vol.242, No.13, pp. 3239–3241

Azevedo, L.S.; Castro, M.C.; Monteiro de Carvalho, D.B.; d'Avila, D.O.; Contieri, F.; Goncalves, R.T.; Manfro, R. & Ianhez, L.E. (2005). Incidence of delayed graft function in cadaveric kidney transplants in Brazil: a multicenter analysis. *Transplant Proc* Vol.37, No.6, pp. 2746 -7

Baumert, H.; Goujon, J.M.; Richer, J.P.; Lacoste, L.; Tillement, J.P.; Eugene, M.; Carretier, M. & Hauet, T. (1999).Renoprotective effects of trimetazidine against ischemia-reperfusion injury and cold storage preservation: a preliminary study. *Transplantation* Vol.27, No.68, pp. 300–303

Baumert, H.; Faure, J.P.; Zhang, K.; Petit, I.; Goujon, J.M.; Dutheil, D.; Favreau, F.; Barriere, M.; Tillement, J.P.; Mauco, G.; Papadopoulos, V. & Hauet, T. (2004). Evidence for a mitochondrial impact of trimetazidine during cold ischemia and reperfusion. *Pharmacology* Vol.71, pp. 25–37

Bayati, A.; Kallskog, O.; Odlind, B. & Wolgast, M. (1988). Plasma elimination kinetics and renal handling of copper/zinc superoxide dismutase in the rat. *Acta Physiol Scand* Vol.134, No.1, pp. 65-74

Bradford, M.M. (1976). A rapid and sensitive method for the quantitation of microgram quantities of protein utilizing the principle of protein–dye binding. *Anal. Biochem.* Vol.72, pp. 248–254.

Caraceni, P.; Domenicali, M.; Vendemiale, G.; Grattagliano, I.; Pertosa, A.; Nardo, B.; Morselli-Labate, A.M.; Trevisani, F.; Palasciano, G.; Altomare, E. & Bernardi, M. (2005). The reduced tolerance of rat fatty liver to ischemia - reperfusion is associated with mitochondrial oxidative injury. *J. Surg. Res.* Vol.124, pp. 160–168

Carter, J.T.; Chan, S.; Roberts, J.P. & Feng, S. (2005). Expanded criteria donor kidney allocation: marked decrease in cold ischemia and delayed graft function at a single center. *Am J Transplant*Vol.5, pp. 2745-53

Catroux, P.; Benchekroun, N.; Robert, J. & Cambar, J. (1990). Influence of trimetazidine on deleterious effect of oxygen radical species in post-ischemic acute renal failure in the rat. *Cardiovasc. Drugs Ther.* Vol.4, pp. 816–817

Chien, C.T.; Lee, P.H.; Chen, C.F.; Ma, M.C.; Lai, M.K. & Hsu, S.M. (2001). De novo demonstration and co-localization of free - radical production and apoptosis formation in kidney subjected to ischemia/reperfusion. *J. Am. Soc. Nephrol.* Vol.12, pp. 973–977

Chouker, A.; Martignoni, A.; Schauer, R.J.; Rau, H.G.; Volk, A.; Heizmann, O.; Dugas, M.; Messmer, K.; Peter, K. & Thiel, M. (2005). Ischemic preconditioning attenuates portal venous plasma concentrations of purines following warm liver ischemia in man. *Eur Surg Res* Vol.37, No.3, pp. 144-152

Colpaert, E.E. & Lefebvre, R.A. (2000). Interaction of hypoxanthine/xanthine oxidase with nitrergic relaxation in the porcine gastric fundus. *Br. J. Pharmacol.* Vol.130, pp. 359–366

Corner, J.A.; Berwanger, C.S. & Stansby, G. (2003). Preservation of vascular tissue under hypothermic conditions. *J Surg Res* Vol.113, pp. 21-5

Crapo, J.D.; Oury, T.D.; Rabouille, C.; Slot, J.W. & Chang, L.Y. (1992). Copper, zinc superoxide dismutase is the primarily a cytosolic protein in human cells. *Proc Natl Acad Sci USA* Vol.89, No.21, pp. 10405-9

Cruthirds, D.L.; Saba, H. & MacMillan-Crow, L.A. (2005). Overexpression of manganese superoxide dismutase protects against ATP depletion-mediated cell death of proximal tubule cells. *Arch. Biochem. Biophys.* Vol.437, pp. 96–105

Davies, S.J.; Reichardt-Pascal, S.Y.; Vaughan, D. & Russell, G.I. (1995). Differential effect of ischemia-reperfusion injury on anti oxidant enzyme activity in the rat kidney. *Exp. Nephrol.* Vol.3, pp. 348–54

Dimmeler, S.; Hermann, C.; Galle, J. & Zeiher, A.M. (1999). Upregulation of superoxide dismutase and nitric oxide synthase mediates the apoptosis-supressive effects of shear stress on endothelial cells. *Arterioscler Thromb Vasc Biol* Vol.19, No.3, pp. 656-64

Dobashi, K.; Ghosh, B.; Orak, J.K.; Singh, I. & Singh, A.K. (2000). Kidney ischemia-reperfusion: Modulation of antioxidant defenses. *Mol. Cell. Biochem.* Vol.205, pp. 1–11

Dowell, F.J.; Hamilton, C.A.; McMurray, J. & Reid, J.L. (1993). Effects of a xanthine oxidase/hypoxanthine free radical and reactive oxygen species generating system on endothelial function in New Zealand white rabbit aortic rings. *J Cardiovasc Pharmacol* Vol.22, pp. 792-797

Elsner, R.; Oyasaeter, S.; Almaas, R. & Saugstad, O.D. (1998). Diving seals, ischemia-reperfusion and oxygen radicals. *Comp. Biochem. Physiol. A Mol. Integr. Physiol.* Vol.119, pp. 975–980

Emerit, I.; Filipe, P.; Freitas, J.; Fernandes, A.; Garban, F. & Vassy, J. (2002). Assaying binding capacity of Cu, ZnSOD and MnSOD: demonstration of their localization in cells and tissues. *Meth Enzymol* Vol.349, pp. 321-327

Facundo, H.T.; de Paula, J.G. & Kowaltowski, A.J. (2005). Mitochondrial ATP-sensitive K+ channels prevent oxidative stress, permeability transition and cell death. *J. Bioenerg. Biomembr.* Vol.37, pp. 75–82

Fattman, C.H.; Schaefer, L.M. & Oury, T.D. (2003). Extracellular superoxide dismutase in biology and medicine. *Free Rad Biol Med* Vol.35, No.3, pp. 236-256.

Foltz, R.J. & Carpo, J.D. (1994). Extracellular superoxide dismutase (SOD3): tissue-specific expression, genomic characterization and computer-assisted sequence analysis of human EC SOD gene. *Genomics* Vol.22, p. 162

Galat, J.A.; Robinson, A.V. & Rhodes, R.S. Oxygen free radical mediated renal dysfunction. (1989). *J Surg Res* Vol.46, pp. 520-525

Gilligan, B.J.; Woo, H.M.; Kosieradzki, M.; Torrealba, J.R.; Southard, J.H. & Mangino, M.J. (2004). Prolonged hypothermia causes primary nonfunction in preserved canine renal allografts due to humoral rejection. *Am J Transplant* Vol.4, pp. 1266-1273

Gnaiger, E.; Rieger, G.; Stadlmann, S.; Amberger, A.; Eberl, T. & Margreiter, R. (1999). Mitochondrial defect in endothelial cold ischemia/reperfusion injury. *Transpl Proc* Vol.31, No.1-2, pp. 994-995

Grinyo, J.M. (2001). Role of ischemia–reperfusion injury in the development of chronic renal allograft damage.*Transpl. Proc.* Vol.33, pp. 3741–3743

Guieu, R.; Dussol, B.; Devaux, C.; Sampol, J.; Brunet, P.; Rochat, H.; Bechis, G. & Berland, Y.F. (1998). Interactions between cyclosporine A and adenosine in kidney transplant recipients. *Kidney Int* Vol.53, No.1, pp. 200-204

Gulati, S.; Ainol, L.; Orak, J.; Singh, A.K. & Singh, I. (1993). Alterations of peroxisomal function in ischemia-reperfusion injury of rat kidney. *Biochim. Biophys. Acta* Vol. 1182, pp. 291–298

Gulec, B.; Coskun, K.; Oner, K.; Aydin, A.; Yigitler, C.; Kozak, O.; Uzar, A. & Arslan, I. (2006). Effects of perfusion solutions on kidney ischemiareperfusion injury in pigs. *Transplant Proc* Vol.38, pp. 371-374

Hai, S.; Takemura, S.; Minamiyama, Y.; Yamasaki, K.; Yamamoto, S.; Kodai, S.; Tanaka, S.; Hirohashi, K. & Suehiro, S. (2005). Mitochondrial K(ATP) channel opener prevents ischemia-reperfusion injury in rat liver. *Transpl. Proc.* Vol.37, pp. 428–431

Harris, A.G.; Leiderer, R.; Peer, F. & Messmer K. (1996). Skeletal muscle microvascular and tissue injury after varying durations of ischemia. *Am J Physiol* Vol.271, pp. 2388-2398

Hass, M.A. & Massaro, D. (1988). Regulation of the synthesis of superoxide dismutases in rat lungs during oxidant and hyperthermic stresses. *J Biol Chem* Vol.263, No.2, pp. 776-781

Hauet, T.; Baumert, H.; Mothes, D.; Germonville, T.; Caritez, J.C.; Carretier, M.; Journe, F.; Eugene, M. & Tillement, J.P. (1998a). Lipid peroxidation after cold storage and normothermic reperfusion: the effect of trimetazidine. *Transpl. Int.* Vol.11, Suppl. 1, pp. 408–409

Hauet, T.; Mothes, D.; Goujon, J.; Germonville, T.; Caritez, J.C;, Carretier, M.; Eugene, M. & Tillement, J.P. (1998b). Trimetazidine reverses deleterious effects of ischemia-reperfusion in the isolated perfused pig kidney model. *Nephron* Vol.80, pp. 296–304

Hauet, T.; Tallineau, C.; Goujon, J.M.; Carretier, M.; Eugene, M. & Tillement, J.P. (1998c). Efficiency of trimetazidine in renal dysfunction secondary to cold ischemia-reperfusion injury: a proposed addition to University of Wisconsin solution. *Cryobiology* Vol.37, pp. 231–244

Hauet, T.; Goujon, J.M.; Vandewalle, A.; Baumert, H.; Lacoste, L.; Tillement, J.P.; Eugene, M. & Carretier, M. (2000). Trimetazidine reduces renal dysfunction by limiting the cold ischemia/reperfusion injury in autotransplanted pig kidneys. *J. Am. Soc. Nephrol.* Vol.11, pp. 138–148

Hiraoka, K.; Kuroda, Y. & Saitoh, Y. (1993). The importance of adenosine metabolism in ischemically damaged canine pancreas during preservation by the two-layer cold storage method. *Kobe J. Med. Sci.* Vol.39, No.5–6, pp. 183–195

Hirayama, A.; Nagase, S.; Ueda, A.; Oteki, T.; Takada, K.; Obara, M.; Inoue, M.; Yoh, K.; Hirayama, K. & Koyama, A. (2005). In vivo imaging of oxidative stress in ischemia-reperfusion renal injury using electron paramagnetic resonance. *Am. J. Physiol. Renal Physiol.* Vol.288, No.3, pp. 597- 603

Hower, R.; Minor, T.; Scneeberger, H.; Theodorakis, J.; Rembold, S.; Illner, W.D.; Hoffman, G.O.; Fraunberger, P.; Isselhard, W. & Land, W. (1996). Assessment of oxygen radicals during transplantation—effect of radical scavenger. *Transpl. Int.* Vol.9, pp. 479-482

Inci, I.; Dutly, A.; Inci, D.; Boehler, A. & Weder, W. (2001). Recipient treatment with trimetazidine improves graft function and protects energy status after lung transplantation. *J. Heart Lung Transpl.* Vol.20, pp. 1115–1122

Inoue, N.; Ramasamy, S.; Fukai, T.; Nerem, R.M. & Harrison, D.G. (1996). Shear stress modulates expression of Cu/Zn superoxide dismutase in human aortic endothelial cells. *Circ Res* Vol.79, No.1, pp. 32-37

Jassem, W.; Ciarimboli, C.; Cerioni, P.N.; Saba, V.; Norton, S.J. & Principato, G. (1996). Glyoxalase II and glutathione levels in rat liver mitochondria during cold storage in Euro-Collins and University of Wisconsin solutions. *Transplantation* Vol.61, pp. 1416–1420

Jassem, W.; Fuggle, S.V.; Rela, M.; Koo, D.D. & Heaton, N.D. (2002). The role of mitochondria in ischemia/reperfusion injury. *Transplantation* Vol.73, pp. 493–499

Johnson, K.J. & Weinberg, J.M. (1993). Postischemic renal injury due to oxygen radicals. *Curr Opin Nephrol Hypertens* Vol.2, No.4, pp. 625-635

Kaur, H.; Padi, S.S. & Chopra, K. (2003). Attenuation of renal ischemia–reperfusion injury by trimetazidine: evidence of an in vivo antioxidant effect. *Meth. Find. Exp. Clin. Pharmacol.* Vol.25, pp. 803–809

Kelley, K.J.; Baird, N.R. & Greene, A.L. (2001). Induction of stress response proteins and experimental renal ischemia/reperfusion. *Kidney Int.* Vol.59, pp. 1789–1802

Komada, F.; Nishiguchi, K.; Tanigawara, Y.; Iwakawa, S. & Okumura, K. (1999). Effects of secretable SOD delivered by genetically modified cells on xanthine/xanthine oxidase and paraquat-induced cytotoxicity in vitro. *Biol. Pharm. Bull.* Vol.22, pp. 846–853

Kurokawa, T.; Kobayashi, H.; Nonami, T.; Harada, A.; Nakao, A. & Takagi H. (1996). Mitochondrial glutathione redox and energy producing function during liver ischemia and reperfusion. *J Surg Res* Vol.66, No. 1, pp. 1-5

Land, W.; Schneeberger, H.; Schleibner, S.; Illner, W.D.; Abendroth, D.; Rutili, G.; Arfors, K.E. & Messmer, K. (1994). The beneficial effect of human recombinant superoxide dismutase on acute and chronic rejection events in recipients of cadaveric renal transplants. *Transplantation* Vol.57, pp. 211-217

Levanon, D.; Lieman-Hurwitz, J.; Dafni, N.; Wigderson, M.; Sherman, L.; Bernstein, Y.; Laver-Rudich, Z.; Danciger, E.; Stein, O. & Groner, Y. (1985). Architecture and anatomy of the chromosomal locus in human chromosome 21 encoding the Cu/Zn superoxide dismutase. *EMBO J* Vol.4, No.1, pp. 77-84

Li, J.M.; Fenton, R.A.; Cutler, B.S. & Dobson, J.G. Jr. (1995). Adenosine enhances nitric oxide production by vascular endothelial cells. *Am J Physiol* Vol.269, pp. 519-523

Linas, S.L.; Whittenburg, D. & Repine, J.E. (1990). Role of xanthine oxidase in ischemia/reperfusion injury. *Am J Physiol* Vol.258, pp. 711-716

Lookene, A.; Stenlund, P. & Tibell, L.A. (2000). Characterization of heparin binding of human extracellular superoxide dismutase. *Biochemistry* Vol.39, No.1, pp. 230-236

Lopez-Marti, J.; Sola, A.; Pi, F.; Alfaro, V.; Marco, A. & Hotter G. (2003). Nucleotides modulate renal ischaemia-reperfusion injury by different effects on nitric oxide and superoxide. *Clin Exp Pharmacol Physiol* Vol.30, pp. 242-248

Marklund, S.L. (1984). Extracellular superoxide dismutase in human tissues and human cell lines. *J Clin Invest* Vol.74, No.4, pp. 1398-1403

Marklund, S.L. (1984). Extracellular superoxide dismutase and other superoxide dismutase isoenzymes in tissues from nine mammalian species. *Biochem J* Vol.222, No.3, pp. 649-655

Marklund, S.L. (1992). Regulation by cytokines of extracellular superoxide dysmutase and other superoxide dismutase isoenzymes in fibroblasts. *J Biol Chem* Vol.267, No.10, pp. 6696-6701

Maupoil, V.; Rochette, L.; Tabard, A.; Clauser, P. & Harpey, C. (1990). Evolution of free radical formation during low-flow ischemia and reperfusion in isolated rat heart. *Cardiovasc. Drugs Ther.* Vol.4, pp. 791–795

Monteiro, P.; Duarte, A.I.; Goncalves, L.M.; Moreno, A. & Providencia, L.A, (2004). Protective effect of trimetazidine on myocardial mitochondrial function in an ex vivo model of global myocardial ischemia. *Eur. J. Pharmacol.* Vol.503, pp. 123–128

Muzakova, V.; Kandar, R.; Vojtisek, P.; Skalicky, J. & Cervinkova, Z. (2000) Selective antioxidant enzymes during ischemia/reperfusion in myocardial infarction. *Physiol. Res.* Vol.49, pp. 315–322

Ostrowski, M.; Romanowski, R.; Domanski, L.; Szydłowski, Ł.; Kempińska, A.; Kamiński, M.; Sulikowski, T.; Sieńko, J. & Mizerski, A. (2004). Application of termovision camera in assessment of reperfusion of the transplanted kidney. *Transplant Asia 2004, Singapore,* 1–4 December, Abstr TA 007–8

Oury, T.D; Day B.J. & Crapo, J.D. (1996) Extracellular superoxide dismutase: a regulator of nitric oxide bioavailability. *Lab Invest* Vol.75, No.5, pp. 617-636

Ozden, A.; Aybek, Z.; Saydam, N.; Calli, N.; Saydam, O.; Duzcan, E. & Guner, G. (1998). Cytoprotective effect of trimetazidine on 75 min warm renal ischemia–reperfusion injury in rats. *Eur. Surg. Res.* Vol.30, pp. 227–234

Paller, M.S.; Hoidal, J.R. & Ferris T.F. (1984). Oxygen free radicals in ischemic acute renal failure in the rat. *J. Clin. Invest.* Vol.74, pp. 1156–1164

Pechan, I.; Danova, K.; Olejarova, I.; Halcak, L.; Rendekova, V. & Fabian, J. (2003). Oxidative stress and antioxidant defense systems in patients after heart transplantation. *Wien. Klin. Wochenschr.* Vol.115, pp. 648–651

Petersen, S.V.; Oury, T.D.; Valnickova, Z.; Thøgersen, I.B.; Højrup, P.; Crapo, J.D. & Enghild, J.J. (2003). The dual nature of human extracellular superoxide dismutase: one sequence and two structures. *PNAS* Vol.100, No.24, pp. 13875-13880

Pincemail, J.; Defraigne, J.O.; Franssen, C.; Bonnet, P.; Deby-Dupont, G.; Pirenne, J.; Deby, C.; Lamy, M.; Limet, M. & Meurisse, M. (1993). Evidence for free radical formation during human kidney transplantation. *Free Rad. Biol. Med.* Vol.15, pp. 343–348

Rabb, H.; O'Meara, Y.M.; Maderna, P.; Coleman, P. & Brady, H.R. (1997). Leukocytes, cell adhesion molecules and ischemic acute renal failure. *Kidney Int* Vol.51, pp. 1463-1468

Radi, R.; Rubbo, H.; Bush, K. & Freeman B.A. (1997). Xanthine oxidase binding to glycosaminoglycans: kinetics and superoxide dismutase interactions of immobilized xanthine oxidase-heparin complexes. *Arch Biochem Biophys* Vol.339, No.1, pp. 125-135

Saiki, S.; Yamaguchi, K.; Chijiiwa, K.; Shimizu, S.; Hamasaki, N. & Tanaka, M. (1997). Phosphoenolpyruvate prevents the decline in hepatic ATP and energy charge after ischemia and reperfusion injury in rats. *J. Surg. Res.* Vol.73, pp. 59–65

Sermet, A.; Tasdemir, N.; Deniz, B. & Atmaca M. (2000). Time-dependent changes in superoxide dismutase, catalase, xanthine dehydrogenase and oxidase activities in focal cerebral ischaemia. *Cytobios* Vol.102, No.401, pp. 157-172
Singh, D. & Chopra, K. (2004). Effect of trimetazidine on renal ischemia/reperfusion injury in rats. *Pharmacol. Res.* Vol.50, pp. 623–629
Singh, I.; Gulati, S.; Orak, J.K. & Singh, A.K. (1993). Expression of antioxidant enzymes in rat kidney during ischemia-reperfusion injury. *Mol. Cell. Biochem.* Vol.125, pp. 97–104
Simon, N.; Tillement, J.P.; Albengres, E.; Jaber, K.; Hestin, D.; Roux, F.; Olivier, P.; d'Athis, P.; Kessler, M.; Berland, Y. & Crevat, A. (1997). Potential interest of anti-ischemic agents for limiting cyclosporin A nephrotoxicity. *Int. J. Clin. Pharmacol. Res.* Vol.17, pp. 133–142
Skrzycki, M. & Czeczot, H. (2004). Extracellular superoxide dismutase (EC-SOD)*structure, properties and functions. *Postepy Hig Med Dosw* Vol.58, pp. 301-11
Smolenski, R.T.; Skladanowski, A.C.; Perko, M. & Zydowo, M.M. (1989). Adenylate degradation products release from the human myocardium during open heart surgery. *Clin Chim Acta* Vol.182, pp. 63-74
Smolenski, R.T.; Lachno, D.R.; Ledingham, S.J. & Yacoub, M.H. (1990). Determination of sixteen nucleotides, nucleosides and bases using high-performance liquid chromatography and its application to the study of purine metabolism in hearts for transplantation. *J. Chromatogr.* Vol.527, pp. 414–420
Stralin, P. & Marklund, S.L. (1994). Effects of oxidative stress on expression of extracellular superoxide dysmutase, CuZn-superoxide dismutase and Mn-superoxide dismutase in human dermal fibroblasts. *Biochem J* Vol.298, No.2, pp. 347-352
Sun, K.; Kiss, E.; Bedke, J.; Stojanovic, T.; Li, Y.; Gwinner, W. & Grone, H.J. (2004). Role of xanthine oxidoreductase in experimental acute renal-allograft rejection. *Transplantation* Vol.77, pp. 1683–1692
Tibell, L.A.E.; Sethson, I. & Buevich, A.V. (1997). Characterization of the heparin-binding domain of human extracellular superoxide dismutase. *Biochim Bioph Acta* Vol.1340, No1., pp. 21-32
Tilney, N.L.; Paz, D.; Ames, J.; Gasser, M.; Laskowski, I. & Hancock, W.W. (2001). Ischemia-reperfusion injury. *Transpl. Proc.* Vol.33, pp. 843–844
Vlessis, A.A. & Mela-Riker, L. (1989). Potential role of mitochondrial calcium metabolism during reperfusion injury. *Am. J. Physiol.* Vol.256, pp. 1196–1206
Vigues, F.; Ambrosio, S.; Franco, E. & Bartrons R. (1993). Assessment of purine metabolism in human renal transplantation. *Transplantation* Vol.55, pp. 733-736
Welsh, D.G. & Lindinger, M.I. (1997). Metabolite accumulation increases adenine nucleotide degradation and decreases glycogenolysis in ischaemic rat skeletal muscle. *Acta Physiol. Scand.* Vol.161, pp. 203–210
Woodle, E.S.; Alloway, R.R.; Buell, .JF.; Alexander, J.W.; Munda, R.; Roy-Chaudhury, P., First, M.R.; Cardi, M. & Trofe, J. (2005). Multivariate analysis of risk factors for acute rejection in early corticosteroid cessation regimens under modern immunosuppression. Am J Transplant Vol.5, No. 11, pp. 2740-2744
Yin, M.; Wheeler, M.D.; Connor, H.D.; Zhong, Z.; Bunzelendahl, H.; Dikalova, A.; Smulski, R.J.; Schoonhoven, R.; Mason, R.P.; Swenberg, J.A. & Thuman, R.G. (2001). Cu/Zn-superoxide dismutase gene attenuates ischemia-reperfusion injury in the rat kidney. *J. Am. Soc. Nephrol.* Vol.12, No.12, pp. 2691-2700

Yoo, H.Y.; Chang, M.S. & Rho, H.M. (1999). The activation of the rat copper/zinc superoxide dismutase gene by hydrogen peroxide through the hydrogen peroxide-responsive element and by paraquat and heat shock through the same heat shock element. *J. Biol. Chem.* Vol.274, pp. 23887–23892

Yoshikawa, T.; Minamiyama, Y.; Ichikawa, H.; Takahashi, S.; Naito, Y. & Kondo M. (1997). Role of lipid peroxidation and antioxidants in gastric mucosal injury induced by the hypoxanthine-xanthine oxidase system in rats. *Free Radic Biol Med* Vol.23, No.2, pp. 243-250

Zager, R.A. & Gmur, D.J. (1989). Effects of xanthine oxidase inhibition on ischemic acute renal failure in the rat. *Am J Physiol* Vol.257, pp. 953-958

Zelko, I.N.; Mariani, T.J. & Folz R.J. (2002). Superoxide dismutase multigene family: a comparison of the CuZn-SOD (SOD1), Mn-SOD (SOD2) and EC-SOD (SOD3) gene structures, evolution and expression. *Free Rad Biol Med* Vol.33, No.3, pp. 337-349

13

Chemical Oxygenation of Pancreatic Tissue Prior to Islet Isolation and Transplantation

Heide Brandhorst, Paul R. V. Johnson and Daniel Brandhorst
Nuffield Department of Surgical Sciences, Islet Transplantation Research Group, University of Oxford, Oxford, UK

1. Introduction

Islet transplantation has been established as a promising treatment for patients suffering from life-threatening hypoglycemic episodes (Shapiro et al., 2000, Shapiro et al., 2006). Apart from the achievement of insulin independence, islet transplantation has been shown to improve metabolic control (Meyer et al., 1998), renal and cardiovascular function (Fiorina et al., 2003a, Fiorina et al., 2003b) and to ameliorate the progression of diabetic complications such as retinopathy (Thompson et al., 2008, Warnock et al., 2008). With regard to long-term posttransplant outcome islet transplantation alone has now reached equivalent function rates when compared to pancreas transplantation alone (Bellin et al., 2008, Vantyghem et al., 2009, Maffi et al., 2011). However, the broad application of this treatment on diabetic patients is limited with respect to the number of suitable islet preparations required to induce long-term insulin independence in recipients of islet allografts (Guignard et al., 2004, Kempf et al., 2005).

In order to reduce costs and save donor resources by increasing the efficancy of the technically challenging procedure for human islet isolation, several collaborative networks have been established between geographically distant donor centers and a core facility long-term experienced in producing high-quality islets (Brunicardi et al., 1995, Rydgard et al., 2001, Berney et al., 2004, Goss et al., 2004). Nevertheless, organ shipment between centers is frequently associated with prolonged ischemia. Since approximately 10% of the normal metabolic activity is still operative in ischemic tissue stored at 4°C, hypothermic organ perfusion and subsequent immersion in various preservation solutions such as University of Wisconsin solution (UWS) or Histidine-Tryptophan-Ketoglutarate (HTK) do not completely prevent irreversible pancreas injury once a critical period of cold ischemia is exceeded (Lakey et al., 1995). This can be explained by the specific preference of islets for the respiratory pathway of glucose breakdown providing more than 95% of the total islet ATP production (Erecinska et al., 1992) if an adequate supply oxygen for cellular energy generation is provided (Hellman et al., 1975, Malaisse et al., 1988, Sekine et al., 1994, Tamarit-Rodriguez et al., 1998). Although islets represent only 1% of the pancreatic tissue, they receive more than 12% of the total pancreatic blood flow (Lifson et al., 1980, Jansson and Hellerstrom, 1983). As a consequence, any ischemic situation has dramatic effects on the energy generation of islets (Hellman et al., 1969) which affects energy-sensitive mechanisms such as the sodium-potassium ATPase. Since this enzyme is essentially required to counteract the intracellular osmotic pressure derived from intracellular proteins and impermeable anions, any suppression results in significant cell swelling (Belzer and Southard, 1988). Nevertheless, among other organs the exocrine pancreas has the capability to produce low amounts of energy during ischemia utilizing the Pasteur effect i.e. the increased anaerobic generation of ATP via glycolysis (Hellman et al., 1975). The increased production of lactate causes intracellular acidosis which is one of the main potential triggers of the premature intracellular auto-activation of trypsinogen in acinar cells (Gorelick and Otani, 1999). Another key factor for activation of autolytic processess within the pancreas is the increase of intracellular calcium levels related to the suppression of calcium ATPases by hypoxic conditions. These enzymes are localized in the plasma membrane as well as in mitochondrial and endoplasmatic membranes and maintain low cytoplasmatic calcium concentrations that are essentially required for intracellular signaling (Arnould et al., 1992, Raraty et al., 1999). Since 90% of the proteins that are synthesized by acinar cells are digestive enzymes, also short periods of ischemia provide ideal conditions to trigger autolytic processes in the pancreas (Steer, 1999, Piton et al., 2010). Although the Pasteur effect does not seem to be relevant for islets (Sekine et al., 1994, Tamarit-Rodriguez et al., 1998), it is quite likely that extensive autolysis affects the functional and morphological integrity of adjacent islets (Tanioka et al., 1997a). Analysis of more than 150 diabetic recipients revealed that achievement of insulin independence after islet allotransplantation correlates with short cold ischemia times (CITR, 2009).

Several approaches have been performed to improve oxygen supply of retrieved organs during cold storage: (1) Continuous hypothermic machine perfusion (HMP) (Wight et al., 2003, Schold et al., 2005, Treckmann et al., 2011). Modifications of this preservation procedure include the use of continuously oxygenated perfusion media as demonstrated in different animal models (Manekeller et al., 2005, Maathuis et al., 2007, Stegemann et al., 2009). First attempts to use HMP for pancreas preservation prior to islet isolations were successfully performed in the pig pancreas (Taylor et al., 2010). Nevertheless, with regard to its high costs and its low availability for a maximum of 20% of transplanted organs in the United States (Maathuis et al., 2007) or less than 4% worldwide (Opelz and Dohler, 2007), the relevance of hypothermic machine perfusion is still under discussion (Watson et al., 2010). (2) Persufflation. The continuous gaseous supply of humidified oxygen via the vessels of explanted kidneys or livers represents another approach to improve oxidative energy metabolism during ischemia (Minor and Isselhard, 1996, Pegg et al., 1989, Minor et al., 2002). Recently, a pilot study was performed to utilize persufflation to rescue marginal donor livers for transplantation into patients (Treckmann et al., 2008). Although the principles of retrograde persufflation has been established in 1972 (Isselhard et al., 1972) first pilot trials in human and porcine pancreases have been reported just recently (Scott et al., 2010). However, the concerns that have been raised regarding the logistical disadvantages of hypothermic machine perfusion and costs related to complex equipment for controlled oxygen generation and additional personnel needed for continuous supervision seems also to be valid for persufflation (Feng, 2010). (3) The incubation of organs in oxygen-precharged perfluorocarbons. One member of this chemical group, perfluorodecalin, has been extensively investigated in pancreases obtained from different species. (4) The perfusion of retrieved organs utilizing oxygen-charged emulsions. In the present chapter we focus primarily on the latter two items.

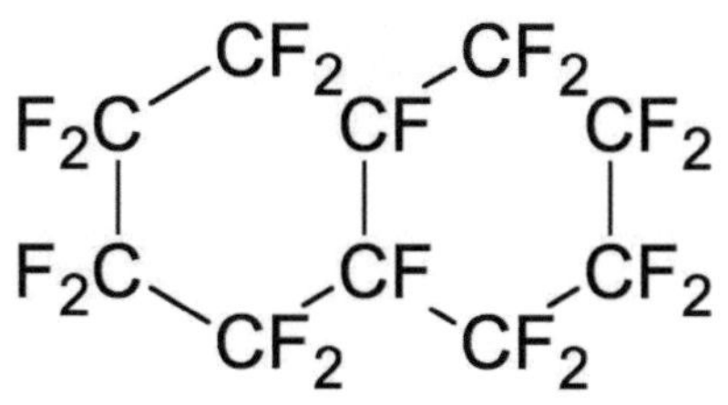

Fig. 1. Chemical structure of perfluorodecalin.

2. Tissue oxygenation prior to solid organ transplantation

Perfluorodecalin (PFD) is a hydrocarbon of bicyclic structure in which all hydrogen atoms are replaced by fluorine atoms (Fig. 1). As a consequence of the high number of carbon-fluorine bonds the specific gravity of PFD is close to 2.0 g/mL (Wong and Lois, 2000). For its use as oxygen carrier it is important that this substance is characterized by a high oxygen dissolving capacity of 45 - 50% (vol./vol.) but at the same time it has a negligible binding constant for oxygen which allows to release oxygen more efficiently into tissue than hemoglobin (Matsumoto and Kuroda, 2002).

First attempts to use PFD for pancreas oxygenation during cold storage prior to autotransplantation were performed in 1988 utilizing canine pancreases (Kuroda et al., 1988). This procedure was established as two-layer method (TLM) because tissue is generally floating on the high gravity PFD and has to be covered by organ preservation solution such as Euro-Collins (Kuroda et al., 1990b) or UWS (Kuroda et al., 1992b) forming a second layer on the inmiscible PFD (Fig. 2). During cold storage the oxygen carrier is continuously gased with 95% oxygen and 5% carbondioxide CO_2 from the bottom of the storage container which results in a partial oxygen pressure (pO_2) of approximately 600 mm Hg (Matsumoto and Kuroda, 2002). As shown in canine (Kuroda et al., 1992a, Matsumoto et al., 1996b) and human pancreases (Kuroda et al., 1992b) this supranormal pO_2 seems to be effective to stimulate the mitochondrial ATP synthesis within the cold-stored pancreatic tissue. The efficiency of this process can be further increased when adenosine is supplied as ATP precursors (Kuroda et al., 1994a, Hiraoka et al., 1994). However, an ongoing ATP synthesis seems to be important not only to preserve pancreatic endocrine function during prolonged cold storage (Kuroda et al., 1991) but also for recovery of ischemically damaged pancreases (Kuroda et al., 1993b).

Inspite of the amazing results that were obtained after autotransplantation of canine pancreases long-term stored for up to 72 and 96 hours (Kawamura et al., 1989, Kuroda et al., 1992c) or exposed to 90 min of warm ischemia time (Kuroda et al., 1993a) only one study to perform TLM prior to clinical pancreas transplantation has been reported so far. Although an improvement in tissue quality and posttransplant function was observed, these differences were not significant when compared to storage in UWS (Matsumoto et al., 2000).

The failure to establish TLM for clinical pancreas transplantation may be related to its complex arrangement which complicates transportation of retrieved organs.

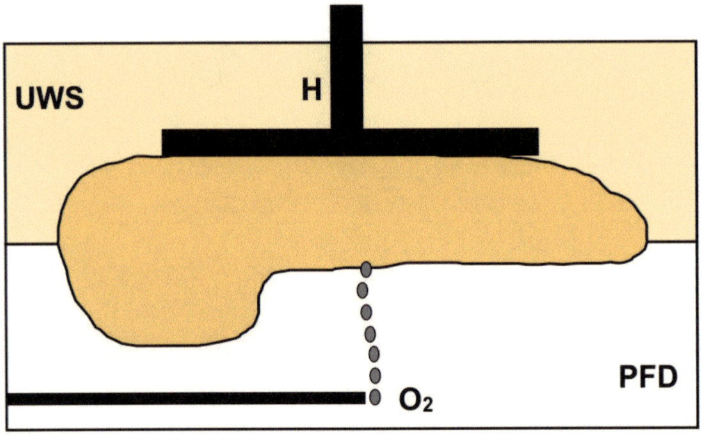

Fig. 2. Pancreas oxygenation utilizing the TLM. The pancreas is floating at the interface between Unversity of Wisconsin solution (UWS) and perfluorodecalin (PFD) and continuously gased with oxygen (O_2). The high gravity of PFD is counteracted utilizing a holder (H) to press the pancreas under the surface of the oxygen carrier.

The practicability of TLM was therefore doubted soon after its introduction. In order to simplify TLM, experiments were performed to assess the efficiency of oxygenation when ischemic pancreases are completely immersed in PFD. It was demonstrated that canine pancreases can be successfully preserved for 48 hours utilizing a one-layer method (OLM) by removing the top-layer consisting of Euro-Collins or UWS (Kuroda et al., 1990a). However, when the cold storage time was prolonged to 96 hours, efficiency of OLM appeared to be inferior compard to TLM (Kin et al., 1993). In contrast, comparative experiments in rats revealed that pancreas preservation for 48 or 72 hours is significantly improved using OLM in comparison to TLM (Urushihara et al., 1992, Urushihara et al., 1994). The principle of OLM was revived some years later in order to improve pig pancreas preservation prior to islet isolation. In agreement with Urushihara´s studies it was found that islet tissue isolated after prolonged cold storage is characterized by a significantly higher potency in terms of insulin secretory capacity, membrane integrity, mitochondrial activity, ATP generation and posttransplant function in diabetic nude mice when the organ is completely immersed in PFD and compared to TLM (Brandhorst et al., 2005).

The idea to immerse organs completely in PFD was picked up to improve preservation of cavernous organs after flushing the cavities with UWS. Using this procedure the small intestine retrieved from rats (Kuroda et al., 1996b, Tsujimura et al., 2004b) or dogs (Tsujimura et al., 2002b, Fujino et al., 2003) could be successfully preserved for 24 to 48 hours. In addition, this technique provided also excellent survival rates of 80% after heterotopic transplantation of UW-perfused rat hearts after cold storage for 48 hours in oxygenated PFD (Kuroda et al., 1995). Remarkably, even higher survival rates in recipients were observed after 72 hours of cold ischemia utilizing a gas mixture composed of 90% oxygen and 10% CO_2. When 100% oxygen was used for preservation complete graft failure was observed (Yoshida et al., 2008). The reason for this discrepancy are unknown but it was speculated that a certain percentage of CO_2 decreases the metabolism of cells beyond the level that can be expected according to the storage temperature (Mitsuda et al., 1987). The period of preservation could successfully be extend to 96 hours when the hearts were continuously perfused during oxygenation with Krebs-Henseleit buffer. In the case that the hearts were continuously perfused for 96 hours with UWS the success rate decreased from 80 to 0% (Hatayama et al., 2009).

Only a few reports have been published so far utilizing conventional TLM for oxygenation of organs other than the pancreas. The suitability of this technique for solid organ preservation was recently demonstrated in syngeneic rat kidneys assessing graft posttransplant survival and apoptosis after 24 hours of cold storage in comparison to UWS. It was observed that posttransplant outcome with respect to one-month survival and creatinine levels was significantly improved compared to UWS storage. In addition, histological tissue damage and frequency of apoptosis were significantly reduced after TLM storage (Marada et al., 2010). In contrast, attempts to preserve porcine kidneys utilizing TLM resulted in increased inflammation, tissue injury and reduced renal function which raised the question whether TLM is suitable for organs from species larger than rodents (Hosgood and Nicholson, 2010). Moreover, experiments to successfully preserve rat lungs during 6 hour-storage by means of TLM failed to demonstrate significant improvement of graft survival compared to cold storage in Ringer´s lactate, UWS or Celsior. Lungs transplanted after TLM were characterized by more infiltrates of inflammatory cells compared to the other experimental groups. Surprisingly, TLM-stored lungs continuously oxygenated during 6 hour-storage had the lowest oyxgen saturation of all media assessed (Liu et al., 2007). It can be speculated that the latter finding was made because the organs were not fixed at the UWS-PFD interface and were rather floating in UWS. In agreement, other approaches to preserve functional integrity of rat livers during extensively prolonged cold storage were also not successful when compared to cold storage in modified UWS (Sumimoto et al., 1990). The authors of this study assumed that in addition to the surface-to-volume ratio also the texture and structure of an organ defines whether inner layers of the tissue can efficiently be supplied with oxygen or not.

3. Pancreas oxygenation for subsequent islet transplantation

First approaches to isolate islets after storage in oxygenated PFD were performed in the dog pancreas. Immediately after retrieval, pancreases were placed on continuously oxygenated PFD until islet isolation was initiated after 3 or 24 hours. It was shown that significantly more islets can be isolated utilizing TLM during prolonged cold storage compared to UWS. However, these experiments are difficult to compare with subsequent studies in human pancreases, since retrieved canine pancreases were not perfused with organ preservation solution prior to cold storage (Tanioka et al., 1997b). The setting for first studies in human pancreases was different to subsequent ones because of logistical reasons. In these experiments retrieved pancreases were shipped in UWS to the isolation facility, dissected to remove excessive fat and connective tissue and either immediately processed or oxygenated by TLM for an additional period of cold storage. Nevertheless, inspite of prolonged cold ischemia time significantly more islets could be isolated and recovered after culture compared to storage in UWS (Matsumoto et al., 2002a). These promising results could be confirmed in a similar setting by achieving a significantly higher islet transplantation rate of 71% in pancreases that were oxygenated for additionally 3 hours compared to UWS storage alone (36%) (Tsujimura et al., 2002a). An even more impressing improvement of the success rate from 11% to 53% was obtained in TLM-oxygenated pancreases from marginal donors older than 50 years (Ricordi et al., 2003). However, it should be stressed that in 80% of the organs used in the latter study oxygenation started immediately after retrieval utilizing oxygen-precharged PFD for oxygen supply. In a number of studies static TLM was implemented as routine procedure for oxygenation of human pancreases during shipment and cold storage prior to clinical islet isolation and transplantation (Hering et al., 2004, Hering et al., 2005, Lee et al., 2004, Goss et al., 2004).

Remarkably, in spite of exposing the tissue to supranormal pO_2, the level of reactive oxygen species (ROS) and their products is significantly lower in TLM-stored pancreases compared to UWS-preserved organs (Salehi et al., 2006). One explanation for this phenomenon is that TLM re-initiates production of ATP in mitochondrial pathways by providing sufficient oxygen levels. One can speculate that maintaining the metabolic activity of mitochondria within a certain range seems to be efficient to prevent excessive generation of ROS in mitochondria as main subcellular producers of ROS (Li et al., 2008, Tsujimura et al., 2004a) and to inhibit mitochondrial pathways of apoptotic cell death (Matsuda et al., 2003).

Beside this important aspect, the main function of mitochondria for cellular metabolism is the production of energy. The relevance of this subcellular structures for islet metabolism is demonstrated by an ATP production that is 17-fold higher compared to the glycolytic metabolization of glucose (Erecinska et al., 1992). The Krebs cycle contributes to the highest extent to the ATP synthesis in islets but is more susceptible toward hypothermia than the cytosolic pathway of non-oxidative glucose metabolization (Escolar et al., 1990). It could be demonstrated that an increase of the storage temperature to 20°C allows for significant reduction of the oxygenation time required to resuscitate canine pancreases after exposure to prolonged warm ischemia (Kuroda et al., 1996a, Matsumoto et al., 1996a). This modification bears the potential of increased flexibility in the logistics of pancreas procurement and subsequent islet isolation by facilitating short-term oxygenation after pancreas arrival in the isolation facility prior to initiating the isolation procedure. Experiments in pig pancreases revealed that determinants of successful islet isolation such as islet yield, viability, and morphological integrity were not reduced compared to non-stored pancreases when the oxygenation temperature was increased to 20°C (Iken et al., 2009). Nevertheless, in spite of an ATP generation that was enormously increased when compared to freshly isolated islets or to oxygenation at 4°C, islets isolated after oxygenation at 20°C were characterized by reduced in vitro function and posttransplant outcome after transplantation into diabetic nude mice (Fig. 3).

These findings are in conflict with the widely accepted hypothesis that the pancreatic ATP content correlates with posttransplant graft function (Kuroda et al., 1991, Kuroda et al., 1992a, Kuroda et al., 1993b). They rather suggest that a temperature-stimulated ATP production does neither reflect tissue viability nor predict posttransplant outcome. In contrast, the relevance of an ongoing ATP production for the recovery of pancreatic tissue predamaged by significant warm ischemia was demonstrated in canine pancreas autotransplantation (Kuroda et al., 1993a, Kuroda et al., 1993b, Kuroda et al., 1994a).

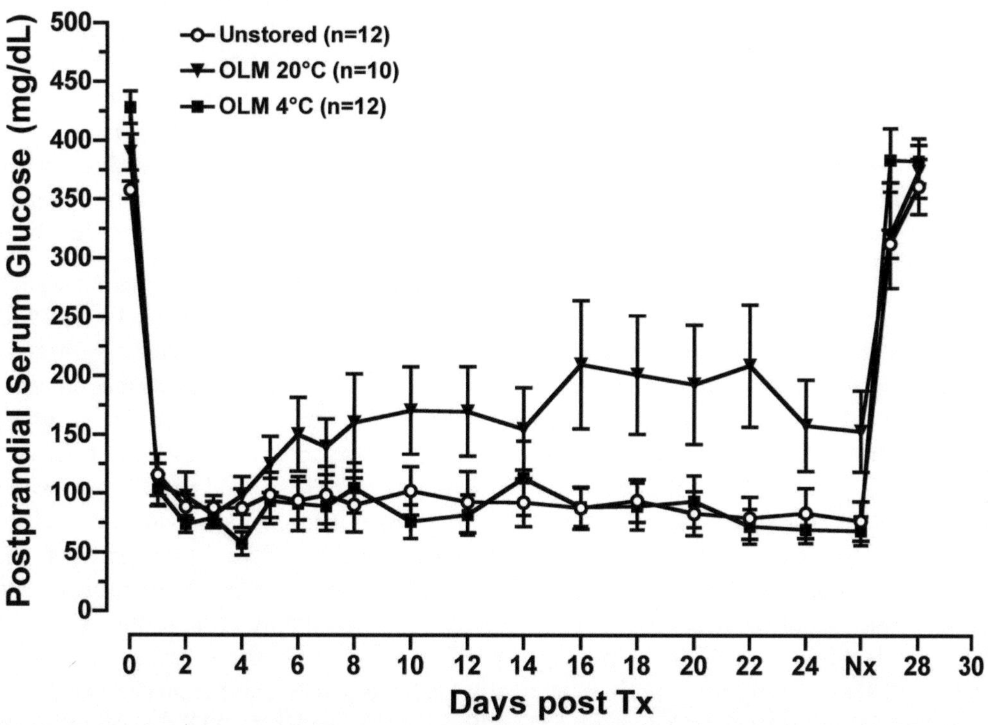

Fig. 3. Non-fasting serum glucose levels in streptozotocin-treated (240 mg/kg) diabetic NMRI nude mice after subcapsular transplantation of pig islets isolated from pancreases (n=3) either immediately procured (unstored, open circles) or subjected to prior oxygenation utilizing the one-layer method (OLM) at 20°C (OLM 20°C, filled triangles) or 4°C (OLM 4°C, filled squares). Graft removal through nephrectomy (Nx) was performed as indicated at day 26 posttransplant.

In agreement, assessment of samples retrieved from cancer patients revealed that TLM increases the ATP content in ischemically predamaged pancreatic tissue (Kuroda et al., 1994b). Islet isolation was not performed in this study. Similarly, a prospective study in adult pigs clearly demonstrated as well that oxygenated PFD can significantly increase the ATP content in islets isolated from pancreases that were pre-exposed to 30 min of warm ischemia. In this study continuous oxygenation for 3 hours did not prevent ischemia-induced deterioration of islet yield and posttransplant function in diabetic nude mice although the ATP content measured after warm ischemia and PFD storage reached the same level as in functioning islets isolated after oxygenation but without warm ischemia time (Brandhorst et al., 2006). This finding is in contradiction with another study in isolated pig islets demonstrating a strong positive correlation between intraislet ATP content and posttransplant function in diabetic nude mice (Kim et al., 2009). Remarkably, the ATP content of the successful (PFD, no warm ischemia) and the failed group (PFD + warm ischemia), as measured in our study, was in a similar range that defined transplant success in Kim´s study. Another approach in isolated pig islets established the ATP-to-

ADP ratio as reliable predictor for posttransplant function using again diabetic nude mice as recipients (Goto et al., 2006). However, another contribution to this ongoing discussion about the relevance of ATP determination in isolated islets clearly preferred the ATP-to-DNA ratio compared to the ATP-to-ADP ratio because of the stability of DNA that favours the preciseness and linearity of this assay (Suszynski et al., 2008). However, as long as no more data are available regarding ischemia, islet ATP production and posttransplant outcome, it can be assumed that oxygen-stimulated ATP synthesis in ischemic pancreases from large mammals does not improve posttransplant islet function.

The scepticisms toward the efficiency of PFD utilized as oxygen carrier for pancreases from large mammals has been additionally supported by two large scale studies which includes more than 350 islet isolations. In contrast to previous experiments that were performed in relatively small numbers of pancreases, these studies clearly revealed that pancreas storage in precharged PFD is unsufficient to increase islet yield, insulin secretory capacity and posttransplant function in recipients when compared to organ storage in UWS (Kin et al., 2006a, Caballero-Corbalan et al., 2007). Several reasons can be discussed for this observation. One important difference that exists between the larger trials and previously published smaller studies concerns the method of oxygenation used. While in the smaller trials pancreases had been subjected to continuous oxygenation for a short period of approximately 3 hours subsequent to cold storage (Tsujimura et al., 2002a, Tsujimura et al., 2004a, Salehi et al., 2006), the large scale trials utilized oxygen-precharged PFD for the entire period of cold ischemia. However, experiments in rats clearly suggested that oxygen-precharged PFD is equivalent to continuously oxygenated PFD with regard to pancreas ATP concentration and isolated islet yield after 24 hours of cold storage (Hiraoka et al., 2001). These findings were confirmed in human pancreases since no difference was observed regarding islet isolation outcome between the static and original TLM (Matsumoto et al., 2002b).

A further technical detail that most likely affects the outcome of pancreas oxygenation is the trimming of the pancreas before incubation in PFD in order to remove non-parenchymatic tissue interfering with oxygen penetration into the pancreatic core. As reported, this was the case for the studies from the Edmonton group (Tsujimura et al., 2002a, Tsujimura et al., 2004a, Salehi et al., 2006, Kin et al., 2006a) but not for the study from the Nordic Network (Caballero-Corbalan et al., 2007). This is of particular relevance when pancreases from obese donors are recovered. These organs are mostly embedded in obstructive quantities of fat aggrevating oxygenation of the tissue (Brandhorst et al., 1995). Apart from these technical considerations it has been doubted that it is physically possible at all to efficiently supply oxygen to a pancreas retrieved from large mammals. pO_2 measurements in different species indicated that the size of a pancreas correlates inversely with the proportion of tissue that can be sufficiently supplied with oxygen following a gradient from the outer surface to the core of the organ. While approximately 80% of a rat pancreas are supplied with oxygen utilizing TLM, this proportion is less than 20% in an averaged-sized pig or human pancreas preserved by the same procedure (Papas et al., 2005, Avgoustiniatos et al., 2006). Since the pancreas volume correlates positively with either body height or body surface area (Goda et al., 2001, de la Grandmaison et al., 2001, Kin et al., 2006b), it can not be excluded that the selection of slim donors has a significant effect on efficiency of pancreas oxygenation during cold storage (Salehi et al., 2006).

4. Alternative oxygen carriers for organ oxygenation

Widely accepted data from canine pancreas autotransplantation suggest a positive correlation between pancreas oxygenation, tissue pO_2, ATP generation and posttransplant graft function (Matsumoto et al., 1996b) but are partially in conflict with findings in human and porcine pancreas preservation as discussed above. The contradiction may be explained, on the one hand, by species-dependent differences with regard to pancreas size, firmness and texture. On the other hand, it has to be discussed whether the hydrophobic and lipophobic character of PFD prevents oxygen penetration into the pancreatic core at all. The solubility of PFD in native olive oil, a parameter for lipophilicity, is only 1.1%. Amphiphilic oxygen carriers, such as perfluorohexyloctan (F6H8), a semifluorinated alkane with a similar oxygen-dissolving capacity as PFD, reach a solubility of 23.4% (Hoerauf et al., 2001). The low lipophobic character of F6H8 can be attributed to the high number of lipophilic CH-groups (Fig. 4), which are completely absent in PFD (Fig. 1). As a result, F6H8 has a much lower specific gravity (1.35 g/cm^3) compared to PFD (1.93 g/cm^3). We hypothesized that oxygenation of ischemic human pancreatic tissue can significantly be improved when lipophilic oxygen carriers are used for shipment from the donor to the recipient center.

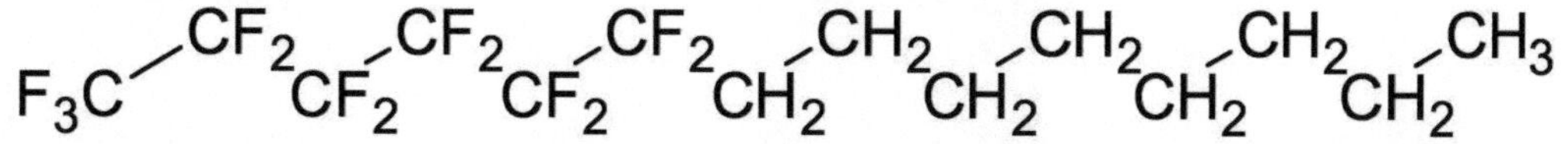

Fig. 4. Chemical structure of perfluorohexyloctan (F6H8).

Initial experiments in rats clearly demonstrated that pancreas oxygenation utilizing the lipophilic compound F6H8 for 24 hours of cold storage significantly improved islet isolation outcome in terms of yield, viability and functional integrity of isolated islets as well as transplant function in diabetic nude mice when compared to PFD (Brandhorst et al., 2009). In agreement with the postulation of Avgoustiniatos (Avgoustiniatos et al., 2006), small organs like rat pancreases can efficently be provided with oxygen regardless of the chemical characteristics of the oxygen carrier used. Utilizing Clark-type microelectrodes probes we found that the pO_2 levels in oxygenated rat pancreases exceeded that of non-stored rat pancreatic tissue by four-fold. Nevertheless, inspite of the extremely increased intrapancreatic pO_2, the ATP content in oxygenated rat pancreases was unexpectedly low when compared to unstored organs. The relatively low ATP production may be explained by the observation that the capacity of oxygenated PFD to stimulated oxidative ATP synthesis in rat pancreases is limited to approximately 12 hours (Scott et al., 2008). It can further be speculated whether a supplementation of fuels such as glucose or pyruvate, which are missing in UWS or HTK, would prevent this energy exhaustion in long-term preserved tissue.

In contrast to the observations made in rats, we demonstrated in porcine and human pancreases that the amphiphilic compound F6H8 is superior for the oxygen supply of pancreatic tissue compared to inert PFD (Fig. 5). To discuss the relevance of these findings for preservation of islet tissue prior to human islet isolation, we have to refer to the extensive work of Carlsson et al. evaluating the pO_2 in native and transplanted islet tissue from rats. According to the findings of this group, the pO_2 in human pancreases oxygenated by means of F6H8 reached only 20 – 25% of native vascularized pancreatic tissue provided that human and rat tissue are similar in blood supply and oxygen consumption (Carlsson et al., 1998, Carlsson et al., 2000). Nevertheless, transplanted human islets can survive for months under hypoxic conditions that correspond to a pO_2 of approximately 5 mm Hg or less (Carlsson et al., 2002). This would mean that the level of oxygenation provided by F6H8 is sufficient to support islet survival during prolonged pancreas cold storage.

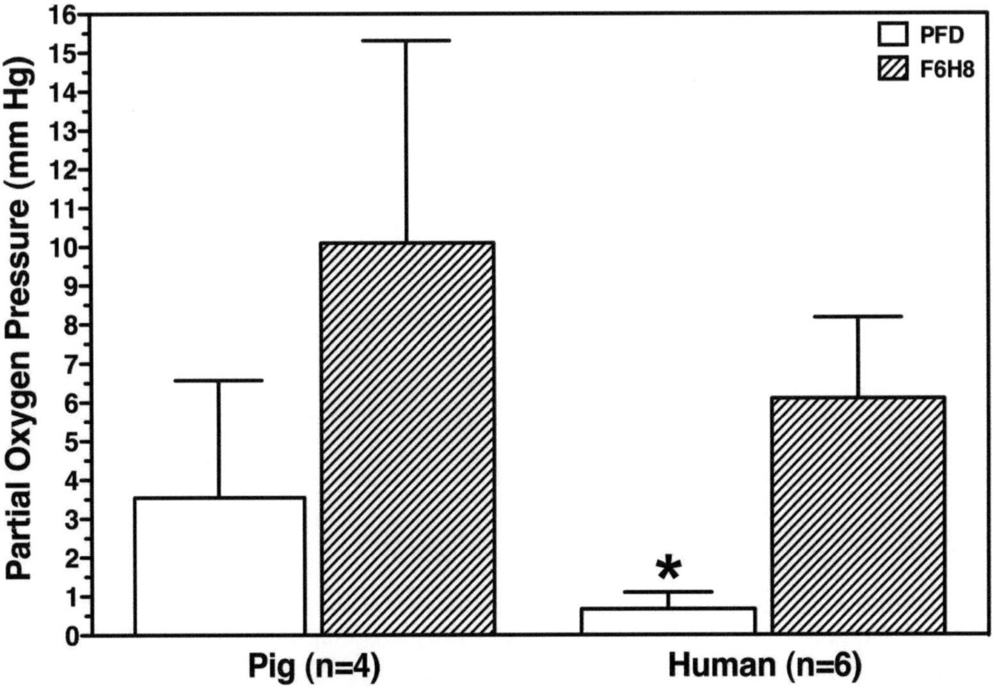

Fig. 5. Intrapancreatic partial oxygen pressure measured in porcine and human pancreases after static oxygenation in PFD (blank bars) or F6H8 (hatched bars) for 8 (pig, n=4) or 24 hours (human, n=6) of cold storage. Pancreas oxygenation was performed utilizing the one-layer method. *P<0.05 by Mann-Whitney test as indicated (mean ± SEM).

The significance of this assumption for human islet isolation outcome was confirmed in human research grade pancreases processed for subsequent islet isolation after storage in oxygen-precharged F6H8 or PFD for at least 24 hours. Compared with PFD, F6H8 significantly increased islet yield, islet cell survival after culture, insulin secretory capacity and posttransplant function in diabetic nude mice (Brandhorst et al., 2010). In agreement, studies in guinea pigs demonstrated improved quality of hearts that were stored for 6 hours of cold ischemia in oxygenated F6H10, another compound belonging to the group of semifluorinated alkanes (Isaka et al., 2005).

Nevertheless, larger organs such as liver or kidney may require vascular supply of oxygen for efficient oxygenation of the entire tissue volume (Hosgood and Nicholson, 2010). As discussed above, the efforts and costs related to continuous perfusion of donor organs with oxygenated preservation solutions are currently limiting the broad implementation of this technique (Opelz and Dohler, 2007). Emulsions made from perfluorocarbon-derived oxygen carriers represent an alternative that is easy to apply during regular organ procurement. We hypothesized that the vascular flush as routinely performed during organ procurement can cover the requirements for both effective tissue preservation and oxygen supply of large organs, if organ preservation solutions combine a high oxygen-dissolving capacity with characteristics of HTK or UWS, vital to prevent cell swelling and maintain tissue viability during cold storage (Belzer and Southard, 1988). However, the chemical requirements to manufacture stable emulsions including a significant percentage of oxygen carrier clearly favour the utilization of semifluorinated alkanes such as F6H8 or F6H10 which possess amphiphilic characteristics in contrast to PFD (Klar et al., 1998, Voiglio et al., 1996).

5. Conclusions

In summary, the prevention of ischemically induced tissue damage in retrieved donor organs during cold ischemia is still a major logistical problem that remains to be solved. This concerns particularly organs with a low ischemic tolerance like the pancreas including the islets of Langerhans. Tissue oxygenation utilizing complex techniques such as continuous machine perfusion or persufflation is more or less established but available only for a limited number of procurement centers. In contrast, the concept to provide oxygen by means of precharged perfluorocarbons for static cold storage is attractive because of its low costs and simplicity. Although the majority of findings obtained in smaller animals clearly indicate that this concept is feasible, efficient oxygenation of organs retrieved from larger species such as humans is difficult because of organ size. One solution to solve the problem of efficient oxygen supply may be provided by utilization of semifluorinated alkanes, lipophilic oxygen carriers that can penetrate into the core of ischemic organs in contrast to inert substances like PFD. Another way to overcome the hurdle to completely oxygenate larger human organs is to use vascular perfusion as routinely performed during organ procurement to administrate oxygen-precharged emulsions. For effective organ preservation these emulsions should ideally combine a high oxygen-dissolving capacity with characteristics of established organ preservation media such as HTK or UWS. Efforts are currently undertaken to evaluate the potential of this new concept in large animal models.

6. Acknowledgements

For the great support and contribution to the experiments presented the authors thank particularly: Marcus Iken from the Dept. of Gastroenterology, Hepatology and Endocrinology, Medical School, Hannover, Germany; and Bernhard Günther, Sonja and Bastian Theisinger from Novaliq GmbH, Heidelberg, Germany.

7. References

Arnould, T., Michiels, C., Alexandre, I. & Remacle, J. (1992). Effect of hypoxia upon intracellular calcium concentration of human endothelial cells. *Journal of Cellular Physiology*, Vol.152, No.1, pp. 215-221.

Avgoustiniatos, E.S., Hering, B.J. & Papas, K.K. (2006). The rat pancreas is not an appropriate model for testing the preservation of the human pancreas with the two-layer method. *Transplantation*, Vol.81, No.10, pp. 1471-1472; author reply 1472.

Bellin, M.D., Kandaswamy, R., Parkey, J., Zhang, H.J., Liu, B., Ihm, S.H., Ansite, J.D., Witson, J., Bansal-Pakala, P., Balamurugan, A.N., Papas, K.K., Sutherland, D.E., Moran, A. & Hering, B.J. (2008). Prolonged insulin independence after islet allotransplants in recipients with type 1 diabetes. *Am J Transplant*, Vol.8, No.11, pp. 2463-2470.

Belzer, F.O. & Southard, J.H. (1988). Principles of solid-organ preservation by cold storage. *Transplantation*, Vol.45, No.4, pp. 673-676.

Berney, T., Benhamou, P.Y., Kessler, L. & Morel, P. (2004). Islet transplantation in multicenter networks: the GRAGIL example. *Current Opinion in Organ Transplantation*, Vol.9, pp. 72-76.

Brandhorst, D., Iken, M., Brendel, M.D., Bretzel, R.G. & Brandhorst, H. (2005). Successful pancreas preservation by a perfluorocarbon-based one-layer method for subsequent pig islet isolation. *Transplantation*, Vol.79, No.4, pp. 433-437.

Brandhorst, D., Iken, M., Bretzel, R.G. & Brandhorst, H. (2006). Pancreas storage in oxygenated perfluorodecalin does not restore post-transplant function of isolated pig islets pre-damaged by warm ischemia. *Xenotransplantation*, Vol.13, No.5, pp. 465-470.

Brandhorst, H., Asif, S., Andersson, K., Theisinger, B., Andersson, H.H., Felldin, M., Foss, A., Salmela, K., Tibell, A., Tufveson, G., Korsgren, O. & Brandhorst, D. (2010). A new oxygen carrier for improved long-term storage of human pancreata before islet isolation. *Transplantation*, Vol.89, No.2, pp. 155-160.

Brandhorst, H., Brandhorst, D., Hering, B.J., Federlin, K. & Bretzel, R.G. (1995). Body mass index of pancreatic donors: a decisive factor for human islet isolation. *Experimental and Clinical Endocrinology and Diabetes*, Vol.103 Suppl 2, pp. 23-26.

Brandhorst, H., Theisinger, B., Yamaya, H., Henriksnas, J., Carlsson, P.O., Korsgren, O. & Brandhorst, D. (2009). Perfluorohexyloctane improves long-term storage of rat pancreata for subsequent islet isolation. *Transpl Int*, Vol.22, No.10, pp. 1017-1022.

Brunicardi, F.C., Atiya, A., Stock, P., Kenmochi, T., Une, S., Benhamou, P.Y., Watt, P.C., Miyamato, M., Wantanabe, Y., Nomura, Y. & et al. (1995). Clinical islet transplantation experience of the University of California Islet Transplant Consortium. *Surgery*, Vol.118, No.6, pp. 967-971; discussion 971-962.

Caballero-Corbalan, J., Eich, T., Lundgren, T., Foss, A., Felldin, M., Kallen, R., Salmela, K., Tibell, A., Tufveson, G., Korsgren, O. & Brandhorst, D. (2007). No beneficial effect of two-layer storage compared with UW-storage on human islet isolation and transplantation. *Transplantation*, Vol.84, No.7, pp. 864-869.

Carlsson, P.O., Liss, P., Andersson, A. & Jansson, L. (1998). Measurements of oxygen tension in native and transplanted rat pancreatic islets. *Diabetes*, Vol.47, No.7, pp. 1027-1032.

Carlsson, P.O., Palm, F., Andersson, A. & Liss, P. (2000). Chronically decreased oxygen tension in rat pancreatic islets transplanted under the kidney capsule. *Transplantation*, Vol.69, No.5, pp. 761-766.

Carlsson, P.O., Palm, F. & Mattsson, G. (2002). Low revascularization of experimentally transplanted human pancreatic islets. *J Clin Endocrinol Metab*, Vol.87, No.12, pp. 5418-5423.

CITR (2009). 2007 Update on Allogeneic Islet Transplantation from the Collaborative Islet Transplant Registry (CITR). *Cell Transplantation*,

de la Grandmaison, G.L., Clairand, I. & Durigon, M. (2001). Organ weight in 684 adult autopsies: new tables for a Caucasoid population. *Forensic Science International*, Vol.119, No.2, pp. 149-154.

Erecinska, M., Bryla, J., Michalik, M., Meglasson, M.D. & Nelson, D. (1992). Energy metabolism in islets of Langerhans. *Biochimica et Biophysica Acta*, Vol.1101, No.3, pp. 273-295.

Escolar, J.C., Hoo-Paris, R., Castex, C. & Sutter, B.C. (1990). Effect of low temperatures on glucose-induced insulin secretion and glucose metabolism in isolated pancreatic islets of the rat. *J Endocrinol*, Vol.125, No.1, pp. 45-51.

Feng, S. (2010). Donor intervention and organ preservation: where is the science and what are the obstacles? *Am J Transplant*, Vol.10, No.5, pp. 1155-1162.

Fiorina, P., Folli, F., Bertuzzi, F., Maffi, P., Finzi, G., Venturini, M., Socci, C., Davalli, A., Orsenigo, E., Monti, L., Falqui, L., Uccella, S., La Rosa, S., Usellini, L., Properzi, G., Di Carlo, V., Del Maschio, A., Capella, C. & Secchi, A. (2003a). Long-term beneficial effect of islet transplantation on diabetic macro-/microangiopathy in type 1 diabetic kidney-transplanted patients. *Diabetes Care*, Vol.26, No.4, pp. 1129-1136.

Fiorina, P., Folli, F., Zerbini, G., Maffi, P., Gremizzi, C., Di Carlo, V., Socci, C., Bertuzzi, F., Kashgarian, M. & Secchi, A. (2003b). Islet transplantation Is associated with improvement of renal function among uremic patients with type I diabetes mellitus and kidney transplants. *J Am Soc Nephrol*, Vol.14, pp. 2150-2158.

Fujino, Y., Kakinoki, K., Suzuki, Y., Li, S., Tanaka, T., Tanioka, Y., Sakai, T., Ku, Y. & Kuroda, Y. (2003). Successful 24-hour preservation of ischemically damaged canine small intestine by the cavitary two-layer method. *Transplantation*, Vol.76, No.5, pp. 777-780.

Goda, K., Sasaki, E., Nagata, K., Fukai, M., Ohsawa, N. & Hahafusa, T. (2001). Pancreatic volume in type 1 and type 2 diabetes mellitus. *Acta Diabetologica*, Vol.38, No.3, pp. 145-149.

Gorelick, F.S. & Otani, T. (1999). Mechanisms of intracellular zymogen activation. *Baillieres Best Pract Res Clin Gastroenterol*, Vol.13, No.2, pp. 227-240.

Goss, J.A., Goodpastor, S.E., Brunicardi, F.C., Barth, M.H., Soltes, G.D., Garber, A.J., Hamilton, D.J., Alejandro, R. & Ricordi, C. (2004). Development of a human pancreatic islet-transplant program through a collaborative relationship with a remote islet-isolation center. *Transplantation*, Vol.77, No.3, pp. 462-466.

Goto, M., Holgersson, J., Kumagai-Braesch, M. & Korsgren, O. (2006). The ADP/ATP ratio: A novel predictive assay for quality assessment of isolated pancreatic islets. *Am J Transplant*, Vol.6, No.10, pp. 2483-2487.

Guignard, A.P., Oberholzer, J., Benhamou, P.Y., Touzet, S., Bucher, P., Penfornis, A., Bayle, F., Kessler, L., Thivolet, C., Badet, L., Morel, P. & Colin, C. (2004). Cost analysis of human islet transplantation for the treatment of type 1 diabetes in the Swiss-French Consortium GRAGIL. *Diabetes Care*, Vol.27, No.4, pp. 895-900.

Hatayama, N., Yoshida, Y. & Seki, K. (2009). A study on the perfusion preservation, resuscitation, and transplantation of a rat heart isolated for 96 hours. *Cell Transplantation*, Vol.18, No.5, pp. 529-534.

Hellman, B., Idahl, L.A. & Danielsson, A. (1969). Adenosine triphosphate levels of mammalian pancreatic B cells after stimulation with glucose and hypoglycemic sulfonylureas. *Diabetes*, Vol.18, No.8, pp. 509-516.

Hellman, B., Idahl, L.A., Sehlin, J. & Taljedal, I.B. (1975). Influence of anoxia on glucose metabolism in pancreatic islets: lack of correlation between fructose-1,6-diphosphate and apparent glycolytic flux. *Diabetologia*, Vol.11, No.6, pp. 495-500.

Hering, B.J., Kandaswamy, R., Ansite, J.D., Eckman, P.M., Nakano, M., Sawada, T., Matsumoto, I., Ihm, S.H., Zhang, H.J., Parkey, J., Hunter, D.W. & Sutherland, D.E. (2005). Single-donor, marginal-dose islet transplantation in patients with type 1 diabetes. *Jama*, Vol.293, No.7, pp. 830-835.

Hering, B.J., Kandaswamy, R., Harmon, J.V., Ansite, J.D., Clemmings, S.M., Sakai, T., Paraskevas, S., Eckman, P.M., Sageshima, J., Nakano, M., Sawada, T., Matsumoto, I., Zhang, H.J., Sutherland, D.E. & Bluestone, J.A. (2004). Transplantation of Cultured Islets from Two-Layer Preserved Pancreases in Type 1 Diabetes with Anti-CD3 Antibody. *Am J Transplant*, Vol.4, No.3, pp. 390-401.

Hiraoka, K., Kuroda, Y., Tanioka, Y., Matsumoto, S., Fujino, Y., Morita, A., Ku, Y. & Saitoh, Y. (1994). Adenosine is a key component in preservation of ischemically damaged canine pancreas by the two-layer cold storage method. *Transplant Proc*, Vol.26, No.2, pp. 953-955.

Hiraoka, K., Trexler, A., Eckman, E., Stage, A., Nevile, S., Sageshima, J., Shibata, S., Sutherland, D.E. & Hering, B.J. (2001). Successful pancreas preservation before islet isolation by the simplified two-layer cold storage method. *Transplantation Proceedings*, Vol.33, No.1-2, pp. 952-953.

Hoerauf, H., Kobuch, K., Dresp, J. & Menz, D.H. (2001). Combined use of partially fluorinated alkanes, perfluorocarbon liquids and silicone oil: an experimental study. *Graefes Arch Clin Exp Ophthalmol*, Vol.239, No.5, pp. 373-381.

Hosgood, S.A. & Nicholson, M.L. (2010). The Role of Perfluorocarbon in Organ Preservation. *Transplantation*, Vol.89, No.10, pp. 1169-1175.

Iken, M., Brandhorst, H., Korsgren, O. & Brandhorst, D. (2009). Pig pancreas oxygenation at 20 degrees C increases islet ATP generation but deteriorates islet function. *Cell Transplantation*, Vol.18, No.7, pp. 745-751.

Isaka, M., Imamura, M., Sakuma, I., Shiiya, N., Fukushima, S., Nakai, K., Kitabatake, A. & Yasuda, K. (2005). Cardioprotective effect of perfluorochemical emulsion for cardiac preservation after six-hour cold storage. *Asaio J*, Vol.51, No.4, pp. 434-439.

Isselhard, W., Berger, M., Denecke, H., Witte, J., Fischer, J.H. & Molzberger, H. (1972). Metabolism of canine kidneys in anaerobic ischemia and in aerobic ischemia by persufflation with gaseous oxygen. *Pflugers Archiv. European Journal of Physiology*, Vol.337, No.2, pp. 87-106.

Jansson, L. & Hellerstrom, C. (1983). Stimulation by glucose of the blood flow to the pancreatic islets of the rat. *Diabetologia*, Vol.25, No.1, pp. 45-50.

Kawamura, T., Kuroda, Y., Suzuki, Y., Fujiwara, H., Fujino, Y., Yamamoto, K. & Saitoh, Y. (1989). Seventy-two-hour preservation of the canine pancreas by the two-layer (Euro-Collins' solution/perfluorochemical) cold storage method. *Transplantation*, Vol.47, No.5, pp. 776-778.

Kempf, M.C., Andres, A., Morel, P., Benhamou, P.Y., Bayle, F., Kessler, L., Badet, L., Thivolet, C., Penfornis, A., Renoult, E., Brun, J.M., Atlan, C., Renard, E., Colin, C., Milliat-Guittard, L., Pernin, N., Demuylder-Mischler, S., Toso, C., Bosco, D. & Berney, T. (2005). Logistics and transplant coordination activity in the GRAGIL Swiss-French multicenter network of islet transplantation. *Transplantation*, Vol.79, No.9, pp. 1200-1205.

Kim, J.H., Park, S.G., Lee, H.N., Lee, Y.Y., Park, H.S., Kim, H.I., Yu, J.E., Kim, S.H., Park, C.G., Ha, J., Kim, S.J. & Park, K.S. (2009). ATP measurement predicts porcine islet transplantation outcome in nude mice. *Transplantation*, Vol.87, No.2, pp. 166-169.

Kin, S., Stephanian, E., Gores, P., Mass, A., Flores, H., Nakai, I., Tamura, K., Gruessner, R. & Sutherland, D.E. (1993). 96-hour cold-storage preservation of the canine pancreas with oxygenation using perfluorochemical. *Transplantation*, Vol.55, No.1, pp. 229-230.

Kin, T., Mirbolooki, M., Salehi, P., Tsukada, M., O'Gorman, D., Imes, S., Ryan, E.A., Shapiro, A.M. & Lakey, J.R. (2006a). Islet isolation and transplantation outcomes of pancreas preserved with University of Wisconsin solution versus two-layer method using preoxygenated perfluorocarbon. *Transplantation*, Vol.82, No.10, pp. 1286-1290.

Kin, T., Murdoch, T.B., Shapiro, A.M. & Lakey, J.R. (2006b). Estimation of pancreas weight from donor variables. *Cell Transplantation*, Vol.15, No.2, pp. 181-185.

Klar, E., Kraus, T., Reuter, P., Mehrabi, A., Fernandes, L.P., Angelescu, M., Gebhard, M.M. & Herfarth, C. (1998). Oxygenated perfusion for liver preservation: a perfluorodecalin-UW emulsion is not feasible. *Transplant Proc*, Vol.30, No.7, pp. 3707-3710.

Kuroda, Y., Fujino, Y., Kawamura, T., Suzuki, Y., Fujiwara, H. & Saitoh, Y. (1990a). Excellence of perfluorochemical with simple oxygen bubbling as a preservation medium for simple cold storage of canine pancreas. *Transplantation*, Vol.49, No.3, pp. 648-650.

Kuroda, Y., Fujino, Y., Kawamura, T., Suzuki, Y., Fujiwara, H. & Saitoh, Y. (1990b). Mechanism of oxygenation of pancreas during preservation by a two-layer (Euro-Collins' solution/perfluorochemical) cold-storage method. *Transplantation*, Vol.49, No.4, pp. 694-696.

Kuroda, Y., Fujino, Y., Morita, A., Ku, Y. & Saitoh, Y. (1991). Correlation between high adenosine triphosphate tissue concentration and good posttransplant outcome for the canine pancreas graft after preservation by the two-layer cold storage method. *Transplantation*, Vol.52, No.6, pp. 989-991.

Kuroda, Y., Fujino, Y., Morita, A., Tanioka, Y., Ku, Y. & Saitoh, Y. (1992a). The mechanism of action of the two-layer (Euro-Collins' solution/perfluorochemical) cold-storage method in canine pancreas preservation--the effect of 2,4 dinitrophenol on graft viability and adenosine triphosphate tissue concentration. *Transplantation*, Vol.53, No.5, pp. 992-994.

Kuroda, Y., Fujino, Y., Morita, A., Tanioka, Y., Ku, Y. & Saitoh, Y. (1992b). Oxygenation of the human pancreas during preservation by a two-layer (University of Wisconsin solution/perfluorochemical) cold-storage method. *Transplantation*, Vol.54, No.3, pp. 561-562.

Kuroda, Y., Fujino, Y., Morita, A., Tanioka, Y., Suzuki, Y., Kawamura, T., Ku, Y. & Saitoh, Y. (1992c). Successful 96-hour preservation of the canine pancreas. *Transpl Int*, Vol.5 Suppl 1, pp. S388-390.

Kuroda, Y., Hiraoka, K., Tanioka, Y., Matsumoto, S., Morita, A., Fujino, Y., Suzuki, Y., Ku, Y. & Saitoh, Y. (1994a). Role of adenosine in preservation by the two-layer method of ischemically damaged canine pancreas. *Transplantation*, Vol.57, No.7, pp. 1017-1020.

Kuroda, Y., Kawamura, T., Suzuki, Y., Fujiwara, H., Yamamoto, K. & Saitoh, Y. (1988). A new, simple method for cold storage of the pancreas using perfluorochemical. *Transplantation*, Vol.46, No.3, pp. 457-460.

Kuroda, Y., Kawamura, T., Tanioka, Y., Morita, A., Hiraoka, K., Matsumoto, S., Kim, Y., Fujino, Y., Suzuki, Y., Ku, Y. & et al. (1995). Heart preservation using a cavitary two-layer (University of Wisconsin solution/perfluorochemical) cold storage method. *Transplantation*, Vol.59, No.5, pp. 699-701.

Kuroda, Y., Matsumoto, S., Fujita, H., Tanioka, Y., Sakai, T., Hamano, M., Hiraoka, K., Kim, Y., Suzuki, Y., Ku, Y. & Saitoh, Y. (1996a). Resuscitation of ischemically damaged pancreas during short-term preservation at 20 degrees C by the two-layer (University of Wisconsin solution/perfluorochemical) method. *Transplantation*, Vol.61, No.1, pp. 28-30.

Kuroda, Y., Morita, A., Fujino, Y., Tanioka, Y., Ku, Y. & Saitoh, Y. (1993a). Restoration of pancreas graft function preserved by a two-layer (University of Wisconsin solution/perfluorochemical) cold storage method after significant warm ischemia. *Transplantation*, Vol.55, No.1, pp. 227-228.

Kuroda, Y., Morita, A., Fujino, Y., Tanioka, Y., Ku, Y. & Saitoh, Y. (1993b). Successful extended preservation of ischemically damaged pancreas by the two-layer (University of Wisconsin solution/perfluorochemical) cold storage method. *Transplantation*, Vol.56, No.5, pp. 1087-1090.

Kuroda, Y., Sakai, T., Suzuki, Y., Tanioka, Y., Matsumoto, S., Kim, Y., Fujita, H., Hamano, M., Hasegawa, Y., Ku, Y. & Saitoh, Y. (1996b). Small bowel preservation using a cavitary two-layer (University of Wisconsin solution/perfluorochemical) cold storage method. *Transplantation*, Vol.61, No.3, pp. 370-373.

Kuroda, Y., Tanioka, Y., Morita, A., Hiraoka, K., Matsumoto, S., Fujino, Y., Ku, Y., Saitoh, Y., Sugihara, J., Okumura, S. & et al. (1994b). The possibility of restoration of human pancreas function during preservation by the two-layer (University of Wisconsin solution/perfluorochemical) method following normothermic ischemia. *Transplantation*, Vol.57, No.2, pp. 282-285.

Lakey, J.R., Rajotte, R.V., Warnock, G.L. & Kneteman, N.M. (1995). Human pancreas preservation prior to islet isolation. Cold ischemic tolerance. *Transplantation*, Vol.59, No.5, pp. 689-694.

Lee, T.C., Barshes, N.R., Brunicardi, F.C., Alejandro, R., Ricordi, C., Nguyen, L. & Goss, J.A. (2004). Procurement of the human pancreas for pancreatic islet transplantation. *Transplantation*, Vol.78, No.3, pp. 481-483.

Li, N., Frigerio, F. & Maechler, P. (2008). The sensitivity of pancreatic beta-cells to mitochondrial injuries triggered by lipotoxicity and oxidative stress. *Biochem Soc Trans*, Vol.36, No.Pt 5, pp. 930-934.

Lifson, N., Kramlinger, K.G., Mayrand, R.R. & Lender, E.J. (1980). Blood flow to the rabbit pancreas with special reference to the islets of Langerhans. *Gastroenterology*, Vol.79, No.3, pp. 466-473.

Liu, C.C., Hsu, P.K., Huang, W.C., Huang, M.H. & Hsu, H.S. (2007). Two-layer method (UW solution/perfluorochemical plus O2) for lung preservation in rat lung transplantation. *Transplantation Proceedings*, Vol.39, No.10, pp. 3019-3023.

Maathuis, M.H., Manekeller, S., van der Plaats, A., Leuvenink, H.G., t Hart, N.A., Lier, A.B., Rakhorst, G., Ploeg, R.J. & Minor, T. (2007). Improved kidney graft function after preservation using a novel hypothermic machine perfusion device. *Ann Surg*, Vol.246, No.6, pp. 982-988; discussion 989-991.

Maffi, P., Scavini, M., Socci, C., Piemonti, L., Caldara, R., Gremizzi, C., Melzi, R., Nano, R., Orsenigo, E., Venturini, M., Staudacher, C., Del Maschio, A. & Secchi, A. (2011). Risks and benefits of transplantation in the cure of type 1 diabetes: whole pancreas versus islet transplantation. A single center study. *Rev Diabet Stud*, Vol.8, No.1, pp. 44-50.

Malaisse, W.J., Rasschaert, J., Zahner, D. & Sener, A. (1988). Hexose metabolism in pancreatic islets: the Pasteur effect. *Diabetes Res*, Vol.7, No.2, pp. 53-58.

Manekeller, S., Leuvenink, H., Sitzia, M. & Minor, T. (2005). Oxygenated machine perfusion preservation of predamaged kidneys with HTK and Belzer machine perfusion solution: an experimental study in pigs. *Transplant Proc*, Vol.37, No.8, pp. 3274-3275.

Marada, T., Zacharovova, K. & Saudek, F. (2010). Perfluorocarbon improves post-transplant survival and early kidney function following prolonged cold ischemia. *European Surgical Research*, Vol.44, No.3-4, pp. 170-178.

Matsuda, T., Suzuki, Y., Tanioka, Y., Toyama, H., Kakinoki, K., Hiraoka, K., Fujino, Y. & Kuroda, Y. (2003). Pancreas preservation by the 2-layer cold storage method before islet isolation protects isolated islets against apoptosis through the mitochondrial pathway. *Surgery*, Vol.134, No.3, pp. 437-445.

Matsumoto, S., Kandaswamy, R., Sutherland, D.E., Hassoun, A.A., Hiraoka, K., Sageshima, J., Shibata, S., Tanioka, Y. & Kuroda, Y. (2000). Clinical application of the two-layer

(University of Wisconsin solution/perfluorochemical plus O2) method of pancreas preservation before transplantation. *Transplantation*, Vol.70, No.5, pp. 771-774.

Matsumoto, S. & Kuroda, Y. (2002). Perfluorocarbon for organ preservation before transplantation. *Transplantation*, Vol.74, No.12, pp. 1804-1809.

Matsumoto, S., Kuroda, Y., Fujita, H., Tanioka, Y., Kim, Y., Sakai, T., Hamano, M., Suzuki, Y., Ku, Y. & Saitoh, Y. (1996a). Resuscitation of ischemically damaged pancreas by the two-layer (University of Wisconsin solution/perfluorochemical) mild hypothermic storage method. *World J Surg*, Vol.20, No.8, pp. 1030-1034.

Matsumoto, S., Kuroda, Y., Hamano, M., Kim, Y., Suzuki, Y., Ku, Y. & Saitoh, Y. (1996b). Direct evidence of pancreatic tissue oxygenation during preservation by the two-layer method. *Transplantation*, Vol.62, No.11, pp. 1667-1670.

Matsumoto, S., Qualley, S.A., Goel, S., Hagman, D.K., Sweet, I.R., Poitout, V., Strong, D.M., Robertson, R.P. & Reems, J.A. (2002a). Effect of the two-layer (University of Wisconsin solution-perfluorochemical plus O_2) method of pancreas preservation on human islet isolation, as assessed by the Edmonton Isolation Protocol. *Transplantation*, Vol.74, No.10, pp. 1414-1419.

Matsumoto, S., Rigley, T.H., Qualley, S.A., Kuroda, Y., Reems, J.A. & Stevens, R.B. (2002b). Efficacy of the oxygen-charged static two-layer method for short-term pancreas preservation and islet isolation from nonhuman primate and human pancreata. *Cell Transplant*, Vol.11, No.8, pp. 769-777.

Meyer, T., Buhler, C., Czub, S., Beutner, U., Otto, C., Thiede, A. & Ulrichs, K. (1998). Selection of donor pigs for pancreatic islet transplantation may depend on the expression level of connective tissue proteins in the islet capsule. *Transplantation Proceedings*, Vol.30, No.5, pp. 2471-2473.

Minor, T. & Isselhard, W. (1996). Synthesis of high energy phosphates during cold ischemic rat liver preservation with gaseous oxygen insufflation. *Transplantation*, Vol.61, No.1, pp. 20-22.

Minor, T., Olschewski, P., Tolba, R.H., Akbar, S., Kocalkova, M. & Dombrowski, F. (2002). Liver preservation with HTK: salutary effect of hypothermic aerobiosis by either gaseous oxygen or machine perfusion. *Clinical Transplantation*, Vol.16, No.3, pp. 206-211.

Mitsuda, H., Azuma, Y. & Ueno, S. (1987). Effect of Carbon-Dioxide on Conservation of Physiological Activities of Animal-Tissues .1. Hyperthermic Potassium Contracture of Rat Skeletal-Muscle (Musculus-Soleus). *Proceedings of the Japan Academy Series B-Physical and Biological Sciences*, Vol.63, No.9, pp. 336-339.

Opelz, G. & Dohler, B. (2007). Multicenter analysis of kidney preservation. *Transplantation*, Vol.83, No.3, pp. 247-253.

Papas, K.K., Hering, B.J., Gunther, L., Rappel, M.J., Colton, C.K. & Avgoustiniatos, E.S. (2005). Pancreas oxygenation is limited during preservation with the two-layer method. *Transplant Proc*, Vol.37, No.8, pp. 3501-3504.

Pegg, D.E., Foreman, J., Hunt, C.J. & Diaper, M.P. (1989). The mechanism of action of retrograde oxygen persufflation in renal preservation. *Transplantation*, Vol.48, No.2, pp. 210-217.

Piton, G., Barbot, O., Manzon, C., Moronval, F., Patry, C., Navellou, J.C., Belle, E. & Capellier, G. (2010). Acute ischemic pancreatitis following cardiac arrest: a case report. *Jop*, Vol.11, No.5, pp. 456-459.

Raraty, M.G., Petersen, O.H., Sutton, R. & Neoptolemos, J.P. (1999). Intracellular free ionized calcium in the pathogenesis of acute pancreatitis. *Baillieres Best Pract Res Clin Gastroenterol*, Vol.13, No.2, pp. 241-251.

Ricordi, C., Fraker, C., Szust, J., Al-Abdullah, I., Poggioli, R., Kirlew, T., Khan, A. & Alejandro, R. (2003). Improved human islet isolation outcome from marginal donors following addition of oxygenated perfluorocarbon to the cold-storage solution. *Transplantation*, Vol.75, No.9, pp. 1524-1527.

Rydgard, K.J., Song, Z., Foss, A., Ostraat, O., Tufveson, G., Wennberg, L., Lundgren, T., Tibell, A., Groth, C. & Korsgren, O. (2001). Procurement of human pancreases for islet isolation-the initiation of a Scandinavian collaborative network. *Transplantation Proceedings*, Vol.33, No.4, pp. 2538.

Salehi, P., Mirbolooki, M., Kin, T., Tsujimura, T., Shapiro, A.M., Churchill, T.A. & Lakey, J.R. (2006). Ameliorating injury during preservation and isolation of human islets using the two-layer method with perfluorocarbon and UW solution. *Cell Transplant*, Vol.15, No.2, pp. 187-194.

Schold, J.D., Kaplan, B., Howard, R.J., Reed, A.I., Foley, D.P. & Meier-Kriesche, H.U. (2005). Are we frozen in time? Analysis of the utilization and efficacy of pulsatile perfusion in renal transplantation. *Am J Transplant*, Vol.5, No.7, pp. 1681-1688.

Scott, W.E., 3rd, Matsumoto, S., Tanaka, T., Avgoustiniatos, E.S., Graham, M.L., Williams, P.C., Tempelman, L.A., Sutherland, D.E., Hering, B.J., Hammer, B.E. & Papas, K.K. (2008). Real-time noninvasive assessment of pancreatic ATP levels during cold preservation. *Transplant Proc*, Vol.40, No.2, pp. 403-406.

Scott, W.E., 3rd, Weegman, B.P., Ferrer-Fabrega, J., Stein, S.A., Anazawa, T., Kirchner, V.A., Rizzari, M.D., Stone, J., Matsumoto, S., Hammer, B.E., Balamurugan, A.N., Kidder, L.S., Suszynski, T.M., Avgoustiniatos, E.S., Stone, S.G., Tempelman, L.A., Sutherland, D.E., Hering, B.J. & Papas, K.K. (2010). Pancreas oxygen persufflation increases ATP levels as shown by nuclear magnetic resonance. *Transplantation Proceedings*, Vol.42, No.6, pp. 2011-2015.

Sekine, N., Cirulli, V., Regazzi, R., Brown, L.J., Gine, E., Tamarit-Rodriguez, J., Girotti, M., Marie, S., MacDonald, M.J., Wollheim, C.B. & et al. (1994). Low lactate dehydrogenase and high mitochondrial glycerol phosphate dehydrogenase in pancreatic beta-cells. Potential role in nutrient sensing. *J Biol Chem*, Vol.269, No.7, pp. 4895-4902.

Shapiro, A.M., Lakey, J.R., Ryan, E.A., Korbutt, G.S., Toth, E., Warnock, G.L., Kneteman, N.M. & Rajotte, R.V. (2000). Islet transplantation in seven patients with type 1 diabetes mellitus using a glucocorticoid-free immunosuppressive regimen. *N Engl J Med*, Vol.343, No.4, pp. 230-238.

Shapiro, A.M., Ricordi, C., Hering, B.J., Auchincloss, H., Lindblad, R., Robertson, R.P., Secchi, A., Brendel, M.D., Berney, T., Brennan, D.C., Cagliero, E., Alejandro, R., Ryan, E.A., DiMercurio, B., Morel, P., Polonsky, K.S., Reems, J.A., Bretzel, R.G., Bertuzzi, F., Froud, T., Kandaswamy, R., Sutherland, D.E., Eisenbarth, G., Segal, M.,

Preiksaitis, J., Korbutt, G.S., Barton, F.B., Viviano, L., Seyfert-Margolis, V., Bluestone, J. & Lakey, J.R. (2006). International trial of the Edmonton protocol for islet transplantation. *N Engl J Med*, Vol.355, No.13, pp. 1318-1330.

Steer, M.L. (1999). Early events in acute pancreatitis. *Baillieres Best Pract Res Clin Gastroenterol*, Vol.13, No.2, pp. 213-225.

Stegemann, J., Hirner, A., Rauen, U. & Minor, T. (2009). Gaseous oxygen persufflation or oxygenated machine perfusion with Custodiol-N for long-term preservation of ischemic rat livers? *Cryobiology*, Vol.58, No.1, pp. 45-51.

Sumimoto, R., Jamieson, N.V. & Kamada, N. (1990). Attempted application of the two-layer storage method to liver preservation. *Transplantation*, Vol.49, No.5, pp. 1027-1028.

Suszynski, T.M., Wildey, G.M., Falde, E.J., Cline, G.W., Maynard, K.S., Ko, N., Sotiris, J., Naji, A., Hering, B.J. & Papas, K.K. (2008). The ATP/DNA ratio is a better indicator of islet cell viability than the ADP/ATP ratio. *Transplant Proc*, Vol.40, No.2, pp. 346-350.

Tamarit-Rodriguez, J., Idahl, L.A., Gine, E., Alcazar, O. & Sehlin, J. (1998). Lactate production in pancreatic islets. *Diabetes*, Vol.47, No.8, pp. 1219-1223.

Tanioka, Y., Hering, B.J., Sutherland, D.E., Kronson, J.W., Kuroda, Y., Gilmore, T.R., Aasheim, T.C., Rusten, M.C. & Leone, J.P. (1997a). Effect of pancreatic warm ischemia on islet yield and viability in dogs. *Transplantation*, Vol.64, No.12, pp. 1637-1641.

Tanioka, Y., Sutherland, D.E., Kuroda, Y., Gilmore, T.R., Asaheim, T.C., Kronson, J.W. & Leone, J.P. (1997b). Excellence of the two-layer method (University of Wisconsin solution/perfluorochemical) in pancreas preservation before islet isolation. *Surgery*, Vol.122, No.2, pp. 435-441; discussion 441-432.

Taylor, M.J., Baicu, S., Greene, E., Vazquez, A. & Brassil, J. (2010). Islet isolation from juvenile porcine pancreas after 24-h hypothermic machine perfusion preservation. *Cell Transplantation*, Vol.19, No.5, pp. 613-628.

Thompson, D.M., Begg, I.S., Harris, C., Ao, Z., Fung, M.A., Meloche, R.M., Keown, P., Meneilly, G.S., Shapiro, R.J., Ho, S., Dawson, K.G., Al Ghofaili, K., Al Riyami, L., Al Mehthel, M., Kozak, S.E., Tong, S.O. & Warnock, G.L. (2008). Reduced progression of diabetic retinopathy after islet cell transplantation compared with intensive medical therapy. *Transplantation*, Vol.85, No.10, pp. 1400-1405.

Treckmann, J., Minor, T., Saad, S., Ozcelik, A., Malago, M., Broelsch, C.E. & Paul, A. (2008). Retrograde oxygen persufflation preservation of human livers: a pilot study. *Liver Transpl*, Vol.14, No.3, pp. 358-364.

Treckmann, J., Moers, C., Smits, J.M., Gallinat, A., Maathuis, M.H., van Kasterop-Kutz, M., Jochmans, I., Homan van der Heide, J.J., Squifflet, J.P., van Heurn, E., Kirste, G.R., Rahmel, A., Leuvenink, H.G., Pirenne, J., Ploeg, R.J. & Paul, A. (2011). Machine perfusion versus cold storage for preservation of kidneys from expanded criteria donors after brain death. *Transplant International*, Vol.24, No.6, pp. 548-554.

Tsujimura, T., Kuroda, Y., Churchill, T.A., Avila, J.G., Kin, T., Shapiro, A.M. & Lakey, J.R. (2004a). Short-term storage of the ischemically damaged human pancreas by the two-layer method prior to islet isolation. *Cell Transplant*, Vol.13, No.1, pp. 67-73.

Tsujimura, T., Kuroda, Y., Kin, T., Avila, J.G., Rajotte, R.V., Korbutt, G.S., Ryan, E.A., Shapiro, A.M. & Lakey, J.R. (2002a). Human islet transplantation from pancreases with prolonged cold ischemia using additional preservation by the two-layer (UW solution/perfluorochemical) cold-storage method. *Transplantation*, Vol.74, No.12, pp. 1687-1691.

Tsujimura, T., Salehi, P., Walker, J., Avila, J., Madsen, K., Lakey, J., Kuroda, Y. & Churchill, T.A. (2004b). Ameliorating small bowel injury using a cavitary two-layer preservation method with perfluorocarbon and a nutrient-rich solution. *Am J Transplant*, Vol.4, No.9, pp. 1421-1428.

Tsujimura, T., Suzuki, Y., Takahashi, T., Yoshida, I., Fujino, Y., Tanioka, Y., Li, S., Ku, Y. & Kuroda, Y. (2002b). Successful 24-h preservation of canine small bowel using the cavitary two-layer (University of Wisconsin solution/perfluorochemical) cold storage method. *Am J Transplant*, Vol.2, No.5, pp. 420-424.

Urushihara, T., Sumimoto, K., Ikeda, M., Hong, H.Q., Fukuda, Y. & Dohi, K. (1994). A comparative study of two-layer cold storage with perfluorochemical alone and University of Wisconsin solution for rat pancreas preservation. *Transplantation*, Vol.57, No.11, pp. 1683-1686.

Urushihara, T., Sumimoto, K., Ikeda, M., Yamanaka, K., Hong, H.Q., Ito, H., Fukuda, Y. & Dohi, K. (1992). A comparison study of rat pancreas preservation using perfluorochemical and fluorocarbon-emulsion as preservation medium. *Biomater Artif Cells Immobilization Biotechnol*, Vol.20, No.2-4, pp. 933-937.

Vantyghem, M.C., Kerr-Conte, J., Arnalsteen, L., Sergent, G., Defrance, F., Gmyr, V., Declerck, N., Raverdy, V., Vandewalle, B., Pigny, P., Noel, C. & Pattou, F. (2009). Primary graft function, metabolic control, and graft survival after islet transplantation. *Diabetes Care*, Vol.32, No.8, pp. 1473-1478.

Voiglio, E.J., Zarif, L., Gorry, F.C., Krafft, M.P., Margonari, J., Martin, X., Riess, J. & Dubernard, J.M. (1996). Aerobic preservation of organs using a new perflubron/lecithin emulsion stabilized by molecular dowels. *J Surg Res*, Vol.63, No.2, pp. 439-446.

Warnock, G.L., Thompson, D.M., Meloche, R.M., Shapiro, R.J., Ao, Z., Keown, P., Johnson, J.D., Verchere, C.B., Partovi, N., Begg, I.S., Fung, M., Kozak, S.E., Tong, S.O., Alghofaili, K.M. & Harris, C. (2008). A Multi-Year Analysis of Islet Transplantation Compared With Intensive Medical Therapy on Progression of Complications in Type 1 Diabetes. *Transplantation*, Vol.86, No.12, pp. 1762-1766.

Watson, C.J., Wells, A.C., Roberts, R.J., Akoh, J.A., Friend, P.J., Akyol, M., Calder, F.R., Allen, J.E., Jones, M.N., Collett, D. & Bradley, J.A. (2010). Cold machine perfusion versus static cold storage of kidneys donated after cardiac death: a UK multicenter randomized controlled trial. *Am J Transplant*, Vol.10, No.9, pp. 1991-1999.

Wight, J.P., Chilcott, J.B., Holmes, M.W. & Brewer, N. (2003). Pulsatile machine perfusion vs. cold storage of kidneys for transplantation: a rapid and systematic review. *Clinical Transplantation*, Vol.17, No.4, pp. 293-307.

Wong, D. & Lois, N. (2000). Perfluorocarbons and semifluorinated alkanes. *Semin Ophthalmol*, Vol.15, No.1, pp. 25-35.

Yoshida, Y., Hatayama, N., Sekino, H. & Seki, K. (2008). Heterotopic transplant of an isolated rat heart preserved for 72 h in perfluorocarbon with CO2. *Cell Transplantation*, Vol.17, No.1-2, pp. 83-89.

14

Bioartificial Pancreas: Evaluation of Crucial Barriers to Clinical Application

Rajesh Pareta, John P. McQuilling,
Alan C. Farney and Emmanuel C. Opara
Institute for Regenerative Medicine, Wake Forest School of Medicine
USA

1. Introduction

The pancreas is a dual-function organ featuring both endocrine and exocrine tissue. Endocrine functionality is provided by approximately one million cell clusters called the islets of Langerhans. Islets consist of four main cell types, 1) α cells: secrete glucagon (increases glucose in blood); β cells: secrete insulin (decreases glucose in blood); δ cells: secrete somatostatin (regulates α and β cells) and PP cells: secrete pancreatic polypeptide. Thus, the islet plays a diverse role in glucose metabolism and blood glucose homeostasis.

Diabetes mellitus, which results from an insufficiency or total lack of insulin, affects 350 million people worldwide (Serup et al., 2001). Diabetes is classified into two main types: Type 1 diabetes (sometimes called juvenile-onset or insulin dependent diabetes) is usually associated with a complete lack of insulin brought about by autoimmune destruction of the insulin producing beta cells (Eisenbarth et al., 1992; Mathis et al., 2001). Recurrence of Type 1 diabetes after pancreas transplantation between identical twins has been described and is a hallmark of autoimmune disease (recurrent autoimmunity occurs) (Sibley et al., 1985). The inciting events for autoimmune (Type 1) diabetes are unknown, but possibly there are viral or environmental triggers that act upon a genetically susceptible population. Type 2 diabetes (often called adult-onset diabetes) is generally non-insulin dependent (though clinical features of Type 1 and Type 2 diabetes may overlap) and arises from peripheral resistance to insulin and a relative insufficiency of insulin, resulting in an initial attempt by the beta cells to compensate with release of higher than normal amounts of insulin. As Type 2 diabetes progresses, β cells become desensitized to persistently high glucose concentrations, and normal responses to glucose signaling are lost (Costa et al., 2002). In late Type 2 diabetes the islets become hyalinized, beta cell dropout occurs, and there is a state of insulinopenia that can be clinically difficult to distinguish from Type 1 diabetes. Although late stage Type 2 diabetic subjects often require insulin in high doses due to peripheral insulin resistance (Holman & Turner, 1995), Type 1 diabetic patients may also develop significant insulin resistance. A bioartificial pancreas capable of supplying a sufficient amount of insulin could effectively treat both Type 1 and Type 2 diabetes.

2. Therapeutic options for Type 1 diabetes

Prior to the discovery of insulin by Banting and Best (1921), effective treatment of diabetes mellitus was limited to dietary manipulation. Many thought that the ability to administer insulin exogenously would prove to cure diabetes, but the long-term imperfections in glycemic control present even with state of the art insulin management results in the so called secondary complications of diabetes (diabetic nephropathy, retinopathy, neuropathy, and vascular disease) and diminishes life expectancy and quality of life in many patients. The discovery of insulin converted an often rapidly fatal disease to a chronic condition requiring life-long treatment. Current treatment for diabetes, both Type 1 and Type 2, includes exogenous insulin therapy and endocrine replacement by transplantation. Both of these clinical approaches have considerable inherent drawbacks. A theoretical alternative that is being tested in animal and pre-clinical models is the bioartifical pancreas.

2.1 Exogenous insulin treatment

Exogenous insulin administration to control blood glucose has been the standard therapy since the discovery of insulin. In this therapy, the amount of carbohydrates consumed is estimated by measuring food, and this is used to determine the amount of insulin necessary to cover the meal. The calculation is based on a simple open-loop model based on past success. Calculated insulin is then adjusted based on pre-meal blood glucose measurement, such that, insulin bolus is increased for high blood glucose or delayed for low-blood glucose. Insulin is injected or infused subcutaneously and enters the blood stream in approximately 15 min. Then blood glucose can be tested again and adjusted by additional insulin bolus or eating more carbohydrates, until balance is achieved. However, exogenous insulin administration, even via pump, is unable to match the fine control of glucose by the endocrine pancreas. The exaggerated glycemic excursions associated with insulin administration impacts health and quality of life. The poor control of blood glucose levels with this therapy leads to severe secondary complications such as retinopathy, neuropathy, nephropathy, and cardiovascular diseases (Kort et al., 2011; Opara et al., 2010). According to the Diabetes Control and Complications Trial (DCCT, 1993), strict control of blood glucose reduces the risk of developing diabetes-related complications, but may result in an increased incidence of hypoglycemia.

2.2 Pancreas transplantation

Kelly and Lillehei performed the first clinical pancreas transplant at the University of Minnesota in 1966. Currently, pancreas transplantation is the only option therapeutically available that reproducibly achieves normoglycemia. Pancreas transplantation re-establishes endogenous insulin secretion that is responsive to normal feedback regulation. Since 1966, more than 30,000 pancreas transplants have been performed worldwide. According to the 2009 Scientific Registry of Transplant Recipients (SRTR), the 1-year rate of graft survival is 86% when a pancreas and a kidney were transplanted together (SPK), 82% when pancreas is transplanted after kidney (PAK) and 75% when pancreas is transplanted alone (PTA). In that year, 848, 258, and 104 transplants were done in those categories. Most pancreatic grafts are from cadaver donors, though transplantation of a segment of the pancreas donated by a living donor has also been reported (Reynoso et al., 2010). Transplantation, however, requires major surgery and dependence on lifelong immunosuppression to prevent rejection. Most pancreas transplants are performed with immunosuppression induction therapy (usually monoclonal or polyclonal T-cell depleting antibody) and maintenance immunosuppression with a calcineurin inhibitor (cyclosporine or tacrolimus), an antimetabolite (mycophenolic acid) plus or minus coticosteroids (Robertson et al., 2000; Sutherland et al., 2001). Because of the limited availability of human pancreases and the need for immunosuppression, relatively few pancreas transplants are done compared to the entire diabetic population. Improvements in surgical technique or immunotherapy are unlikely to make whole organ pancreas transplantation available to the majority of patients with diabetes.

2.3 Islet transplantation

Islet transplantation promises to be a cure at least as effective as pancreas transplantation, while being much less invasive. The efficiency of islet recovery from the whole organ pancreas and the susceptibility of allogeneic islet to immune attack (both alloimmunity and autoimmunity) are the two major barriers to successful islet transplantation. There are approximately 1 million islets in an adult human pancreas. However, only half or fewer of these are successfully isolated on a consistent basis. Thus, islet transplantation usually requires islets isolated from two or more donor pancreases. Because islet isolation requires manipulation of human tissue, the process must be carried out in a good manufacturing process (GMP) facility, which adds to the expense of the procedure. Islets are transplanted by transfusion into the portal vein and embolization into the liver. The transplanted islets engraft in the distal portal triad (Figure 1).

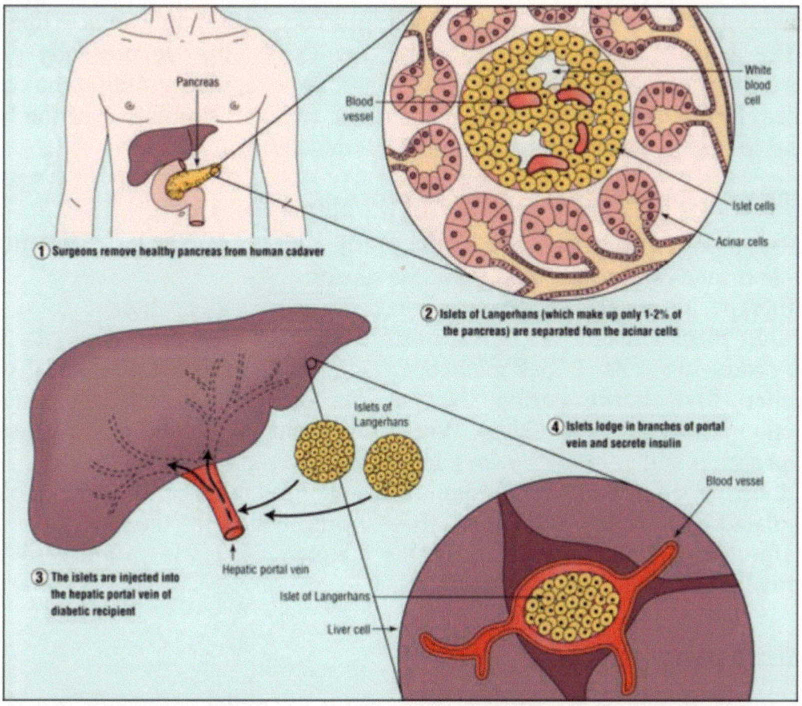

Fig. 1. Illustration of islet transplantation (Serup et al., 2001)(with permission).

Allogeneic human islets have been successfully transplanted using the Edmonton immunosuppression (steroid free) protocol (Shapiro et al., 2000). In investigations with this protocol, glycemic control has been restored for extended periods of greater than 5 years, but at the expense of immunosuppression of the transplant recipient. The necessary life long adherence to an immunosuppression drug regimen is inconvenient and associated with side effects and complications of over-immunosuppression.

Transplantation of the islets isolated from the same individual is referred to as autologous or autotransplantation, transplantation from one individual to another of the same species is referred to as allogenic or allotransplantation, and transplantation from a different species is referred to as xenogenic or xenotransplantation. Autotransplantation of islets is generally done for nondiabetic patients who require a pancreatectomy for benign disease of the pancreas (Farney et al., 1991) As of April 2008, allogeneic islet transplantation had been applied to 325 patients worldwide (CITR 2008). Only limited numbers of xenoislet transplants have been performed in humans and would appropriately be considered experimental.

2.4 Artificial pancreas

In the pancreas, the insulin is released in proportional response to actual blood glucose levels. The insulin gets released into the portal vein, where it predominately flows toward the liver, which is the major organ to store glycogen and about 50% of secreted insulin gets used in the liver. Also, the insulin release is pulsatile which helps to maintain the insulin sensitivity of the hepatic tissue. Owing to severe shortage of human pancreas and the shortcomings of insulin therapy, a lot of effort has been made to develop an artificial pancreas. The artificial pancreas is a technological development to enable Type 1 diabetic patients to automatically control their blood glucose, acting in essence like a healthy pancreas. The goals of the artificial pancreas are: 1) To improve presently popular but inefficient insulin therapy to attain a better glycemic control, thus avoiding the complication due to blood glucose fluctuations, and 2) To mimic normal stimulation of the liver by the pancreas and to normalize carbohydrate and lipid metabolism.

There are various approaches to the artificial pancreas:

1. Medical equipment approach: An insulin pump under closed loop control utilizing real-time data from a continuous blood glucose sensor.
2. Gene therapy approach: Therapeutic infection of a diabetic person by a genetically engineered virus causing a DNA transformation of few intestinal cells to become insulin-producing cells. It has even been suggested to tackle the cause of beta cell destruction itself hence curing the patients before full and irreversible β cells destruction (Rothman et al., 2005). While novel and potentially able to treat diabetes, this approach is still in infancy with a lot of unanswered questions.
3. Bioengineering approach: Development of microcapsules or biocompatible sheet of encapsulated islets. When implanted, these would behave as the native pancreas itself. This approach is the main focus of this chapter, as it has promise to be a good alternative to pancreas transplantation.

3. Bioartificial pancreas

Bioengineering approach to the artificial pancreas is to implant islet, which would secrete insulin, amylin and glucagon in response to host blood glucose without any external interference. Severe shortage of human islets and the associated need for immunosuppression have led to a lot of interest to overcome these barriers using the bioartificial pancreas approach. In Type 1 diabetes, the afflicted individual has pre-existing antibodies and immune cells against β-cell surface epitopes and insulin (Jaeger et al., 2000) and hence a simple islet transplant is not tenable. Therefore, the islets would require a protective coating to preserve their viability and function prior to transplantation. With this approach allo- and xenotransplants can be done safely, thus overcoming the shortage of islets and rejection problem while serving to restore the pancreatic endocrine function. This approach not only benefits the longevity of transplant but also relieves patients from the burden of immunosuppressant drugs.

3.1 Islet isolation

Isolation of pure islets without inflicting any significant damage to islets is key to successful islet transplantation. A critical balance of composition, process and duration of collagenase digestion is required for isolating islets with integrity, viability and high purity with a significant yield. This overall process has tremendous impact on the clinical outcome of islet transplants (Lakey et al., 2002). The pancreas is digested with combined collagenase and protease action, which disintegrates the intercellular matrix of collagen, releasing islets. These islets are isolated, purified, tested for viability, and sometimes cultured before being transplanted in the patient. Collagenase digestion disrupts islet-exocrine tissue adhesive contacts (Wolters et al., 1992). Thus, shorter duration or lower concentration of collagenase would lead to incomplete purification of islets from exocrine tissue, leading to reduced yield on purification. On the other hand, extended duration of incubation or higher concentration of collagenase would adversely affect the islet cell-cell adhesion, leading to loss of islet integrity and viability. Intra-islet cell-cell adhesion is protease-sensitive, while extra-islet cell-matrix adhesion is collagenase sensitive. In the pig, very little periinsular capsule is present and the structural integration of the porcine islet in the exocrine pancreas is almost exclusively cell-cell adhesion. In canine, the islets are almost exclusively encapsulated with very little exocrine-endocrine cell-cell contact. In rodent and human, the situation is intermediate with a tendency towards predominance of cell-matrix adhesion. The presence of protease in the collagenase preparations has been reported to reduce the yield and quality of isolated islets in rats (Vos-Scheperkeuter et al., 1997), however it is more efficient for the isolation of pig islets (Deijnen et al., 1992). Figure 2 shows the effect of transplanted islet mass on short- and long-term glycemic normalization in a rat.

3.2 Biomaterials

Islets are encapsulated in a protective coating for immunoisolation, hence it is very important that not only are the biomaterials used biocompatible, they should also be permeable for hormonal, nutrient and oxygen exchange. Biocompatibility of these devices is mostly assessed for fibrosis at the site of implantation. Use of a smooth outer surface and hydrogels further improves biocompatibility of these devices through absence of interfacial tension, thus reducing protein adsorption and cell adhesion.

Polyacrylonitrile and polyvinylchloride copolymer has been examined for the construction of microcapillaries used with intravascular macrocapsules. Extravascular macrocapsules have been made with various biomaterials, including nitrocellulose acetate, 2-hydroxyethyl methacrylate (HEMA), acrylonitrile, polyacrylonitrile and polyvinylchloride copolymer, sodium methallylsulfonate, and alginate (Narang & Mahato, 2006). Hydrogels are very attractive for making microcapsules as they provide higher permeability for low molecular weight nutrients and metabolites. Furthermore, the soft and pliable features of the gel reduce the mechanical or frictional irritations to surrounding tissue (de Vos et al., 2002). The most commonly applied materials for microencapsulation are alginate (Lim & Sun, 1980), chitosan (Zielinski & Aebischer, 1994), agarose (Iwata et al., 1989), cellulose (Risbud & Bhonde, 2001), poly(hydroxyethylmetacrylate-methyl methacrylate) (HEMA-MMA) (Dawson et al., 1987), copolymers of acrylonitrile (Kessler et al., 1991), and polyethylene glycol (PEG) (Cruise et al., 1999).

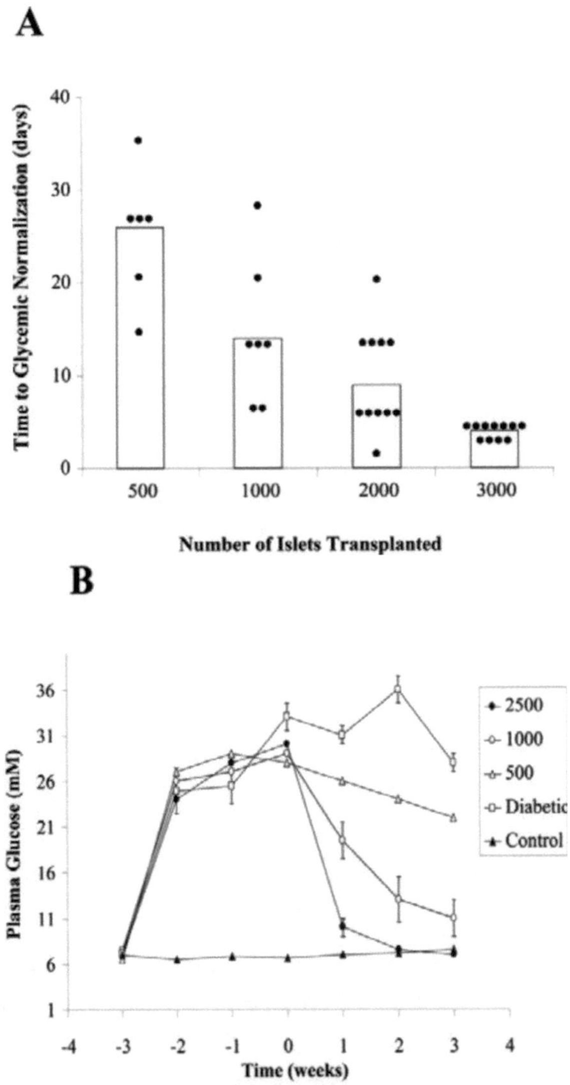

Fig. 2. Effect of transplanted islet mass on short- and long-term glycemic normalization in a rat (Finegood et al., 1992; Bell et al., 1994)(with permission).

3.2.1 Alginate

Alginate is the most studied hydrogel for islet encapsulation, as it provides some major advantages over other encapsulation alternatives. Alginate molecules are linear block co-polymers of β-d-mannuronic (M) and α-l-guluronic acids (G). It forms a gel in the presence of divalent ions like Ca^{2+} and Ba^{2+}. Recent findings have shown that divalent ions crosslink not only G blocks but also blocks of alternating M and G (M-G blocks) (Donati et al., 2005). Mainly calcium is used for gelling, as barium is known to be toxic and concerns have been raised about patients' safety if it is used as the cross-linking agent.

Alginate is one of the few materials that allow islet encapsulation at physiological conditions. The encapsulation can be done at room or body temperature, at physiological pH, and in isotonic solutions. Islets have been shown to more readily and adequately survive when being enveloped in alginate capsules (Sandler et al., 1997). It does not interfere with cellular function of the islets (Fritschy et al., 1991a,b; Haan et al., 2003). It has been shown that alginate capsules provide a microenvironment facilitating functional survival of islets probably because the three-dimensional matrix provides mechanical support for the islets and prevents clumping and fusion of the free islets, thus preserving its organization. Alginate-based capsules have been shown to be stable for years in both animals and human (Soon-Shiong et al., 1994; Sun et al., 1996). Also, since alginates are negatively charged, the attachment of immune cells to the microcapsule is limited due to the negative charge on the cell surface.

3.3 Islet encapsulation

Presently, life-long immunosuppression with drugs is required for islet transplantation, but immunosuppression can be obviated by immunoisolating the islets in a semipermeable membrane to protect them from the host immune system. Immunoisolation by encapsulation would not only allow for successful transplantation of allogeneic islets without immunosuppression (Lim & Sun, 1980) but also transplantation of islets from non-human origin (Omer et al., 2003; Zimmermann et al., 2005).

Islet encapsulation is done in aqueous dispersion with low agitation, in the presence of iso-osmotic salt, glucose and oxygen in the media under physiological pH with a preferably short encapsulation time. Usually the formed beads are post-coated with a cationic poly(amino acid), e.g., PLL or PLO, to provide perm-selectivity and improve capsule integrity (Chaikof, 1999). This is followed by a surface coating of low viscosity alginate, resulting in a microcapsule morphology that presents encapsulated islet(s) in a liquid layer of alginate, followed by PLL/PLO coating and gel layer of alginate on exterior, thus creating an alginate-PLL/PLO-alginate construct known as APA microcapsules. Figure 3 shows encapsulated islets in alginate microcapsules.

Islet encapsulation has been done mainly with one of these techniques: 1) Interfacial precipitation, 2) Phase Inversion, and 3) Polyelectrolyte coacervation. Phase inversion has been used for macrocapsules and would be discussed in that section below while interfacial precipitation would be discussed in the microcapsules section. Polyelectrolyte coacervation is a modification of alginate-calcium interfacial precipitation system, in which complexation of oppositely charged polymers leads to formation of a hydrogel membrane encapsulating the islets (Chaikof, 1999). Encapsulated islets have shown improved graft function and survival in animals compared with unencapsulated islets. Sun et al. reported that the transplantation of encapsulated porcine islets in spontaneously diabetic monkeys induced normoglycemia without immunosuppression for more than 800 days (Sun et al., 1996). Schneider et al. showed survival of encapsulated human and rat xenografts in mice for 7 months without a semi-permeable coating (Schneider et al., 2005). However, generally alginate microcapsules without perm-selectivity have not been shown to be viable in clinical trials (Tuch et al., 2009).

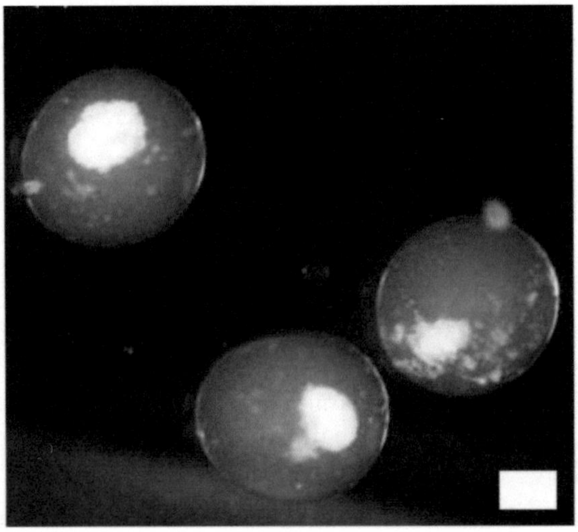

Fig. 3. Encapsulated islets in an alginate microcapsule. Scale=100 μm.

3.3.1 Macroencapsulation

There are two types of macrocapsule systems, based on their transplant location; extravascular and intravascular. Intravascular macrocapsules are based on the principle of "dialysis cartridges". Islets are seeded between hollow fibers that get perfused by blood flow. These hollow fibers are enclosed within a larger tube and implanted into the vessels of the host by vascular anastomoses. These devices have been successful in inducing normoglycemia in various diabetic animal models including rats, dogs and monkeys (Maki et al., 1993; Sun et al., 1977). The use of these devices however requires intense systemic anticoagulation (due to direct contact of foreign material with blood) and thus has the potential for fatal thrombus formation.

Extravascular macrocapsule devices in contrast have the advantage that biocompatibility issues do not pose a serious risk to patient. They have been designed in both flat sheet membrane and hollow fiber forms (Zekorn et al., 1995). A semi-permeable membrane around the sheet allows diffusion of nutrients and secreted hormones but not macrophages. They are usually coated with hydrogels to achieve a smooth outer surface to improve biocompatibility. Initial studies with extravascular macrocapsules have encapsulated multiple islets in one or several large capsules. Islets aggregated in large clumps and these studies were not successful, due to necrosis at the center of the clumps (Lacy et al., 1991). Later, this problem was addressed by solitude immobilization of islets in a matrix before encapsulation. Promising results were observed in animal studies, with survival rate of islets in the device up to 200 days after implantation in the peritoneal cavity of rat but human studies have not been very encouraging (Jain et al., 1999; Scharp et al., 1994).

The major drawback of macrocapsules is relative low surface to volume ratio, which interferes with optimal diffusion of nutrients and oxygen. For adequate nutrients and oxygen the islet density in the macrocapsules is kept quite low (usually 5-10% volume). This makes the macrocapsules rather impractical as large devices have to be implanted to provide sufficient masses of islets and these devices cannot be implanted in conventional transplantation sites (Suylichem et al., 1992). Low surface to volume ratio also interferes with glucose regulation due to slow exchange of glucose and insulin.

3.3.2 Microencapsulation

In most tissues, it has been shown that maximum diffusion distance for effective oxygen and nutrient diffusion from blood capillary to cells is about 200 μm. Absence of this convection inside a capsule induces a nutrient-gradient from the capsule surface to center of islet. Present insights suggest microcapsules as preferable system over macrocapsules due to their high surface to volume ratio for fast exchange of hormones and nutrients. Microencapsulation uses the interfacial precipitation predominantly, where a polyanionic polymer (alginate) gels with a divalent cation (Ca^{2+}, Ba^{2+}). Islets are suspended in an alginate solution and its droplets are generated either by air jet spray method (Wolters et al., 1991), electrostatic generators (Hallé et al., 1994; Hsu et al., 1994), submerged oscillating coaxial extrusion nozzles (Dawson et al., 1987), conformal coatings (Desmangles et al., 2001), and spinning disk atomization (Senuma et al., 2000). Of these methods, the air jet spray method, which uses a two-channel air droplet microencapsulator, is the most commonly used. Two-channel air droplet microencapsulators operate by allowing the alginate cell suspension to drip through an inner channel of the device while the outer channel uses an air jacket to shear off the alginate droplet. Using this method, the diameters of the inner and outer channels, the flow rate of the alginate, and air pressure of the outer channel can be adjusted to vary the microcapsule size (Wolters et al., 1991). In order to prevent hypoxic damage to islet cells, microencapsulation must be done relatively quickly around 4°C.

One major limitation to the current encapsulation devices is that they are incapable of efficiently encapsulating large numbers of islets in a reasonable amount of time. This may result in hypoxic stress and loss of functionality to islets in larger scaled up experiments (de Vos et al., 1997; Opara et al., 2010). A recently proposed alternative microencapsulation method utilizes multichannel air jacket microfluidic devices. These devices have the advantage of rapidly encapsulating large numbers of islets into microcapsules, at speeds in excess of 8 times conventional methods, without effecting the functionality of the islets. Additionally, this microfluidic approach can be easily scaled up to increase production rates, and can be cost effectively produced using rapid prototyping technology (Tendulkar et al., 2011). A reduction in capsule size would benefit the islet and also exponentially decrease the total transplant volume. Therefore, much work has been done with various new technologies to make beads as small as 185 μm (diameter), which is about four times smaller than conventional beads (800 μm). The smaller the diameter of the capsules the better the diffusion of nutrients to the islets, and Omer et al. demonstrated that capsules with a diameter of 600±100 μm showed improved stability in vivo over larger capsules with diameters of 1000±100 μm (Omer et al., 2005). However, there is another factor, with reduction in capsule size the number of capsules containing partially protruding islets also proportionally increases, and this in turn increases the number of capsules affected by an inflammatory response. Decreasing the islet density in alginate can solve this problem. It has been shown that each capsule size has an optimal islet density. Usually this is associated with a slight increase in empty capsules but minimizing protruding islets is of upmost priority. In many cases, the inner alginate bead will be either completely or partially liquefied by the removal of calcium ions with calcium quenching reagents such as sodium citrate, which allows for improved diffusion in the microbeads (Darrabie et al., 2005). Another consideration is the morphology of the microcapsules used for encapsulated islets. Spherical microcapsules are necessary for long term functionality; irregularities or imperfections in the microcapsules can cause an immune response and result in loss of islet functionality (Hobbs et al., 2001).

3.4 Immune barrier

Uncoated non-permselective alginate microbeads have been reported to have a high permeability (>600 kD). Uptake studies with IgG (150 kD) and thyroglobulin (669 kD) suggested they were able to get into these uncoated microbeads. Similarly, uncoated alginate microbeads implanted in the peritoneum were positive for both IgG and C3 component after only 1 week (Lanza et al., 1995). So, small molecules from macrophages and T-cells to smaller cytokine molecules such as IL-1β, TNF-α, and IFN-γ can easily penetrate into the microcapsules and can damage or destroy the encapsulated islets (van Schilfgaarde & de Vos, 1999). To provide immunoisolation for the microcapsules, it is essential to apply a permeability barrier between the encapsulated islets and host immune system. Applying a polyamino acid layer, followed by an additional outer coating of alginate, typically creates this barrier. The positively charged polyamino acid molecules will readily bind to the negatively charged alginate molecules forming a complex membrane (Bystrický et al., 1990; Thu et al., 1996), which significantly reduces the pore size of the microcapsule, and prevents immune cells from entering the microcapsule (Hallé et al., 1994; King et al., 1987; Kulseng et al., 1997). In order to prevent interactions of non-bound polyamines to host tissue, a thin second layer of alginate is added. This polyamino barrier acts as a shell, providing mechanical stability to the microcapsule, allowing for the liquefaction of the inner alginate (Darrabie et al., 2001). The thickness of this barrier can be varied through incubation time and concentration (Gugerli et al., 2002). The most researched perm-selective biomaterial is poly-L-Lysine (PLL) which was the first material used to generate this barrier, however more recent research has shown that poly-L-ornithine had markedly reduced immune response and has been shown to provide more mechanical support to the microcapsules (Lim & Sun, 1980; Darrabie et al., 2001).

In general, we can distinguish the host reaction towards encapsulated islets into two types: 1) Inflammatory reaction against the capsule material. With the present technology these reactions can be successfully prevented by applying purification steps to the materials to be used, and 2) Host response against the allogenic or xenogenic cell-derived bioactive factors or antigens that leak out of the capsules (de Vos et al., 2002). It results in overgrowth by macrophages and lymphocytes on a small portion (~10%) of the capsules and in a humoral immune response against the encapsulated tissue. It has long been known that islets secrete cytokines upon stress (Cardozo et al., 2003). Encapsulated islets have been shown to produce the cytokines MCP-1, MIP, nitric oxide (NO) and IL-6 under stress (stress induced by adding IL-1β and TNF-α), and these cytokines are well known to contribute to the recruitment and activation of inflammatory cells (de-Groot et al., 2001). Also, it has been demonstrated that activated macrophages on the 2-10% microcapsules with overgrowth do secrete the cytokines

IL-1β and TNF-α when cultured with encapsulated islets but not with empty capsules (Vos et al., 2004). This activation of inflammatory cells results in the production of cytokines, which are deleterious not only to the islet cells in the overgrown capsules but also the islets in the vast majority of transplanted, clean, and non-overgrown capsules. Figure 4 shows the manipulation of alginate microcapsules permeability to control cytokine action.

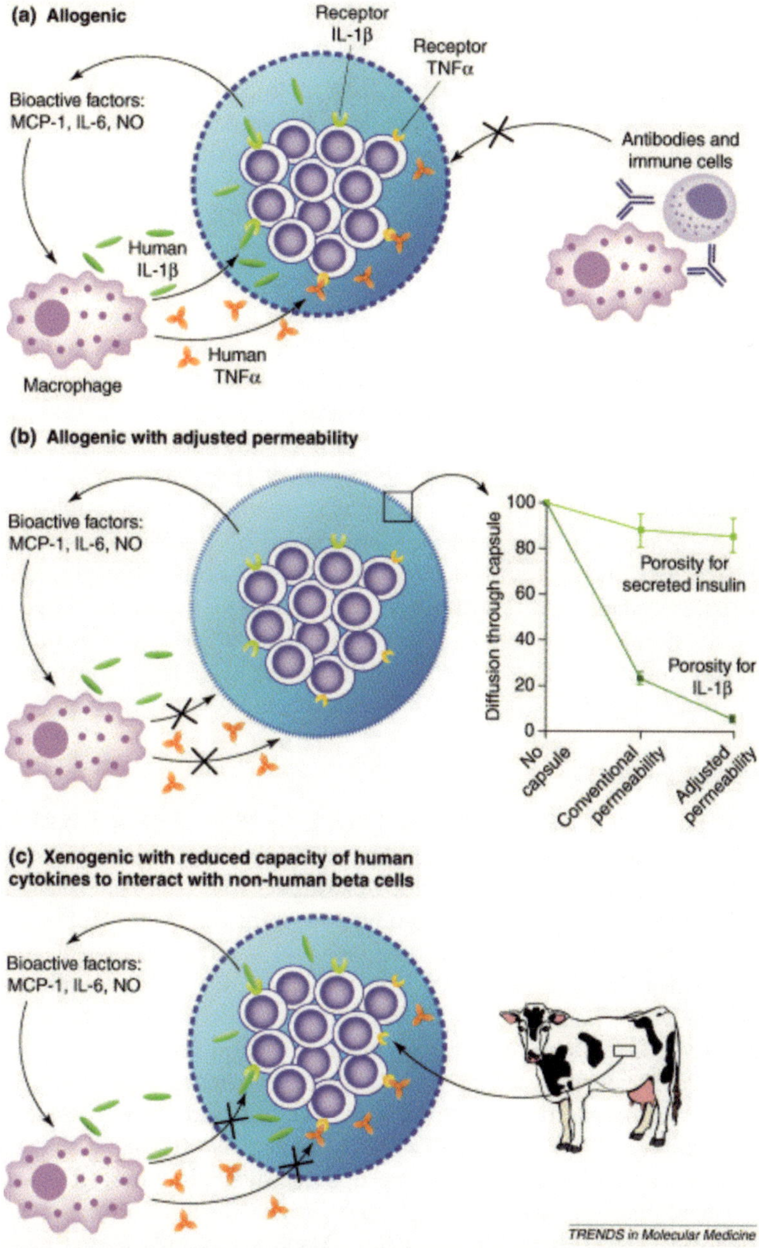

Fig. 4. Manipulation of microcapsules permeability to control cytokine action (de Vos & Marchetti, 2002)(with permission).

3.4.1 Poly-L-Lysine (PLL)

Since the introduction of the concept of microencapsulation of islets, PLL has been routinely used as the selectively-permeable membrane for microcapsules. It makes xenotransplantation of islets a feasible option and provides mechanical stability features required for application in large animals and human. After gelation of the beads in calcium, the beads are suspended in polycation solutions such as PLL, which increases membrane integrity via electrostatic association with the anionic alginate.

Many studies have shown the effectiveness of APA microcapsules in small animals (Chen et al., 1994; Fan et al., 1990; Fritschy et al., 1991a; Lim & Sun, 1980; Lum et al., 1992; O'Shea & Sun, 1986; O'Shea et al., 1984; Sun et al., 1984), large animals (Kendall et al., 2001; Soon-Shiong et al., 1992; Sun et al., 1996; Wang et al., 2008), and humans (Calafiore et al., 2006; Elliott et al., 2000; Sun et al., 1996). However, unbound PLL has been shown to cause an inflammatory response and result in fibrotic over growth over microcapsules (Strand et al., 2001; Thu et al., 1996b). This fibrotic overgrowth can severely affect islet functionality and viability by significantly reducing the rate of diffusion into the capsule (de Vos et al., 2006). Recent studies which have examined the alginate–PLL interface have found that the PLL does not form a distinct membrane separate from the alginate as originally thought, rather the PLL is found within 30 μm of the alginate (Strand et al., 2003; Thu et al., 1996a). These results indicate that even in capsule systems which use an outer alginate core, PLL is still present to some extent on the surface of the capsules. This could increase the chance of triggering an inflammatory reaction and fibrotic overgrowth (Clayton et al., 1991; King et al., 1987; Strand et al., 2001). An additional problem caused by the PLL layer is an increase in surface roughness, and one study by de Vos et al. (1999) showed that implanted alginate-PLL microcapsules made with ultra-pure alginate still caused significant fibrotic overgrowth. Also, atomic force microscopy indicated that these capsules had an increased surface roughness due to the PLL molecules (Bunger et al., 2003). However when PLL is properly bound, the implanted capsules can avoid an inflammatory response.

3.4.2 Poly-L-Ornithine (PLO)

One well-investigated alternative to PLL is PLO. Like PLL, PLO is a positively charged polyamine which, when applied to alginate microcapsules, forms a semi-permeable membrane which significantly reduces the porosity of the microcapsules, allowing for immuno-isolation without impairing oxygen and nutrient diffusion. Unlike PLL, PLO has been shown to evoke less of an immune response and has been shown to have improved mechanical properties (Brunetti et al., 1991; Calafiore et al., 1997; Calafiore et al., 2004; Kizilel et al., 2005). When compared to alginate-PLL microcapsules, alginate-PLO microcapsules have been shown to better resist swelling and bursting under osmotic stress (Darrabie et al., 2005). Bead swelling is an important factor to take into consideration because it can lead to increased in pore size, permeability, and shear stress, which leads to decreased islet viability (Thu et al., 1996a). It has been hypothesized that the improved mechanical properties of alginate-PLO microcapsules over alginate-PLL microcapsules is due to the improved bonding of PLO to alginate owing to the shorter monomer structure of PLO (Darrabie et al., 2005; Inaki et al., 1997). Also, while PLL seems to bind to M-G sequences, PLO has been shown to prefer M-M sequences (Calafiore et al., 2006). Long-term studies, where empty alginate-PLO microcapsules were injected intraperitoneally in rodents, dogs, or pigs have always resulted in retrieval of intact and overgrowth-free microcapsules up to one year post-implant (de Vos et al., 2006).

3.5 Transplantation site

It is necessary for clinical application to find a site where encapsulated islets are in close contact with the blood stream. Unfortunately, it is difficult to find such a site since it should combine the capacity to bear a large graft volume in the immediate vicinity of blood vessels. Implantation of islets is most commonly done intraperitoneally, as it offers the advantages of laparoscopic implantation or through injection, and allows ample room to implant numerous microcapsules (Calafiore et al., 2006; Elliott et al., 2000). However, there are several disadvantages to this site. The most significant disadvantage is that microcapsules that are implanted intraperitoneally are vulnerable to an immune response from intra-peritoneal T-cells and macrophages (de Groot et al., 2004; de Vos et al., 1999; de Vos et al., 2003; Safley et al., 2005), and have less access to the vasculature (de Vos and Marchetti, 2002; de Vos et al., 1999). This results in an increased likelihood of fibrotic growth over encapsulated islets, a loss of graft functionality, and a delay in insulin uptake into the blood circulation (de Vos et al., 1996). Consequently, alternative transplantation sites have been investigated, including transplanting into the liver (Toso et al., 2005), kidney capsule (Dufrane et al., 2006a), subcutaneously (Dufrane et al., 2006b), and into an omentum pouch (Kin et al., 2003; Kobayashi et al., 2006; Moya et al., 2010(a,b); Opara et al., 2010). In a study conducted by Toso et al., microcapsules were injected into the portal veins of rats; however, the results of the study showed that immunosuppressants are necessary to prevent fibrotic overgrowth (Toso et al., 2005), and the risk of hepatic thrombosis makes this approach impractical. Studies by Dufrane et al. investigated implant sites such as subcutaneous and the kidney capsule, and the results indicated that encapsulated islets implanted in these two sites had less cellular overgrowth compared to encapsulated islets implanted intraperitoneally. Additional studies demonstrated the functionality of encapsulated islets implanted within the kidney capsule of primates (Dufrane et al., 2006a); however, for clinical applications the limited space within this site may be a problem (de Vos et al., 2002). Studies have also investigated using the omentum as pouch for implanting encapsulated islets, which, like the kidney capsules, offers a well vascularized site for transplantation but has more space for microcapsules and is easier to access (Kin et al., 2003).

3.5.1 Omentum pouch

The use of an omentum pouch as a site for islet transplantation has also been investigated, and early studies (Ferguson & Scothorne, 1977; Yasunami et al., 1983) demonstrated the ability of unencapsulated islet grafts to survive within an omental pouch. More recent research has shown that encapsulated islets implanted into the omentum pouch have increased periods of functionality than encapsulated islets implanted intraperitoneally (Aomatsu et al., 1999; Kobayashi et al., 2006). In a study by Aomatsu et al. diabetic Balb/c mice were implanted with 1000 agarose microencapsulated islets in both the peritoneal cavity and omentum pouch; the results indicated that graft functionality was significantly longer in the omentum pouch (27.1±5.5 days) than the peritoneal cavity (12.5±12.5 days) (Aomatsu et al., 1999). In one long-term study, agarose microencapsulated islets were implanted into the omentum pouch of diabetic NOD mice and evaluated up to 400 days post transplantation. Results from this study indicated that the islets were able to maintain normoglycemia for up to 100 days; however, a portion of islets evaluated at 400 days showed signs of central necrosis (Kobayashi et al., 2006). Omentum pouches are generally created by exposing the greater omentum and running a suture along the perimeter of the omental pouch; capsules are then placed in the center of the omental tissue, and the suture is then pulled up and tied, creating the pouch (Kin et al., 2003). Figure 5 shows encapsulated islets in an omentum pouch created in a Lewis rat (Opara et al., 2010).

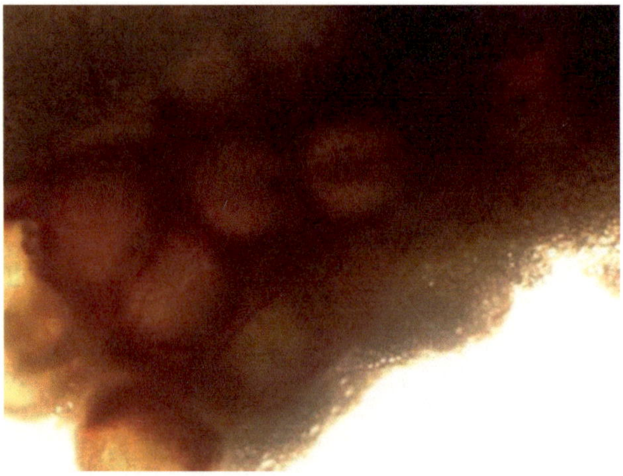

Fig. 5. Alginate microcapsules implanted within an omentum pouch and retrieved after 1 week in vivo (Opara et al., 2010).

3.6 Vascularization

While considerable research has improved the quality of the microcapsules and found suitable implantation sites, there is still a limit to long-term islet survival (de Vos et al., 2004; Opara et al., 2010). A major cause for the long-term failure of grafts is lack of appropriate vascularization to deliver oxygen and nutrients. Islets require functional vasculature to support normal function, as evident by the fact that they receive up to 10-12% of pancreatic blood flow to the pancreas while they account for only about 1-2% of the organ mass (Lifson et al., 1980; Jansson & Hellerstrom, 1983). Deficiencies in vascularization results in hypoxia causing islet dysfunction and death, and, in cases of implanted microencapsulated islets, severe damage has been caused by hypoxia within three days of implantation (Davalli et al., 1996). One approach to this problem is to redesign the microcapsule to provide for the controlled release of angiogenic proteins, such as growth factor fibroblast growth factor 1 (FGF-1) as recently suggested (Opara et al., 2010).

3.6.1 Angiogenesis

During the islet isolation, the vascular supply is disrupted causing rapid endothelial fragmentation and compromises perfusion to the core of islets. Thus, it is very crucial to revascularize the islets for their post-transplantation survival and function (Brissova et al., 2004). Successful islet grafts have been observed to regenerate the microvasculature in about 10-14 days post-transplantation (Beger et al., 1998; Furuya et al., 2003; Menger et al., 1994; Merchant et al., 1997; Vajkoczy et al., 1995). The proportion of islets that restore their original vasculature determines the long term graft survival and function. In encapsulated islets, islets depend on the diffusion of oxygen and nutrients from the periphery. Lower oxygen and nutrient supply leads to hypoxia and eventual cell death in the inner core of islets which is predominantly comprised of insulin-secreting β-cells (Vasir et al., 1998). Research has shown that the application of angiogenic growth factors such as vascular endothelial growth factor (VEGF), nerve growth factor (NGF), and FGF-1 improved graft functionality of naked islets as a result of increased angiogenesis (Lai et al., 2005; Miao et al., 2005; Rivas-Carrillo et al., 2006). However, bolus administration of growth factors has been shown to result in abnormal and unsustainable vasculature formation. It has also been shown that sustained release of FGF-1, however, allows for normal blood vessel growth, but this growth can actually be limited to the site of implantation (Moya et al., 2009). Using this information, studies have shown that microbeads can be used for a controlled localized delivery of FGF-1 for improved angiogenesis (Moya et al., 2010a). Additionally methods for generating alginate-PLO-alginate microbeads for sustained release of FGF-1 have been investigated (Khanna et al., 2010) and have been shown to cause significant angiogenesis over controls when implanted into the omentum pouches of rats for two weeks (Opara et al., 2011).

3.6.2 Antioxidants

Another concern for the survival of encapsulated islets is the protection from oxidative stress in vivo. Islets are exposed to oxidative stress during the isolation process and after implantation when exposed to activated immune cells, which release free radicals. β cells in particular, are highly vulnerable to oxidative stress (Rabinovitch & Suarez-Pinzon, 1998) and encapsulated islets have been shown to be damaged as a result of oxidative stress (Wiegand et al., 1993). The application of free radical scavengers is an established solution to this problem. Oxidative stress is caused when the amount of oxygen free radicals present within a tissue or cell exceeds the ability of that tissue or cell to neutralize these free radicals (Opara, 2006). These oxygen radicals are most commonly superoxide oxygen (O_2^-), hydrogen peroxide (H_2O_2), hydroxyl radicals (OH^-) and peroxynitrite ($ONOO^-$) and are generally referred to as reactive oxygen species (ROS) (Opara, 2002). This process can occur intracellularly and extracellularly as well as from exogenous sources. Intracellular sources of ROS include normal cellular metabolism, and extracellular ROS are generated from the immune system during the destruction of foreign bodies (Opara, 2006). Several studies have found that the addition of traditional antioxidants such as the free radical scavenger Catalase, or Trolox (a water soluble derivative of vitamin E) have improved islet functionality following isolation (Stiegler et al., 2010) and during encapsulation. Other studies have investigated the use of hemoglobin as an antioxidant for encapsulated islets (Chae et al., 2004).

3.7 Functionality studies

The technique of microencapsulation of islets prior to transplantation has shown promise in both large animal trials and pilot clinical trials (Table 1). Multiple canine and primate studies have been conducted and have demonstrated the ability of encapsulated islets to maintain insulin independence (Dufrane et al., 2006a,b; Kendall et al., 2001; Soon-Shiong et al., 1992; Wang et al., 2008). A study conducted by Sun Y. et al. demonstrated the ability of encapsulated islet xenografts to reverse diabetes for periods of time greater than 800 days (Sun et al., 1996). A more recent study by Dufrane et al. demonstrated the ability of encapsulated islets to survive and produce insulin in the kidney capsule of *Cynomolgus macacus* for up to six months (Dufrane et al., 2006a).

Several pilot clinical studies (Calafiore et al., 2006; Elliott et al., 2007) have been conducted on humans. While these trials have failed to establish long-term insulin independence in any of the subjects, they have established that the implantation of viable encapsulated islets can stabilize blood glucose levels and reduce the required amount of exogenous insulin required. In a study by Soon-Shiong et al., a long-term Type 1 diabetic patient was implanted with 15,000 encapsulated islet equivalents per kilogram body weight and evaluated for up to 9 months post-transplantation. In this study average blood glucose levels were maintained at 135mg/dl, and daily insulin requirements decreased from 0.69±0.01 U/kg to 0 U/kg, and hyperglycemic episodes (>200 mg/dl) decreased from 11.7% to 6.14% at nine months. Furthermore, the patient's quality of life was evaluated and shown to have greatly improved over the duration of the study (Soon-Shiong et al., 1994). Another human study by Calafiore et al. evaluated two individuals 60 days after receiving encapsulated allografts. Although insulin independence was not attained, there was a significant reduction in the daily insulin requirements as well as a significant reduction in the number of hypoglycemic events (Calafiore et al., 2006). A third human study by Elliot RB et al., evaluated the effectiveness of porcine xenograft encapsulated islets up to 9.5 years after implantation. In this study, immediately after implantation, the daily insulin dosage was reduced by 30% and C-peptide was present in urine samples up to 14 months post transplantation. Retrieval of the capsules 9.5 years later revealed that the islets were still capable of producing insulin, however the levels of insulin were significantly reduced and C-peptide could not be measured (Elliott et al., 2007).

Study	Model	Type of Graft	Islet Equivalents (IEQ/Kg body weight)	Duration of insulin independence
(Soon-Shiong et al., 1992)	Canine	Allograft		63-107 days
(Sun et al., 1996)	Primate	Xenograft (porcine)	7,500-17,500	120-803 days
(Dufrane et al., 2006a)	Primate	Xenograft (porcine)	15,000	
(Wang et al., 2008)	Canine	Allograft	55,270-87,031	50-214 days
(Kendall et al., 2001)	Primate	Xenograft (porcine)	15,000	up to 9 months
(Soon-Shiong et al., 1994)	Human	Allograft	15,000	9 months
(Calafiore et al., 2006)	Human	Allograft	400,000-600,000 total IEQ	
(Elliott et al., 2007)	Human	Xenograft (porcine)	15,000	

Table 1. Summary of large animal and human studies. With the exception of Dufrane et al. (2006a), where encapsulated islets were implanted within the kidney capsule, all studies implanted encapsulated islets intra-peritonealy with either PLL or PLO barriers.

In addition to these small pilot trials, larger clinical trials are underway in New Zealand and Russia by Living Cell Technologies Limited (LCT). LCT is currently undergoing phase I and II clinical trials on DIABECELL® which are encapsulated neonatal porcine islets that are injected into the peritoneal cavity via laparoscopy at doses of 10,000-20,000 islet equivalents/kg. Currently the short-term and long-term safety and effectiveness as well as proper dosage are being evaluated (Zukerman, 2010).

4. Conclusion

In spite of the simplicity of the concept of microencapsulation and the urgent need for alternatives to immunosuppression in transplantation, the progress in the field during the past decades has not met the high expectations. Causal factors for this situation include insufficient knowledge of the microcapsule structure, immunoisolation technology and biomaterial properties, and their combined effect relative to biocompatibility. Most of the prematurely failed grafts had one or more flaws such as unpurified alginate, surface exposure of PLL, rough external surface, low surface to volume ratio, and other issues. Recent studies have indicated that it is important to have absolutely no overgrowth on the transplanted microcapsules to ensure its longevity. Another limiting factor in the progress of the microencapsulated islet technology has been the dearth of high-throughput devices for making encapsulated islets. When dealing with high numbers of islets (~500,000 islets, as expected in human studies), at present capabilities, it would take a multitude of hours to encapsulate this number of islets and islet viability would suffers immensely. Recent developments in encapsulation devices allow scaling up the process such that encapsulation time can be exponentially reduced from hundreds of hours to less an hour (Tendulkar et al., 2011).

Barriers to Microcapsule Transplantation	Strategies for Clinical Success
Loss of viability during islet isolation and encapsulation	Improved enzymatic blends and process control to maximize pure islet yield
	Culture media for long-term in-vitro culture and encapsulation
	Scalable microfluidic encapsulation devices
Failure to revascularize on transplantation	Better vascularized implant site
	Co-encapsulation with angiogenic factors to promote revascularization
	Co-encapsulation with antioxidants to counter oxidative stress
Inflammatory reaction	Good hydrogel coating
	Immunoisolation barriers with no surface exposure
Inadequate islet mass	Xenotransplants
	Stem cell and gene therapy based approaches

Table 2. Barriers to clinical success of encapsulated islet transplantation and counter-strategies.

It is also very important to have sufficient islet mass to achieve normoglycemia for long-term graft survival and function (Rickels et al., 2005). When inadequate numbers of islets are transplanted, increased metabolic demand and persistent hyperglycemia may lead to islet apoptosis and hence graft failure (Leahy et al., 1992; Rossetti et al., 1990). Since the life span of a β cell is approximately 3 months (Finegood et al., 1992), success in encapsulated islet graft studies over a long period suggests that regeneration of islet cells occurs in capsules. Indeed, β cell replication has been shown to be 10-fold higher in encapsulated islets compared to the native pancreas (van Schilfgaarde & de Vos, 1998). Inadequate islet supply issues are being addressed by regeneration therapy and xenotransplantation. Various strategies are being explored to improve islet graft outcomes, including immunoisolation using semipermeable biocompatible polymeric capsules, induction of immune tolerance, enhanced vascularization of transplant sites, and reduction of oxidative stress induced by the islet isolation process using antioxidants, as well as the use of adequate number of islets. Furthermore, synergistic application of more than one strategy maybe required to improve the success of islet transplantation. Table 2 summarizes the crucial barriers and strategies to achieve clinical success.

5. Acknowledgements

Research studies in our laboratory described in this chapter have been made possible by generous financial support from the National Institutes of Health (RO1DK080897) and the Vila Rosenfeld Estate, NC.

6. References

Alejandro, R., Barton, F. B., Hering, B. J., & Wease, S. (2008). Update from Collaborative Islet Transplant Registry. *Transplantation,* Vol.86, No.12, pp. 1783-1788, ISSN 0041-1337.

Aomatsu, Y., Nakajima, Y., Kin, T., Ohyama, T., Kanehiro, H., Hisanaga, M., et al. (1999). Omental pouch site for microencapsulated islet transplantation. *Japanese Journal of Transplantation,* Vol.34, No.4, pp. 14-21, ISSN 0041-1345.

Beger, C., Cirulli, V., Vajkoczy, P., Halban, P. A., & Menger, M. D. (1998). Vascularization of purified pancreatic islet-like cell aggregates (pseudoislets) after syngeneic transplantation. *Diabetes,* Vol.47, No.4, pp. 559-565, ISSN 0012-1797.

Bell, R. C., Khurana, M., Ryan, E. A., & Finegood, D. T. (1994). Gender differences in the metabolic response to graded numbers of transplanted islets of Langerhans. *Endocrinology, 135*(6), 2681-2687, ISSN 0013-7227.

Brissova, M., Fowler, M., Wiebe, P., Shostak, A., Shiota, M., Radhika, A., et al. (2004). Intraislet endothelial cells contribute to revascularization of transplanted pancreatic islets. *Diabetes,* Vol.53, No.5, pp. 1318-1325, ISSN 0012-1797.

Brunetti, P., Basta, G., Faloerni, A., Calcinaro, F., Pietropaolo, M., & Calafiore, R. (1991). Immunoprotection of pancreatic islet grafts within artificial microcapsules. *Int J Artif Organs,* Vol.14, No.12, pp. 789-791, ISSN 0391-3988.

Bunger, C. M., Gerlach, C., Freier, T., Schmitz, K. P., Pilz, M., Werner, C., et al. (2003). Biocompatibility and surface structure of chemically modified immunoisolating alginate-PLL capsules. *J Bio Mat Res A,* Vol.67, No.4, pp. 1219-1227, ISSN 0021-9304.

Bystrický, S., Malovíková, A., & Sticzay, T. (1990). Interaction of alginates and pectins with cationic polypeptides. *Carbohydrate Poly,* Vol.13, No.3, pp. 283-294, ISSN 0144-8617.

Calafiore, R., Basta, G., Boselli, C., Bufalari, A., Giustozzi, G. M., Luca, G., et al. (1997). Effects of alginate/polyaminoacidic coherent microcapsule transplantation in adult pigs. *Transplant Proc,* Vol.29, No.4, pp. 2126-2127, ISSN 0041-1345.

Calafiore, R., Basta, G., Luca, G., Calvitti, M., Calabrese, G., Racanicchi, L., et al. (2004). Grafts of microencapsulated pancreatic islet cells for the therapy of diabetes mellitus in non-immunosuppressed animals. *Biotechnol Appl Biochem,* Vol.39, No.2, pp. 159-164, ISSN 0885-4513 .

Calafiore, R., Basta, G., Luca, G., Lemmi, A., Montanucci, M. P., Calabrese, G., et al. (2006). Microencapsulated Pancreatic Islet Allografts Into Nonimmunosuppressed Patients With Type 1 Diabetes. *Diab Care,* Vol.29, No.1, pp. 137-138, ISSN 0149-5992.

Cardozo, A. K., Proost, P., Gysemans, C., Chen, M. C., Mathieu, C., & Eizirik, D. L. (2003). IL-1beta and IFN-gamma induce the expression of diverse chemokines and IL-15 in human and rat pancreatic islet cells, and in islets from pre-diabetic NOD mice. *Diabetologia,* Vol.46, No.2, pp. 255–266, ISSN 0012-186X.

Chae, S. Y., Lee, M., Kim, S. W., & Bae, Y. H. (2004). Protection of insulin secreting cells from nitric oxide induced cellular damage by crosslinked hemoglobin. *Biomaterials,* Vol.25, No.5, pp. 843-850, ISSN 0142-9612.

Chaikof, E. L. (1999). Engineering and material considerations in islet cell transplantation. *Annual Review of Biomedical Engineering,* Vol.1, No.1, pp. 103-127, ISSN 1523-9829.

Chen, C. F., Chern, H. T., Leu, F. J., Chang, T. M., Shian, L. R., & Sun, A. M. (1994). Xenotransplantation of microencapsulated canine islets into diabetic rats. *Artif Organs,* Vol.18, No.3, pp. 193-197, ISSN 0160-564X.

Clayton, H. A., London, N. J., Colloby, P. S., Bell, P. R., & James, R. F. (1991). The effect of capsule composition on the biocompatibility of alginate-poly-l-lysine capsules. *J Microencapsul,* Vol.8, No.2, pp. 221-233, ISSN 0265-2048 .

Costa, A., Conget, I., & Gomis, R. (2002). Impaired glucose tolerance: is there a case for pharmacologic intervention? *Treat Endocrinol,* Vol.1, pp. 205-210, ISSN 1175-6349.

Cruise, G. M., Hegre, O. D., Lamberti, F. V., S.R. Hager, R. H., & al., D. S. S. e. (1999). In vitro and in vivo performance of porcine islets encapsulated in interfacially photopolymerized poly(ethylene glycol) diacrylate membranes. *Cell Transplantation,* Vol.8, No.3, pp. 293–306, ISSN 0963-6897.

Darrabie, M., Freeman, B. K., Kendall, W. F., Jr., Hobbs, H. A., & Opara, E. C. (2001). Durability of sodium sulfate-treated polylysine-alginate microcapsules. *J Biomed Mater Res,* Vol.54, No.3, pp. 396-399, ISSN 0021-9304.

Darrabie, M. D., Kendall, W. F., & Opara, E. C. (2005). Characteristics of poly-L-ornithine-coated alginate microcapsules. *Biomaterials,* Vol.26, No.34, pp. 6846-6852, ISSN 0142-9612.

Davalli, A. M., Scaglia, L., Zangen, D. H., Hollister, J., BonnerWeir, S., & Weir, G. C. (1996). Vulnerability of islets in the immediate posttransplantation period - Dynamic changes in structure and function. *Diabetes,* Vol.45, No.9, pp. 1161-1167, ISSN 0012-1797.

Dawson, R. M., Broughton, R. L., Stevenson, W. T., & Sefton, M. V. (1987). Microencapsulation of CHO cells in a hydroxyethyl methacrylate-methyl methacrylate copolymer. *Biomaterials,* Vol.8, No.5, pp. 360–366, ISSN 0142-9612.

DCCT Group (1993). The effect of intensive treatment of diabetes on the development and progression of long-term complications in insulin-dependent diabetes mellitus. *N Engl J Med*, Vol.329, pp. 977-986, ISSN 0028-4793.

de Groot, M., Keizer, P. P. M., de Haan, B. J., Schuurs, T. A., Leuvenink, H. G. D., van Schilfgaarde, R., et al. (2001). Microcapsules and their ability to protect islets against cytokine-mediated dysfunction. *Transplantation Proceedings*, Vol.33, No.1-2, pp. 1711-1712, ISSN 0041-1345.

de Groot, M., Schuurs, T. A., & van Schilfgaarde, R. (2004). Causes of limited survival of microencapsulated pancreatic islet grafts. *J of Surl Res*, Vol.121, No.1, pp. 141-150, ISSN 0022-4804.

de Vos, P., de Haan, B. J., de Haan, A., van Zanten, J., & Faas, M. M. (2004). Factors influencing functional survival of microencapsulated islet grafts. *Cell Transplantation*, Vol.13, No.5, pp. 515-524, ISSN 0963-6897.

de Vos, P., de Haan, B. J., & VanSchilfgaarde, R. (1997). Upscaling the production of microencapsulated pancreatic islets. *Biomaterials*, Vol.18, No.16, pp. 1085-1090, ISSN 0142-9612.

de Vos, P., Faas, M. M., Strand, B., & Calafiore, R. (2006). Alginate-based microcapsules for immunoisolation of pancreatic islets. *Biomaterials*, Vol.27, No.32, pp. 5603-5617, ISSN 0142-9612.

de Vos, P., Hamel, A. F., & Tatarkiewicz, K. (2002). Considerations for successful transplantation of encapsulated pancreatic islets. *Diabetologia*, Vol.45, No.2, pp. 159-173, ISSN 0012-186X.

de Vos, P., & Marchetti, P. (2002). Encapsulation of pancreatic islets for transplantation in diabetes: the untouchable islets. *Trends in Mol Med*, Vol.8, No.8, pp. 363-366 ISSN 1471-4914.

de Vos, P., Smedema, I., van Goor, H., Moes, H., van Zanten, J., Netters, S., et al. (2003). Association between macrophage activation and function of micro-encapsulated rat islets. *Diabetologia*, Vol.46, No.5, pp. 666-673, ISSN 0012-186X.

de Vos, P., Van Straaten, J. F., Nieuwenhuizen, A. G., de Groot, M., Ploeg, R. J., de Haan, B. J., et al. (1999). Why do microencapsulated islet grafts fail in the absence of fibrotic overgrowth? *Diabetes*, Vol.48, No.7, pp. 1381-1388, ISSN 0012-1797.

de Vos, P., Vegter, D., de Haan, B. J., Strubbe, J. H., Bruggink, J. E., & VanSchilfgaarde, R. (1996). Kinetics of intraperitoneally infused insulin in rats - Functional implications for the bioartificial pancreas. *Diabetes*, Vol.45, No.8, pp. 1102-1107, ISSN 0012-1797.

Deijnen, J. H. M., Hulstaert, C. E., Wolters, G. H. J., & Schilfgaarde, R. (1992). Significance of the peri-insular extracellular matrix for islet isolation from the pancreas of rat, dog, pig, and man. *Cell and Tissue Research*, Vol.267, No.1, pp. 139-146, ISSN 0302-766X.

Desmangles, A. I., Jordan, O., & Marquis-Weible, F. (2001). Interfacial photopolymerization of beta-cell clusters: approaches to reduce coating thickness using ionic and lipophilic dyes. *Biotechnol Bioeng*, Vol.72, No.6, pp. 634-641, ISSN 0006-3592.

Donati, I., Holtan, S. v., MÃ¸rch, Y. A., Borgogna, M., & Dentini, M. (2005). New hypothesis on the role of alternating sequences in calcium alginate gels. *Biomacromolecules*, Vol.6, No.2, pp. 1031-1040, ISSN 1525-7797.

Dufrane, D., Goebbels, R. M., Saliez, A., Guiot, Y., & Gianello, P. (2006a). Six-month survival of microencapsulated pig islets and alginate biocompatibility in primates: Proof of concept. *Transplantation*, Vol.81, No.9, pp. 1345-1353, ISSN 0041-1337.

Dufrane, D., Steenberghe, M., Goebbels, R. M., Saliez, A., Guiot, Y., & Gianello, P. (2006b). The influence of implantation site on the biocompatibility and survival of alginate encapsulated pig islets in rats. *Biomaterials,* Vol.27, No.17, pp. 3201-3208, ISSN 0142-9612.

Eisenbarth, G. S., Jackson, R. A., & Pugliese, A. (1992). Insulin autoimmunity: the rate limiting factor in pre-Type 1 diabetes. *J Autoimmun,* Vol.5, Suppl.A, pp. 241-246, ISSN 0896-8411.

Elliott, R. B., Escobar, L., Garkavenko, O., Croxson, M. C., Schroeder, B. A., McGregor, M., et al. (2000). No evidence of infection with porcine endogenous retrovirus in recipients of encapsulated porcine islet xenografts. *Cell Transplant,* Vol.9, No.6, pp. 895-901, ISSN 0963-6897.

Elliott, R. B., Escobar, L., Tan, P. L., Muzina, M., Zwain, S., & Buchanan, C. (2007). Live encapsulated porcine islets from a Type 1 diabetic patient 9.5 yr after xenotransplantation. *Xenotransplantation,* Vol.14, No.2, pp. 157-161, ISSN 0908-665X.

Fan, M. Y., Lum, Z. P., Fu, X. W., Levesque, L., Tai, I. T., & Sun, A. M. (1990). Reversal of diabetes in BB rats by transplantation of encapsulated pancreatic islets. *Diabetes,* Vol.39, No.4, pp. 519-522, ISSN 0012-1797.

Farney, A. C., Najarian, J. S., Nakhleh, R. E., Lloveras, G., Field, M. J., Gores, P. F., & Sutherland, D. E. (1991). Autotransplantation of dispersed pancreatic islet tissue combined with total or near-total pancreatectomy for treatment of chronic pancreatitis. *Surgery,* Vol.110, No.2, pp. 427-437, ISSN 0039-6060.

Ferguson, J., & Scothorne, R. J. (1977). Further studies on the transplantation of isolated pancreatic islets. *J Anat,* Vol.124, Pt.1, pp. 9-20, ISSN 0021-8782.

Finegood, D., Tobin, B. W., & Lewis, J. T. (1992). Dynamics of glycemic normalization following transplantation of incremental islet masses in streptozotocin-diabetic rats. *Transplantation,* Vol.53, No.5, pp. 1033-1037, ISSN 0041-1337.

Fritschy, W. M., Strubbe, J. H., Wolters, G. H., & van Schilfgaarde, R. (1991a). Glucose tolerance and plasma insulin response to intravenous glucose infusion and test meal in rats with microencapsulated islet allografts. *Diabetologia,* Vol.34, No.8, pp. 542-547, ISSN 0012-186X.

Fritschy, W. M., Wolters, G. H., & Schilfgaarde, R. V. (1991b). Effect of alginate-polylysine-alginate microencapsulation on in vitro insulin release from rat pancreatic islets. *Diabetes,* Vol.40, No.1, pp. 37–43, ISSN 0012-1797.

Furuya, H., Kimura, T., Murakami, M., Katayama, K., Hirose, K., & Yamaguchi, A. (2003). Revascularization and function of pancreatic islet isografts in diabetic rats following transplantation. *Cell Tran,* Vol.12, No.5, pp. 537-544, ISSN 0963-6897.

Group, T. D. P. (2006). Incidence and trends of childhood Type 1 diabetes worldwide 1990–1999. *Diabetic Medicine,* Vol.23, No.8, pp. 857-866, ISSN 0742-3071.

Gugerli, R., Cantana, E., Heinzen, C., von Stockar, U., & Marison, I. W. (2002). Quantitative study of the production and properties of alginate/poly-L-lysine microcapsules. *J Microencapsul,* Vol.19, No.5, pp. 571-590, ISSN 0265-2048.

Haan, B. J. D., Faas, M. M., & Vos, P. D. (2003). Factors influencing insulin secretion from encapsulated islets. *Cell Transplantation,* Vol.12, No.6, pp. 617–625, ISSN 0963-6897.

Hallé, J., Leblond, F., Pariseau, J., Jutras, P., Brabant, M., & Lepage, Y. (1994). Studies on small (< 300 microns) microcapsules: II--Parameters governing the production of alginate beads by high voltage electrostatic pulses. *Cell Transplant*, Vol.3, No.5, pp. 365-372, ISSN 0963-6897.

Hobbs, H. A., Kendall, W. F., Jr., Darrabie, M., & Opara, E. C. (2001). Prevention of morphological changes in alginate microcapsules for islet xenotransplantation. *J Investig Med*, Vol.49, No.6, pp. 572-575, ISSN 1081-5589.

Holman, R. R., & Turner, R. C. (1995). Insulin therapy in Type II diabetes. *Diabetes Research and Clinical Practice*, Vol. 28, Supplement 1, pp. S179-S184, ISSN 0168-8227.

Hsu, B. R., Chen, H. C., Fu, S. H., Huang, Y. Y., & Huang, H. S. (1994). The use of field effects to generate calcium alginate microspheres and its application in cell transplantation. *J Formos Med Assoc*, Vol.93, No.3, pp. 240-245, ISSN 0929-6646.

Inaki, Y., Tohnai, N., Miyabayashi, K., & Miyata, M. (1997). Isopoly-L-ornithine derivative as nucleic acid model. *Nucleic Acids Symp. Ser.*, No.37, pp.25-26, ISSN 0261-3166.

Iwata, H., Amemiya, H., Matsuda, T., Takano, H., Hayashi, R., & Akutsu, T. (1989). Evaluation of microencapsulated islets in agarose gel as bioartificial pancreas by studies of hormone secretion in culture and by xenotransplantation. *Diabetes*,Vol.38, Suppl.1, pp. 224–225, ISSN 0012-1797.

Jaeger, C., Brendel, M. D., Eckhard, M., & Bretzel, R. G. (2000). Islet autoantibodies as potential markers for disease recurrence in clinical islet transplantation. *Exp Clin Endocrinol Diabetes*, Vol.108, No.05, pp. 328,333, ISSN 0947-7349.

Jain, K., Asina, S., Yang, H., Blount, E. D., Smith, B. H., Diehl, C. H., et al. (1999). Glucose control and long-term survival in biobreeding/worcester rats after intraperitoneal implantation of hydrophilic macrobeads containing porcine islets without immunosuppression. *Transplantation*, Vol.68, No.11, pp. 1693-1700, ISSN 0041-1337.

Jansson, L., & Hellerstrom, C. (1983). Stimulation by glucose of the blood flow to the pancreatic islets of the rat. *Diabetologia*, Vol.25, No.1, pp. 45-50, ISSN 0012-186X.

Kendall, W. F., Jr., Collins, B. H., & Opara, E. C. (2001). Islet cell transplantation for the treatment of diabetes mellitus. *Expert Opin Biol Ther*, Vol.1, No.1, pp. 109-119, ISSN 1471-2598.

Kessler, L., Pinget, M., Aprahamian, M., Dejardin, P., & Damgé, C. (1991). In vitro and in vivo studies of the properties of an artificial membrane for pancreatic islet encapsulation. *Horm Metab Res*, Vol.23, No.7, pp.312, ISSN 0018-5043.

Khanna, O., Moya, M. L., Opara, E. C., & Brey, E. M. (2010). Synthesis of multilayered alginate microcapsules for the sustained release of fibroblast growth factor-1. *Journal of Biomed Materials Research Part A*, Vol.95A, No.2, 632-640, ISSN 1549-3296.

Kin, T., Korbutt, G. S., & Rajotte, R. V. (2003). Survival and metabolic function of syngeneic rat islet grafts transplanted in the omental pouch. *Am J Transplant*, Vol.3, No.3, pp. 281-285, ISSN 1600-6135.

King, G. A., Daugulis, A. J., Faulkner, P., & Goosen, M. F. A. (1987). Alginate-polylysine microcapsules of controlled membrane molecular weight cutoff for mammalian cell culture engineering. *Biotechnology Prog*, Vol.3, No.4, pp. 231-240, ISSN 1520-6033.

Kizilel, S., Garfinkel, M., & Opara, E. (2005). The bioartificial pancreas: Progress and challenges. *Diabetes Technol Ther*, Vol.7, No.6, pp. 968-985, ISSN 1520-9156.

Kobayashi, T., Aomatsu, Y., Iwata, H., Kin, T., Kanehiro, H., Hisanga, M., et al. (2006). Survival of microencapsulated islets at 400 days posttransplantation in the omental pouch of NOD mice. *Cell Trans*, Vol. 15, No. 4, pp. 359-365, ISSN 0963-6897.

Kort, H. d., Koning, E. J. d., Rabelink, T. J., Bruijn, J. A., & Bajema, I. M.. (2011). Islet transplantation in Type 1 diabetes. *BMJ*, Vol. 342, pp. d217, ISSN 0959-8146.

Kulseng, B., Thu, B., Espevik, T., & Skjak-Braek, G. (1997). Alginate polylysine microcapsules as immune barrier: permeability of cytokines and immunoglobulins over the capsule membrane. *Cell Trans*, Vol.6, No.4, pp. 387-394, ISSN 0963-6897.

Lacy, P. E., Hegre, O. D., Gerasimidi-Vazeou, A., Gentile, F. T. & Dionne, K. E. (1991). Maintenance of normoglycemia in diabetic mice by subcutaneous xenografts of encapsulated islets. *Science*, Vol.254, pp. 1782–1784, ISSN 0036-8075.

Lai, Y., Schneider, D., Kidszun, A., Hauck-Schmalenberger, I., Breier, G., Brandhorst, D., et al. (2005). Vascular endothelial growth factor increases functional beta-cell mass by improvement of angiogenesis of isolated human and murine pancreatic islets. *Transplantation*, Vol.79, No.11, pp. 1530-1536, ISSN 0041-1337.

Lakey, J. R. T., Tsujimura, T., Shapiro, A. M. J., & Kuroda, Y. (2002). Preservation of the human pancreas before islet isolation using a two-layer (UW solution-perfluorochemical) cold storage method. *Transplantation*, Vol.74, No.12, pp. 1809-1811, ISSN 0041-1337.

Lanza, R. P., Kuhtreiber, W. M., Ecker, D., Staruk, J. E., & Chick, W. L. (1995). Xenotransplantatton of porcine and bovine islets without immunosuppression using uncoated alginate microspheres. *Transplantation*, Vol.59, No.10, pp. 1377-1384, ISSN 0041-1337.

Leahy, J. L., Bonner-Weir, S., & Weir, G. C. (1992). Beta-cell dysfunction induced by chronic hyperglycemia: Current ideas on mechanism of impaired glucose-induced insulin secretion. *Diabetes Care*, Vol.15, No.3, pp. 442-455, ISSN 0149-5992.

Lifson, N., KG, K., RR, M., & EJ, L. (1980). Blood flow to the rabbit pancreas with special reference to the islets of Langerhans. *Gastroenterology*, Vol.79, No.33, pp. 466-473, ISSN 0016-5085.

Lim, F., & Sun, A. M. (1980). Microencapsulated islets as bioartificial endocrine pancreas. *Science*, Vol.210, No.4472, pp. 908-910, ISSN 0036-8075.

Lum, Z. P., Krestow, M., Tai, I. T., Vacek, I., & Sun, A. M. (1992). Xenografts of rat islets into diabetic mice. An evaluation of new smaller capsules. *Transplantation*, Vol.53, No.6, pp. 1180-1183, ISSN 0041-1337.

Maki, T., Lodge, J. P., Carretta, M., et al. (1993). Treatment of severe diabetes mellitus for more than one year using a vascularized hybrid artificial pancreas. *Transplantation*, Vol.55, No.4, pp. 713-717, ISSN 0041-1337.

Mathis, D., Vence, L., & Benoist, C. (2001). [beta]-Cell death during progression to diabetes. *Nature*, Vol.414, No.6865, pp. 792-798, ISSN 0028-0836.

Menger, M. D., Vajkoczy, P., Beger, C., & Messmer, K. (1994). Orientation of microvascular blood flow in pancreatic islet isografts. *The Journal of Clinical Investigation*, Vol.93, No.5, pp. 2280-2285, ISSN 0021-9738.

Merchant, F. A., Diller, K. R., Aggarwal, S. J., & Bovik, A. C. (1997). Angiogenesis in cultured and cryopreserved pancreatic islet grafts. *Transplantation*, Vol.63, No.11, pp. 1652-1660, ISSN 0041-1337.

Miao, G., Mace, J., Kirby, M., Hopper, A., Peverini, R., Chinnock, R., et al. (2005). Beneficial effects of nerve growth factor on islet transplantation. *Transplantation Proceedings*, Vol.37, No.8, pp. 3490-3492, ISSN 0041-1345.

Morrow, C., Cohen, J. I., Sutherland, D. E., & Najarian, J. S. (1984). Chronic pancreatitis: long-term surgical results of pancreatic duct drainage, pancreatic resection and near-total pancreatectomy and islet autotransplantation. *Surgery*, Vol.96, No.4, pp. 608, ISSN 0039-6060.

Moya, M. L., Lucas, S., Francis-Sedlak, M., Liu, X., Garfinkel, M. R., Huang, J. J., et al. (2009). Sustained delivery of FGF-1 increases vascular density in comparison to bolus administration. *Microvasc Res*, Vol.78, No.2, pp. 142-147, ISSN 0026-2862.

Moya, M. L., Garfinkel, M. R., Liu, X., Lucas, S., Opara, E. C., Greisler, H. P., et al. (2010a). Fibroblast growth factor-1 (FGF-1) loaded microbeads enhance local capillary neovascularization. *J Surg Res*, Vol.160, No.2, pp. 208-212, ISSN 0022-4804.

Moya, M. L., Cheng, M. H., Huang, J. J., Francis-Sedlak, M. E., Kao, S. W., Opara, E. C., et al. (2010b). The effect of FGF-1 loaded alginate microbeads on neovascularization and adipogenesis in a vascular pedicle model of adipose tissue engineering. *Biomaterials*, Vol.31, No.10, pp. 2816-2826, ISSN 0142-9612.

Narang, A. S., & Mahato, R. I. (2006). Biological and biomaterial approaches for improved islet transplantation. *Pharm Reviews*, Vol.58, No.2, pp. 194-243, ISSN 0031-6997.

O'Shea, G. M., Goosen, M. F. A., & Sun, A. M. (1984). Prolonged survival of transplanted islets of langerhans encapsulated in a biocompatible membrane. *Biochimica et Biophysica Acta (BBA) - Mol Cell Res*, Vol.804, No.1, pp. 133-136, ISSN 0006-3002.

O'Shea, G. M., & Sun, A. M. (1986). Encapsulation of rat islets of langerhans prolongs xenograft survival in diabetic mice. *Diabetes*, Vol.35, No.8, pp. 943-946, ISSN 0012-1797.

Omer, A., Duvivier-Kali, V. r. F., Trivedi, N., Wilmot, K., Bonner-Weir, S., & Weir, G. C. (2003). Survival and maturation of microencapsulated porcine neonatal pancreatic cell clusters transplanted into immunocompetent diabetic mice. *Diabetes*, Vol.52, No.1, pp. 69-75, ISSN (0012-1797).

Omer, A., Duvivier-Kali, V., Fernandes, J., Tchipashvili, V., Colton, C. K., & Weir, G. C. (2005). Long-term normoglycemia in rats receiving transplants with encapsulated islets. *Transplantation*, Vol.79, No.1, pp. 52-58, ISSN 0041-1337.

McQuilling, J., Arenas-Herrera, J., Childers, C., Pareta, R. A., et al., & Opara, E. C. (2011). New alginate microcapsule system for angiogenic protein delivery and immunoisolation of islets for transplantation. *Transplant. Proceedings,* Vol 43 (#9): 3262-3264, 2011

Opara, E. C. (2002). Oxidative stress, micronutrients, diabetes mellitus and its complications. *J R Soc Promot Health*, Vol.122, No.1, pp. 28-34, ISSN 1466-4240.

Opara, E. C. (2006). Oxidative stress. *Disease-a-month*, Vol.52, No.5, pp. 183-198, ISSN 0011-5029.

Opara, E. C., Mirmalek-Sani, S. H., Khanna, O., Moya, M. L., & Brey, E. M. (2010). Design of a bioartificial pancreas. *J Investig Med*, Vol.58, No.7, pp. 831-837, ISSN 1081-5589.

Rabinovitch, A., & Suarez-Pinzon, W. L. (1998). Cytokines and their roles in pancreatic islet [beta]-cell destruction and insulin-dependent diabetes mellitus. *Biochemical Pharmacology*, Vol.55, No.8, pp. 1139-1149, ISSN 0006-2952.

Reynoso, J. F., Gruessner, C. E., Sutherland, D. E., & Greussner, R. W. (2010). Short- and long-term outcome for living pancreas donors. *J Hepatobiliary Pancreat Sci,* Vol.17, No.2, pp 92 - 96, ISSN 1868-6974.

Rickels, M. R., Schutta, M. H., Markmann, J. F., Barker, C. F., Naji, A., & Teff, K. L. (2005). Beta-cell function following human islet transplantation for Type 1 diabetes. *Diabetes*, Vol.54, No.1, pp. 100-106, ISSN 0012-1797.

Risbud, M. V., & Bhonde, R. R. (2001). Suitability of cellulose molecular dialysis membrane for bioartificial pancreas: In vitro biocompatibility studies. *Journal of Biomedical Materials Research*, Vol.54, No.3, pp. 436-444, ISSN 0021-9304.

Rivas-Carrillo, J. D., Navarro-Alvarez, N., Soto-Gutierrez, A., Okitsu, T., Chen, Y., Tabata, Y., et al. (2006). Amelioration of diabetes in mice after single-donor islet transplantation using the controlled release of gelatinized FGF-2. *Cell Transplantation*, Vol.15, No.10, pp. 939-944, ISSN 0963-6897.

Robertson, R. P. (2000). Successful islet transplantation for patients with diabetes - fact or fantasy? *New England J of Medicine*, Vol.343, No.4, pp. 289-290, ISSN 0028-4793.

Rossetti, L., Giaccari, A., & DeFronzo, R. A. (1990). Glucose toxicity. *Diabetes Care*, Vol.13, No.6, pp. 610-630, ISSN 0149-5992.

Rossini, A. A., Greiner, D. L., & Mordes, J. P. (1999). Induction of immunologic tolerance for transplantation. *Physiological Reviews*, Vol.79, No.1, pp. 99-141, ISSN 0031-9333.

Rothman, S., Tseng, H., & Goldfine, I. (2005). Oral gene therapy: A novel method for the manufacture and delivery of protein drugs. *Diabetes Technology & Therapeutics*, Vol.7, No.3, pp. 549-557, ISSN 1520-9156.

Safley, S. A., Kapp, L. M., Tucker-Burden, C., Hering, B., Kapp, J. A., & Weber, C. J. (2005). Inhibition of cellular immune responses to encapsulated porcine islet xenografts by simultaneous blockade of two different costimulatory pathways. *Transplantation*, Vol.79, No.4, pp. 409-418, ISSN 0041-1337.

Sandler, S., Andersson, A., Eizirik, D. L., Hellerstrom, C., Espevik, T., Kulseng, B., et al. (1997). Assessment of Insulin secretion in vitro from microencapsulated fetal porcine islet-like cell clusters and rat, mouse, and human pancreatic islets. *Transplantation*, Vol.63, No.12, pp. 1712-1718, ISSN 0041-1337.

Scharp, D. W., et. al. (1994). Protection of encapsulated human islets implanted without immunosuppression in patients with Type I or Type II diabetes and in nondiabetic control subjects. *Diabetes*, Vol.43, No.9, pp. 1167–1170, ISSN 0012-1797.

Schneider, S., Feilen, P. J., Brunnenmeier, F., Minnemann, T., Zimmermann, H., Zimmermann, U., et al. (2005). Long-term graft function of adult rat and human islets encapsulated in novel alginate-based microcapsules after transplantation in immunocompetent diabetic mice. *Diabetes*, Vol.54, No.3, pp. 687-693, ISSN 0012-1797.

Senuma, Y., Lowe, C., Zweifel, Y., Hilborn, J. G., & Marison, I. (2000). Alginate hydrogel microspheres and microcapsules prepared by spinning disk atomization. *Biotechnol Bioeng*, Vol.67, No.5, pp. 616-622, ISSN 0006-3592.

Serup, P., Madsen, O., & Mandrup-Poulsen, T. (2001). Islet and stem cell transplantation for treating diabetes. *BMJ*, Vol.322, No.7277, pp. 29-32, ISSN 0959-8138.

Shapiro, A. M. J., Lakey, J. R. T., Ryan, E. A., et al. (2000). Islet transplantation in seven patients with type 1 diabetes mellitus using a glucocorticoid-free immunosuppressive regimen. *N Eng J Med*, Vol.343, No.4, pp. 230-238, ISSN 0028-4793.

Sibley, R. K., Sutherland, D. E., Goetz, F., & Michael, A. F. (1985). Recurrent diabetes mellitus in the pancreas iso- and allograft. A light and electron microscopic and immunohistochemical analysis of four cases. *Lab Invest*, Vol.53, No.2, pp. 132-144, ISSN 0023-6837.

Soon-Shiong, P., Feldman, E., Nelson, R., Komtebedde, J., Smidsrod, O., Skjak-Braek, G., et al. (1992). Successful reversal of spontaneous diabetes in dogs by intraperitoneal microencapsulated islets. *Transplantation*, Vol.54, No.5, pp. 769-774, ISSN 0041-1337.

Soon-Shiong, P., Heintz, R. E., Merideth, N., Yao, Q. X., Yao, Z., Zheng, T., et al. (1994). Insulin independence in a Type 1 diabetic patient after encapsulated islet transplantation. *The Lancet*, Vol.343, No.8903, pp. 950-951, ISSN 0140-6736.

Stiegler, P., Stadlbauer, V., Hackl, F., Schaffellner, S., Iberer, F., Greilberger, J., et al. (2010). Prevention of oxidative stress in porcine islet isolation. *Journal of Artificial Organs*, Vol.13, No.1, pp. 38-47, ISSN 1434-7229.

Strand, B. L., Ryan, T. L., In't Veld, P., Kulseng, B., Rokstad, A. M., Skjak-Brek, G., et al. (2001). Poly-L-Lysine induces fibrosis on alginate microcapsules via the induction of cytokines. *Cell Transplant*, Vol.10, No.3, pp. 263-275, ISSN 0963-6897.

Strand, B. L., Morch, Y. A., Espevik, T., & Skjak-Braek, G. (2003). Visualization of alginate-poly-L-lysine-alginate microcapsules by confocal laser scanning microscopy. *Biotechnol Bioeng*, Vol.82, No.4, pp. 386-394, ISSN 0006-3592.

Sun, A. M., Parisius, W., Healy, G. M., Vacek, I., & Macmorine, H. G. (1977). The use, in diabetic rats and monkeys, of artificial capillary units containing cultured islets of Langerhans (artificial endocrine pancreas). *Diabetes*, Vol.26, No.12, pp. 1136-1139, ISSN 0012-1797.

Sun, A. M., O'Shea, G. M., & Goosen, M. F. (1984). Injectable microencapsulated islet cells as a bioartificial pancreas. *Appl Biochem Biotechnol*, Vol.10, pp. 87-99, ISSN 0273-2289.

Sun, Y., Ma, X., Zhou, D., Vacek, I., & Sun, A. M. (1996). Normalization of diabetes in spontaneously diabetic cynomologus monkeys by xenografts of microencapsulated porcine islets without immunosuppression. *The J of Clin Investigation*, Vol.98, No.6, pp. 1417-1422, ISSN 0021-9738.

Sutherland, D. E. R., Gruessner, R. W. G., & Gruessner, A. C. (2001). Pancreas transplantation for treatment of diabetes mellitus. *World Journal of Surgery*, Vol.25, No.4, pp. 487-496, ISSN 1976-2283.

Suylichem, P. T. R. V., Strubbe, J. H., Houwing, H., Wolters, G. H. J., & Schilfgaarde, R. V. (1992). Insulin secretion by rat islet isografts of a defined endocrine volume after transplantation to three different sites. *Diabetologia*, Vol.35, No.10, pp. 917–923, ISSN 0012-186X.

Tendulkar, S., McQuilling, J. P., Childers, C., Pareta, R. A., Opara, E. C., & Ramasubramanian, M. K. (2011). A scalable microfluidic device for the mass production of microencapsulated islets. *Transplantation Proceedings*, Vol 43 (#9): 3184-3187, 2011

Thu, B., Bruheim, P., Espevik, T., Smidsrod, O., SoonShiong, P., & SkjakBraek, G. (1996a). Alginate polycation microcapsules. I. Interaction between alginate and polycation. *Biomaterials*, Vol.17, No.10, pp. 1031-1040, ISSN 0142-9612.

Thu, B., Bruheim, P., Espevik, T., Smidsrod, O., Soon-Shiong, P., & Skjak-Braek, G. (1996b). Alginate polycation microcapsules. II. Some functional properties. *Biomaterials*, Vol.17, No.11, pp. 1069-1079, ISSN 0142-9612.

Toso, C., Mathe, Z., Morel, P., Oberholzer, J., Bosco, D., Sainz-Vidal, D., et al. (2005). Effect of microcapsule composition and short-term immunosuppression on intraportal biocompatibility. *Cell Transplantation*, Vol.14, No.2-3, pp. 159-167, ISSN 0963-6897.

Tuch, B. E., Keogh, G. W., Williams, L. J., Wu, W., Foster, J. L., Vaithilingam, V., et al. (2009). Safety and viability of microencapsulated human islets transplanted into diabetic humans. *Diabetes Care*, Vol.32, No.10, pp. 1887-1889, ISSN 0149-5992.

Vajkoczy, P., Menger, M. D., Simpson, E. & Messmer, K. (1995). Angiogenesis and vascularization of murine pancreatic islet isografts. *Transplantation*, Vol.60, No.2, pp. 123-127, ISSN 0041-1337.

van Schilfgaarde, R., & de Vos, P. (1998). Factors in success and failure of microencapsulated pancreatic islets. *Transplantation Proceedings*, Vol.30, No.2, pp. 501-502, ISSN 0041-1345.

van Schilfgaarde, R., & de Vos, P. (1999). Factors influencing the properties and performance of microcapsules for immunoprotection of pancreatic islets. *J Mol Med (Berl)*,Vol.77, No.1, pp. 199-205, ISSN 0946-2716.

Vasir, B., Aiello, L. P., Yoon, K. H., Quickel, R. R., Bonner-Weir, S., & Weir, G. C. (1998). Hypoxia induces vascular endothelial growth factor gene and protein expression in cultured rat islet cells. *Diabetes*, Vol.47, No.12, pp. 1894-1903, ISSN 0012-1797.

Vos-Scheperkeuter, G. H., Van Suylichem, P. T. R., Vonk, M. W. A., Wolters, G. H. J., & Van Schilfgaarde, R. (1997). Histochemical analysis of the role of class I and class II clostridium histolyticum collagenase in the degradation of rat pancreatic extracellular matrix for islet isolation. *Cell Transplantation*, Vol.6, No.4, pp. 403-412, ISSN 0963-6897.

Vos, P. D., Haan, B. J. D., Zanten, J. v., & Faas, M. M. (2004). Factors influencing functional survival of microencapsulated islets. *Cell Transplantation*, Vol.13, No.5, pp. 515–524, ISSN 0963-6897.

Wang, T., Adcock, J., Kuhtreiber, W., Qiang, D., Salleng, K. J., Trenary, I., et al. (2008). Successful allotransplantation of encapsulated islets in pancreatectomized canines for diabetic management without the use of immunosuppression. *Transplantation*, Vol.85, No.3, pp. 331-337, ISSN 0041-1337.

White, S. A., Robertson, G. S. M., London, N. J. M., & Dennison, A. R. (2000). Human islet autotransplantation to prevent diabetes after pancreas resection. *Digestive Surgery*, Vol.17, No.5, pp. 439-450, ISSN 0253-4886.

Wiegand, F., Kroncke, K. D., & Kolbbachofen, V. (1993). Macrophage-generated nitric-oxide as cytotoxic factor in destruction of alginate-encapsulated islets-protection of arginine analogs and/or coencapsulated erythrocytes. *Transplantation*, Vol.56, No.5, pp. 1206-1212, ISSN 0041-1337.

Wolters, G. H., Fritschy, W. M., Gerrits, D., & van Schilfgaarde, R. (1991). A versatile alginate droplet generator applicable for microencapsulation of pancreatic islets. *J Appl Biomater*, Vol.3, No.4, pp. 281-286, ISSN 1045-4861.

Wolters, G. H., Vos-Scheperkeuter, G. H., van Deijnen, J. H., & van Schilfgaarde, R. (1992). An analysis of the role of collagenase and protease in the enzymatic dissociation of the rat pancreas for islet isolation. *Diabetologia*, Vol.35, No.8, pp. 735-742, ISSN 0012-186X.

Yasunami, Y., Lacy, P. E., & Finke, E. H. (1983). A new site for islet transplantation -a peritoneal-omental pouch. *Transplant*, Vol.36, No.2, pp. 181-182, ISSN 041-1337.

Zekorn, T., Horcher, A., Siebers, U., Federlin, K., & Bretzel, R. G. (1995). Islet transplantation in immunoseparating membranes for treatment of insulin-dependent diabetes mellitus. *Exp Clin Endocrinol Diabetes*, Vol.103, Suppl.2, pp. 136, ISSN 0947-7349.

Zielinski, B. A., & Aebischer, P. (1994). Chitosan as a matrix for mammalian cell encapsulation. *Biomaterials*, Vol.15, No.13, pp. 1049–1056, ISSN 0142-9612.

Zimmermann, H., Zimmermann, D., Reuss, R., Feilen, P. J., Manz, B., Katsen, A., et al. (2005). Towards a medically approved technology for alginate-based microcapsules allowing long-term immunoisolated transplantation. *J of Mat Sci: Mat in Med*, Vol.16, No.6, pp. 491-501, ISSN 0957-4530.

Zukerman, W. (2010). 'Pig Sushi' diabetes trial brings xenotransplant hope. *New Scientist*.

15

Transcranial Doppler as an Confirmatory Test in Brain Death

Arijana Lovrencic-Huzjan
University Departement of Neurology,
University Hospital Center «Sestre milosrdnice», Referral Center for Neurovascular Disorders of The Ministry of Health and Social Welfare of Republic Croatia
Croatia

1. Introduction

Brain death in a normothermic, nondruged comatose patient with a known irreversible massive brain lesion and no contributing metabolic or hormonal derangements, is declared when brainstem reflexes, motor responses and respiratory drive are absent.

Loss of brain function in a mechanically ventilated patient has been observed since the early days of intensive care units, but criteria for brain death in the United States were not forthcoming until 1968 after publication of a report of the Harvard Medical School ad hoc committee using the neurologic criteria (JAMA 1968.). The report defined totally destroyed unsalvageable brain for the first time, and one of the criteria was the isoelectric, flat electroencephalography (EEG) despite the heartbeat. However, its value became much less important when the clinical picture became defined and the technical difficulties became recognized. Due to a number of confounders that mimic or partly mimic brain death, like hypothermia, intoxication or acute metabolic or endocrine derangements, different ancillary tests to confirm cessation of brain functions by means of electrophysiology or showing the cessation of flow, developed. EEG would show no electrical activity of the cerebral cortex. However, in one consecutive series of patients fulfilling the clinical diagnosis of brain death, 20% of patients had residual EEG activity, and also, considerable artifacts in the intensive care unit can limit interpretation. Somatosensory evoked potentials and auditory brainstem responses should show no brainstem electrical activity, and were tested in small series of patients with brain death, and most patients were found to have no responses. Isotope angiography by rapid intravenous injection of serum albumin labeled with technetium 99m and following by bedside imaging with a portable gamma camera would show absent intracranial radioisotope activity. However, its sensitivity and specificity have not been defined in adults. The same procedure can be performed with technetium-99m hexamethylpropyleneamineoxime (^{99m}Tc-HMPAO), and the sensitivity has been reported to be as low as 94% with a specificity of 100%, but the reproducibility has been tested in only a few patients. Due to high costs and technique is not widely available, expertise is limited. Four vessel angiogram showing absent intracerebral filling at the level of the carotid bifurcation or circle of Willis seemed to be an ideal method showing cessation of the intracranial flow thus confirming cerebral circulatory arrest. Repeated contrast injections may increase the risk of nephrotoxicity and decrease the acceptance rate in organ recipients. Multislice computerized angiography is a more sensible method for assessment of cerebral circulatory arrest, but its disadvantage is that it may show tinny filling of contrast in one of the arteries of the Willis circle, disabling the confirmation of circulatory arrest. In such instances repeated application of contrast injections and imaging is performed until complete cessation of flow. Up to now there is no unified agreement of criteria for assessment of the cerebral circulatory arrest with this method, and nephrotoxicity due to repeated contrast injections is a disadvantage. Transcranial Doppler sonography is an easy bedside method, reporting characteristic signals indicating circulatory arrest. Its disadvantage is that the velocities can be affected by marked changes in pCO_2, hematocrit, cardiac output, it requires considerable practice and skill, and suboptimal temporal bone window may be a problem.

Due to perceived need for standardized clinical examination criteria for the diagnosis of brain death in adults, large differences in practice in performing the apnea test, and controversies over appropriate utilization of confirmatory tests in the year 1995., brain death was selected as a topic for practice parameters (Wijdicks EFM. Neurology 1995.). The committee defined practice parameters that should serve as guidelines in management patients with brain death (Report of the Quality Standards Subcommittee of the American Academy of Neurology. Neurology 1995.). Despite such definition, criteria varies between countries, and guidelines have recently been updated (Wijdicks EFM, et al. Neurology 2010.).

A survey on brain death criteria (Wijdicks EFM. Neurology 2002.) throughout the world revealed uniform agreement on the neurologic examination with exception of the apnea test. Major differences between countries were present between presence of legal standards on organ transplantation, presence of practice guidelines for brain death for adults, number of physicians required to declare brain death, observational period or presence of required expertise of examining physicians. Only 28 of 70 (40%) national practice guidelines require confirmatory testing. Therefore, a necessity of a universal consensus for brain death determination exists, and agreement must be found and set due to medical, legal, and ethical reasons.

2. Recommendations for diagnosing brain death

By recently publiched guidelines (Wijdicks EFM et al. Neurology 2010.), the criteria for the determination of brain death given in the 1995. by American Academy of Neurology practice parameters have not been invalidated by recently published reports of neurologic recovery in patients who fulfille these criteria, so that the guidelines remains the same.

The determination of brain death can be considered to consist of four steps:

1. The clinical evaluation establishing irreversible and proximate cause of coma by history, examination and neuroimaging. Clinical conditions that may confound the clinical assessment must be ruled out like severe electrolyte, acid-base or endocrine disturbances, administration of neuromuscular blocking agents or central nerve system (CNS) depressant drugs by hystory or laboratory tests. Normal core temperature and normal systolic blood pressure should be achieved. The clinical examination must show

absence of brain and brainstem functions, and irreversibiliy by adequate observational period.
2. The clinical evaluation (neurological assessment) must show coma, absence of brainstem reflexes and apnea.
3. Ancillary tests accepted in practice are electroencephalography (EEG), cerebral angiography, nuclear scan, transcranial Doppler (TCD), computerised tomography angiography (CTA) and magnetic resonance imaging/angiography (MRI/MRA), with the expertise in interpretation of each of the tests. In some countries tests are mandatory, in other countries may serve to shorten the observational period. They cannot replace a neurologic examination. Rather than ordering ancillary tests, physicians may decide not to proceed with the declaration of brain death if clinical findings are unreliable.
4. The time of brain death is documented in the medical records. Time of death is the time the arterial pCO_2 reaches the target value. In patients in whom ancillary test has been performed, the time of death is the time the test has been officially interpreted. Federal and state law requires the physician to contact an organ procurement organization following determination of brain death.

3. Transcranial Doppler sonography

Soon after Doppler sonography has been introduced for cerebrovascular evaluation, typical findings for cerebral circulatory arrest were described as oscillating flow or systolic spikes (Yoneda S, et al. Stroke 1974.). The reliability of the method increased with the introduction of TCD, and standardization of the insonating protocol (Ducrocq X, et al. J Neurol Sci 1998.).

Extensive death of brain tissue causes extreme increase of intracranial pressure (ICP). When the ICP equals the diastolic arterial pressure, the brain is perfused only in systole and with further increase of ICP over the systolic arterial pressure, cerebral perfusion will cease. Due to elasticity of the arterial wall and the compliance of the vasculature distal to the recording site, such cerebral circulatory arrest is associated with Doppler evidence of oscillatory movement of blood in the large arteries at the base of the brain. However the net forward flow volume is zero. With time the oscillations decrease in amplitude of spectral spikes until no pulsations are detectable. This development correlates with a more proximal demonstration of the angiographic flow arrest (Hassler W, et al. J Neurosurg 1989.). At the time of angiographic flow arrest at the internal carotid artery, the TCD shows an oscillating flow pattern in the middle cerebral artery, because the contrast medium progresses slowly toward the brain. From the clinical experience from cardiac arrest, such cerebral ischemia of about 10-15 minutes in vivo at normal body temperature, leads to irreversible total loss of brain function.

TCD is actualy evaluating the blood flow velocities from basal cerebral arteries, depending of the sistemic blood pressure (BP) and ICP. Figure 1. represents time course of spectral changes and flow velocities in middle cerebral artery (MCA) from normal condition up to development of cerebral circulatory arrest in relation of ICP with BP. With increase of ICP, a higher pulsatility in basal cerebral arteries can be registred, and with further increase of the ICP over diastolic BP, only forward flow persists in systole.

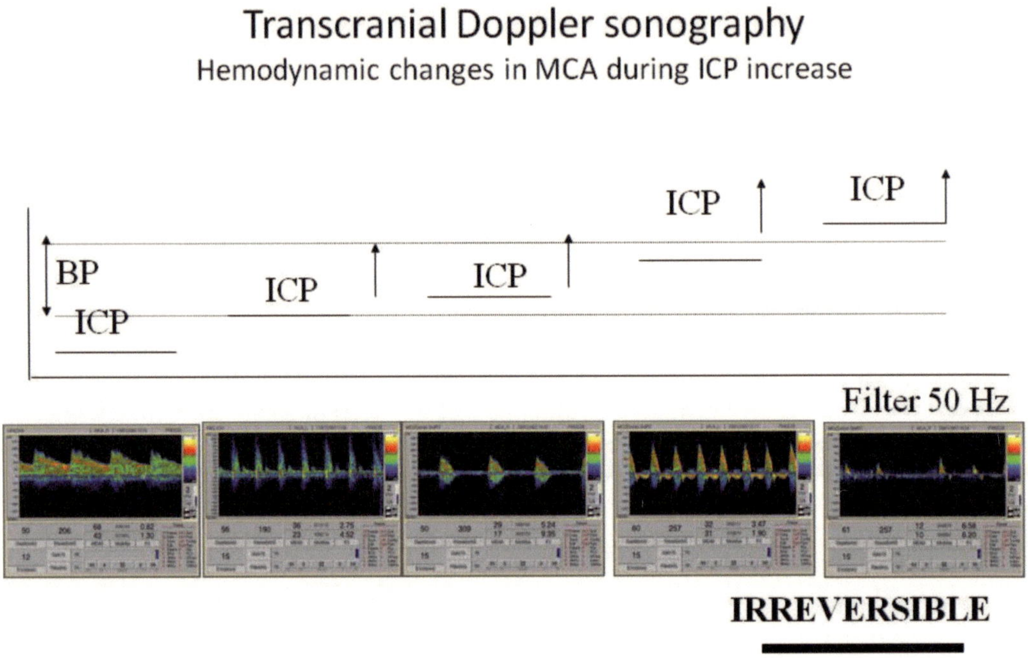

Fig. 1. Hemodynamic changes in middle cerebral artery (MCA) during increase of intracranial pressure (ICP)

With further increase of ICP that equals the systolic BP, reverberating flow with forward and reverse flow are nearly equal and cerebral perfusion cesseases. Net flow is zero when the equality of both flow components are present and if the area under the evelope of the positive and negative deflection is the same. This finding correlates with the angiographic appearance of cerebral circulatory arrest (Hassler W, et al. J Neurosurg 1989.).

With further increace of ICP over the systolic BP, only systolic spikes can be registered, and their amplitudes decreases with time. Such systolic spikes have characteristic pattern for cerebral circulatory arest, but may resemble high resistence pattern with reduction of diastolic flow, the phase before developement of reveberating flow. Due to the usage of high pass filters for elimination of artefacts from wall movement, reverberating flow can be missed. Therefore the filters must be set at its lowest level, at 50 Hz.

With further reduction of blood movement, the further decrease of amplitude can be registered until the complete cessation of signals. Failure to detect flow signals alone as the first finding, may also be a result from ultrasonic transmission problems. In such cases, the extracranial findings showing typical hemodynamic spectra in common carotid arteries (CCA), internal carotid arteries (ICA) and vertebral arteries (VA), represent important criterion (Fig 2., Fig 3., Fig 4.), but cannot replace the intracranial finding. At the same time flow in the external carotid arteries remain patent, with normal hemodynamic spectras. Flow in the ICA can be influenced by flow through the ophthalmic artery, althought the volume of the ophthalmic artery flow plays a minor portion of the ICA flow.

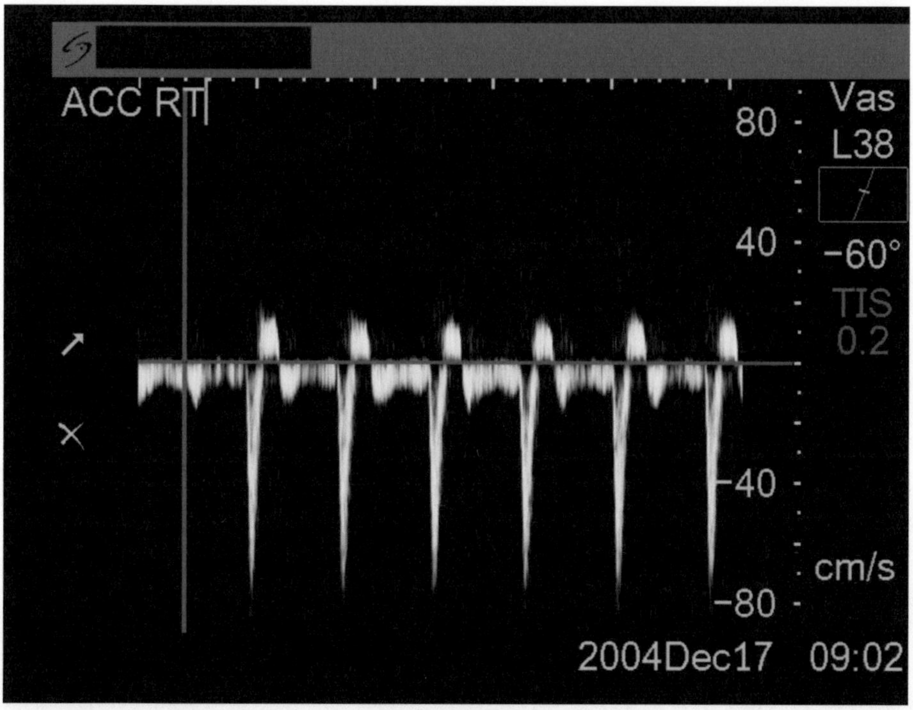

Fig. 2. Reveberating flow in common carotid artery (CCA)

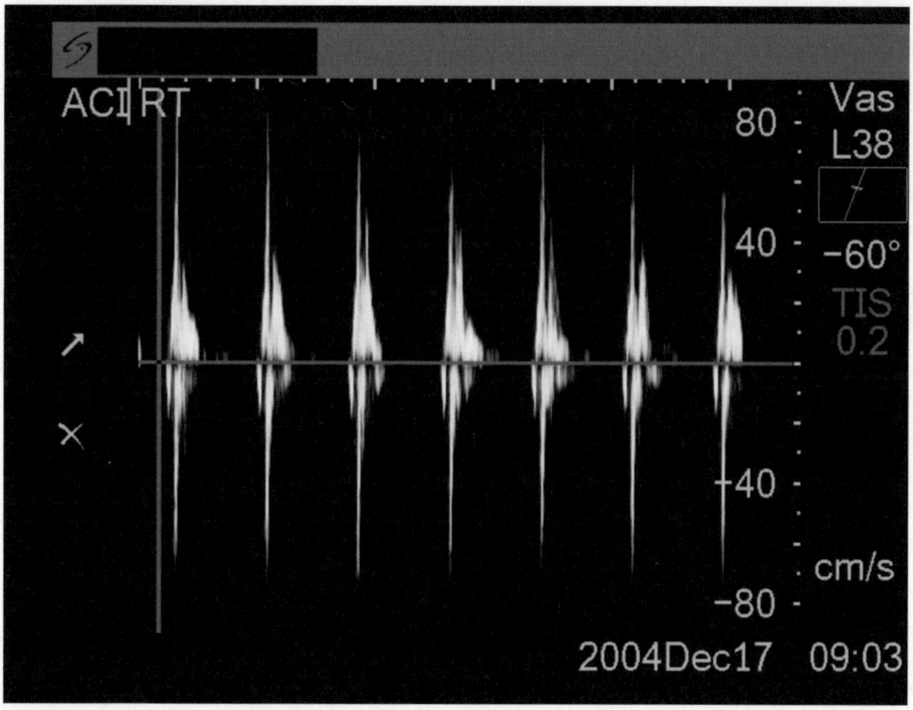

Fig. 3. Systolic spikes in internal carotid artery (ACI)

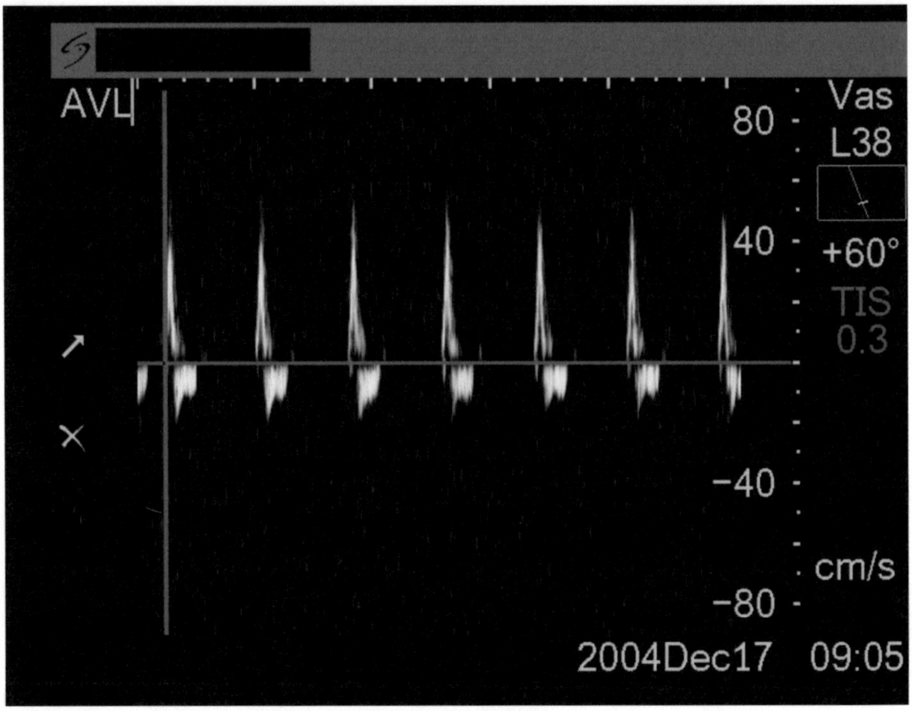

Fig. 4. Reveberating flow in left vertebral artery (AVL)

4. Guidelines for the use of Doppler sonography in brain death

The Neurosonology Research Group (NSRG) of the World Federation of Neurology (WFN) created a Task Force Group in order to evaluate the role of Doppler sonography as a confirmatory test for determining brain death, and created criteria which are defined and guidelines for the use of Doppler-sonography in this setting (Ducrocq X, et al. J Neurol Sci 1998.), and these guidelines were addopted and endorsed by numerous national societies (Demarin V, et al. Acta clin Croat 2005, Lovrencic-Huzjan A, et al. Acta clin Croat 2006., Alexandrov AV, et al. J Neuroimaging 2010., Segura T, et al. Rev Neurosci 2009., Calleja S, et al. Neurologia 2007., Marinoni M, et al. Neurol Sci 2011.).

According to aforementioned findings, Task Force Group of the NSRG WFN, (Ducrocq X, et al. J Neurol Sci 1998.) set guidelines for the use of Doppler sonography as a confirmatory test for cerebral circulatory arrest as follows:

4.1 Prerequisites

Doppler sonography can be used to confirm cerebral circulatory arrest thus confirming brain death only if the following diagnostic prerequisites are fulfilled:

1. The cause of coma has been established and is sufficient to account for a permanent loss of brain function.
2. Other conditions such as intoxication, hypothermia, severe arterial hypotension, metabolic disorders and others have been excluded.

3. Clinical evaluation by two experienced examiners shows no evidence of cerebral and brainstem function.

4.2 Criteria

Cerebral circulatory arrest can be confirmed if the following extra- and intracranial Doppler sonographic findings have been recorded and documented both intra- and extracranially and bilaterally on two examinations at an interval of at least 30 min.

1. Systolic spikes (Fig. 5.) or oscillating flow (Fig. 6.) in any cerebral artery which can be recorded by bilateral transcranial insonation of the ICA and MCA, respectively any branch, or other artery which can be recorded (anterior and posterior circulation). Oscillating flow is defined by signals with forward and reverse flow components in one cardiac cycle exhibiting almost the same area under the envelope of the wave form (to and fro movement). Systolic spikes are sharp unidirectional velocity signals in early systole of less than 200 ms duration, less than 50 cm/s peak systolic velocity, and without a flow signal during the remaining cardiac cycle. Transitory patterns between oscillating flow and systolic spikes may be seen. In order to enable visualisation of the low signals, wall filter must be set at its lowest level (50 Hz).
2. The diagnosis established by the intracranial examination must be confirmed by the extracranial bilateral recording of the CCA, ICA and VA.

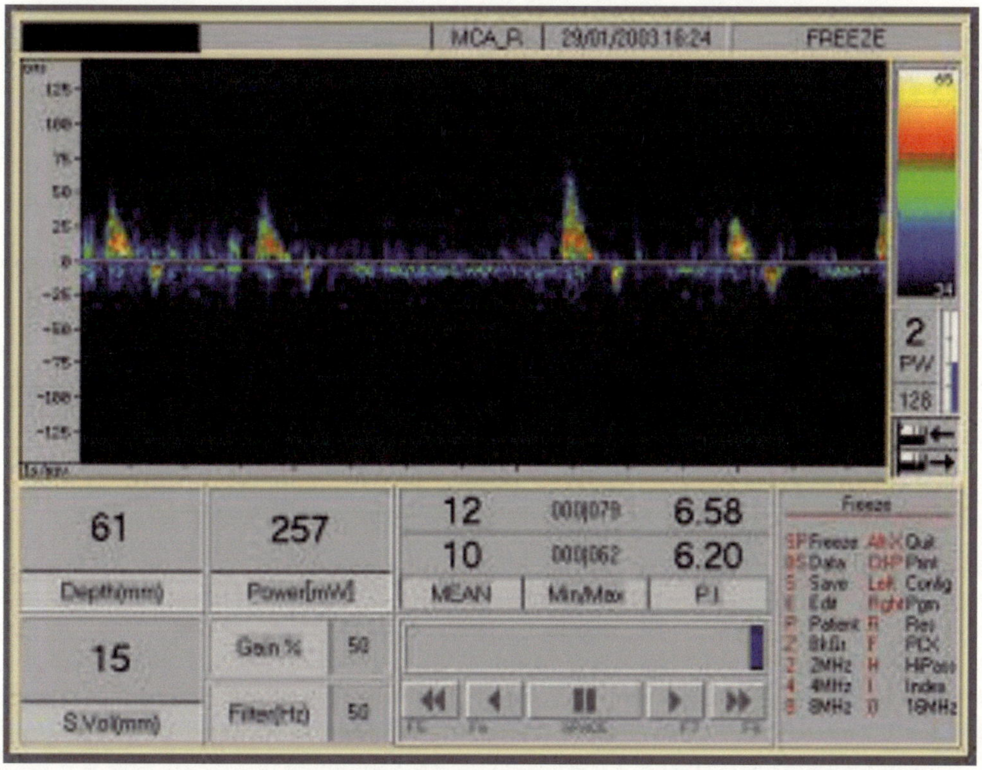

Fig. 5. Systolic spikes in middle cerebral artery (MCA)

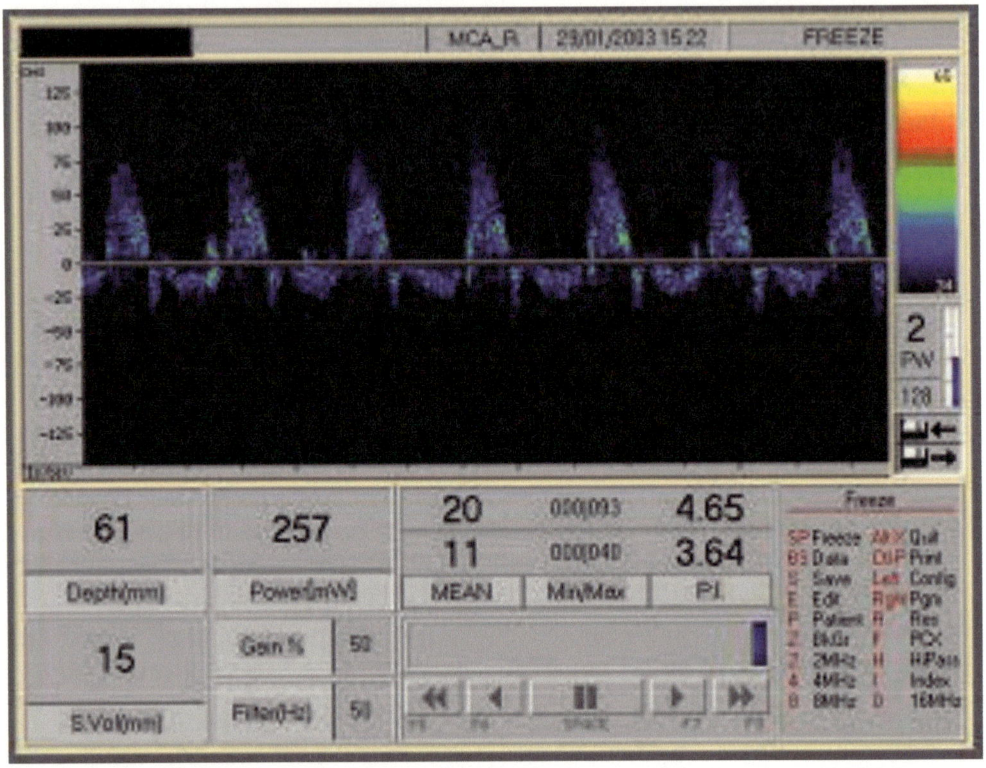

Fig. 6. Oscillating flow in middle cerebral artery (MCA)

3. The lack of signal during transcranial insonation of the basal cerebral arteries is not a reliable finding because this can be due to transmission problems. But the disappearance of intracranial flow signals in conjunction with typical extracranial signals can be accepted as proof of circulatory arrest.
4. Ventricular drains or large openings of the skull like in decompressive craniectomy possibly interfering with the development of the ICP is not present.

If the clinical prerequisites are fulfilled and cerebral circulatory arrest has been documented by Doppler sonography according to the above mentioned criteria, the diagnosis of brain death may be confirmed without further observation time, (Ducrocq X, et al. J Neurol Sci 1998.).

5. False positive and false negative TCD findings

There are no reports of previously published literature of a child or adult patient «surviving» who demonstrated bilateral signals or oscillating flow or systolic spikes in the MCA and ICA for at least half an hour. Only false positive reports with «some flow» in MCA or basilar artery were the result of the skull defects (Zurynski Y, et al. Neurol Res 1991.). Since the TCD registers the blood flow velocities (BFV) in relation to ICP, the skull defects are contraindications for examination (Fig. 1.). Due to the relation of BFV to BP, hypotension should be corrected before starting the examination (Fig. 1.), and during the examination.

5.1 Sonographic condition in which false positive findings can be detected

Acutely raised intracranial pressure due to bleeding or rebleeding from an aneurysm has been observed with transient flow patterns similar to those in cerebral circulatory arrest (Eng CC, et al. Anesthesiology 1993., Grote E & Hassler W. Neurosurgery 1988.). A similar high resistance pattern can occur shortly after cardiac arrest during the «no reflow phase». Both conditions are transient and the flow abnormalities will reverse at least partially within less than 30 minutes. During this initial phase, patients are clinically not brain dead. A proportion of these patients may later deteriorate to brain death.

Since brain death is a clinical condition, the clinical findings must first be fulfilled. In patients with both ICA distal occlusion, only systolic spikes in both ICAs would be detected. These patients would be mistaken if examination of the posterior circulation is not part of the protocal. Aortic insufficiency, especialy in aortic dissection, may also pose problems for interpretation of the flow pattern of the CCA and ICA (Fig.7.,8.,9.,10.,11.,12.,13.), and also in basilar artery (Fig.14.). The reverse component, if present, is smaller than the forward component of the flow signals. If the flow signals transtemporally cannot be registered, the transmission problems can be suspected. Up to 20% of individuals have strong ossification of the temporal bones making the insonation imposible.

An experienced investigator is required. During the developement of cerebral circulatory arrest, marked changes of hemodynamic spectras develop. Therefore, an unexperienced examiner may mistake ECA for ICA, due to patent flow in extracranial circulation, with normal spectrum, and therefore a lower pulsatility than in intracranial circulation (which is contrary to normal situation).

TCD provides indirect information on cerebral blood flow regardless of brainstem status. It is important to fulfill the prerequisites because after excluding the skull opening or low BP, all together three false positive cases were described in the literature. Recently one case reported comatose patient with TCD brain death pattern detected without absence of brainstem reflexes (Wijdicks EFM. 2010.). In the meta-analysis (Monteiro LM, et al. Intensive Care Med 2006.) including ten studies of the usage of TCD in brain death, two false-positive results were reported, but in both patients brain-stem function did show brain death shortly thereafter. In the first (Hadani M, et al. Intensive Care Med 1999.) weak respiratory movements in response to an apnea test persisted for some hours after the first TCD signals of cerebral circulatory arrest were detected. The second (Velthoven van V, et al. Acta Neurochir (Wien) 1988.) a clinically brain-dead patient, with cerebral circulatory arrest by TCD in the basilar artery and the circle of Willis, confirmed by angiography, became iso-electric only several hours later. Ten other false-positive results in literature from that meta-analysis were not in agreement with predefined criteria of a false-positive result, examination of the posterior circulation was not performed, or the changes were transient. Ducrocq et al. described one case with continued spontaneous respiration for some minutes after TCD examination showing typical spectras, but without data available as to which vessels were examined and under which condition TCD examination took place (Ducrocq X, et al. J Neurol Sci 1998.). Since TCD was never meant to be a replacement for clinical investigational, and if the prerequisites are met, it doesn't decrease the reliability of TCD and can be used with high confidelity in assessment of cerebral circulatory arrest.

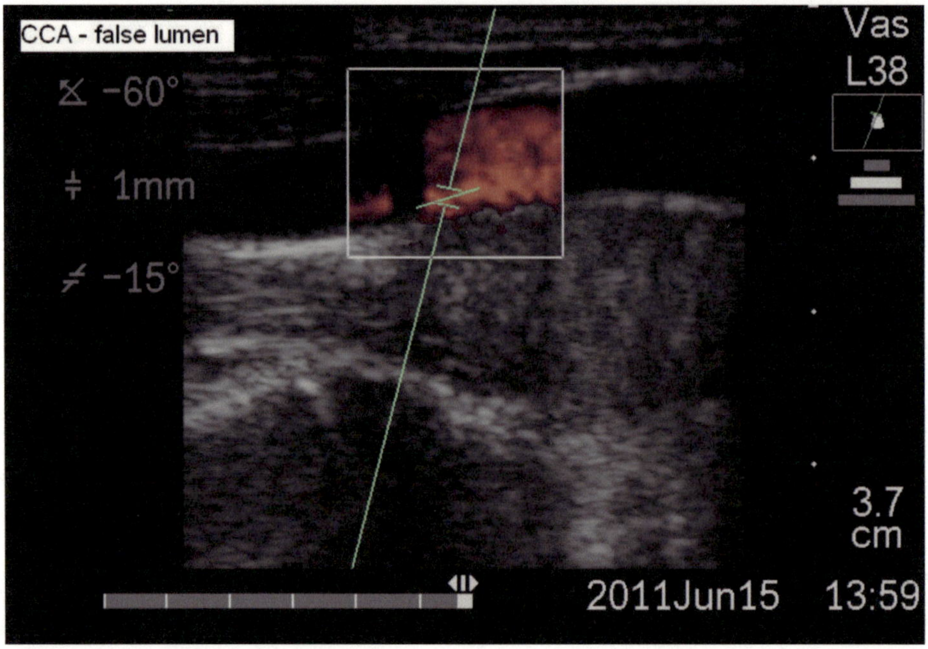

Fig. 7. Dissection of common carotid artery (CCA), measurement of hemodynamic in false lumen (B mod)

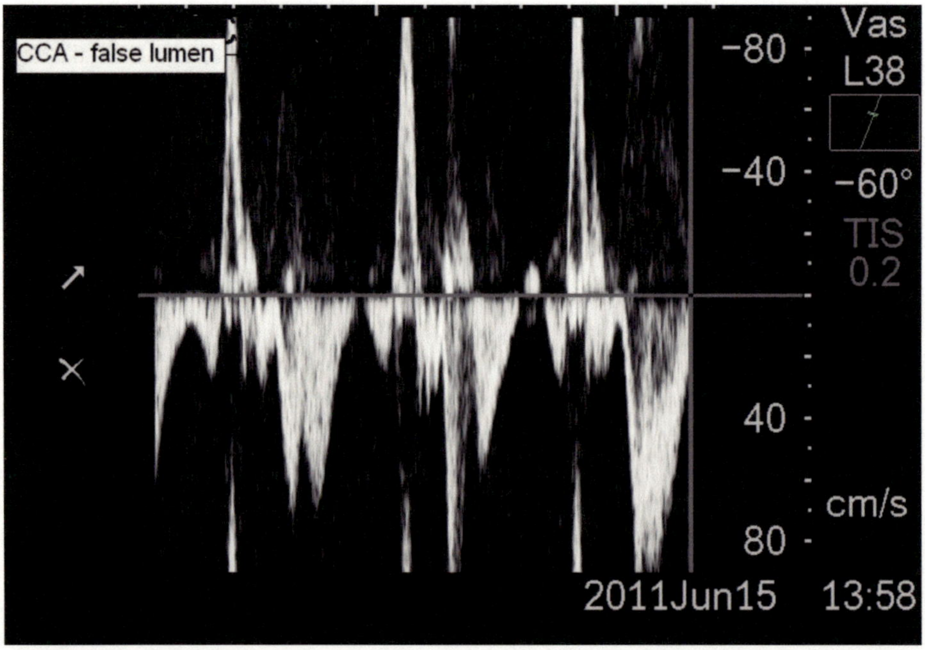

Fig. 8. Reverberating flow in false lumen of common carotid artery (CCA) dissection as a result of aortic insufficiency in aortic dissection

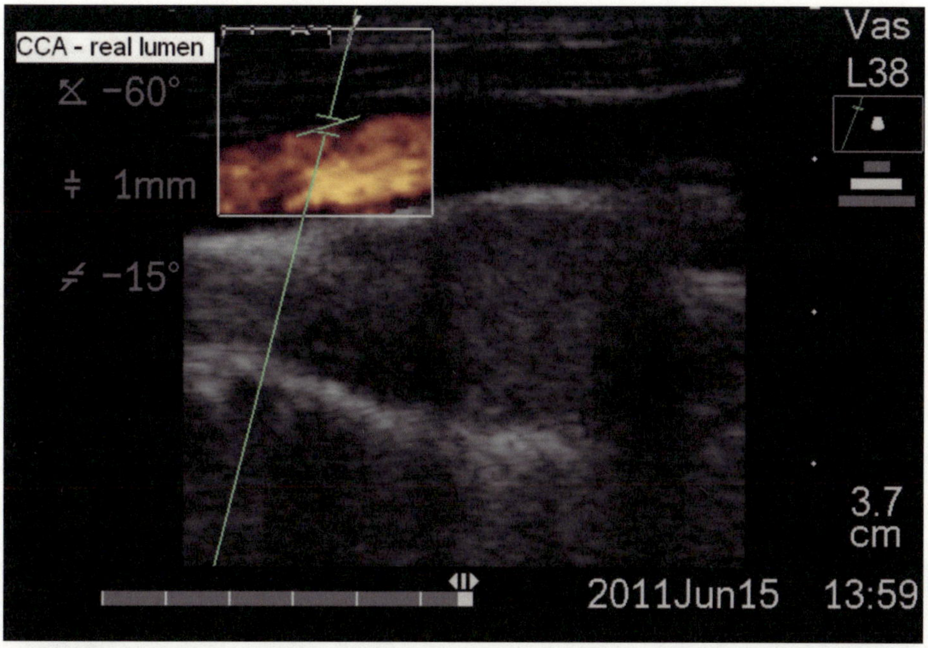

Fig. 9. Dissection of common carotid artery (CCA), measurement of hemodynamic in real lumen (B mod)

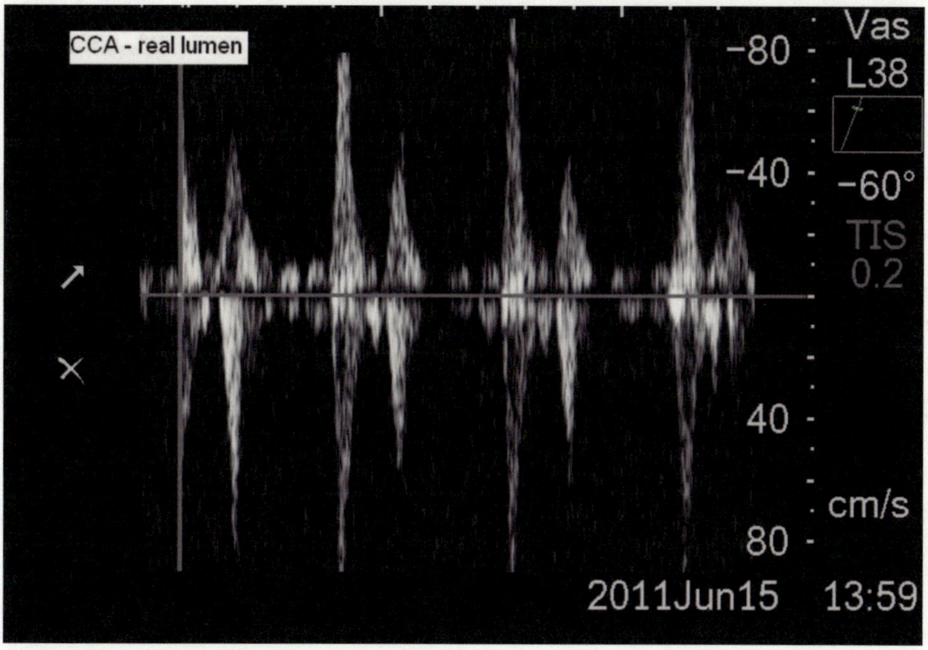

Fig. 10. Reverberating flow in real lumen of common carotid artery (CCA) dissection as a result of aortic insufficiency in aortic dissection

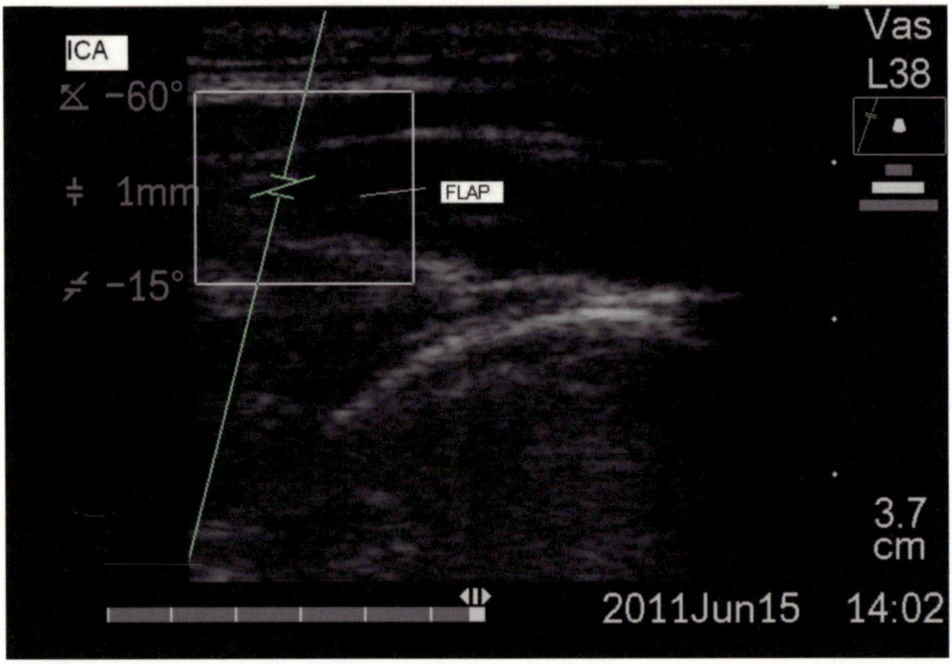

Fig. 11. Dissection of internal carotid artery (ICA) with intimal flap in B mod

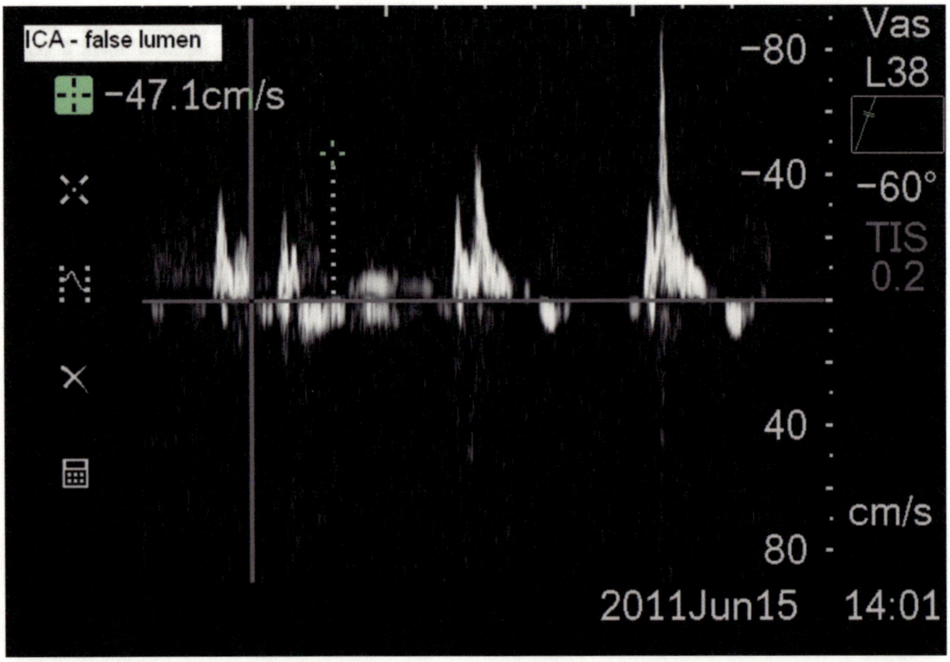

Fig. 12. Systolic spikes in false lumen of internal carotid artery (ICA) as a result of aortic dissection

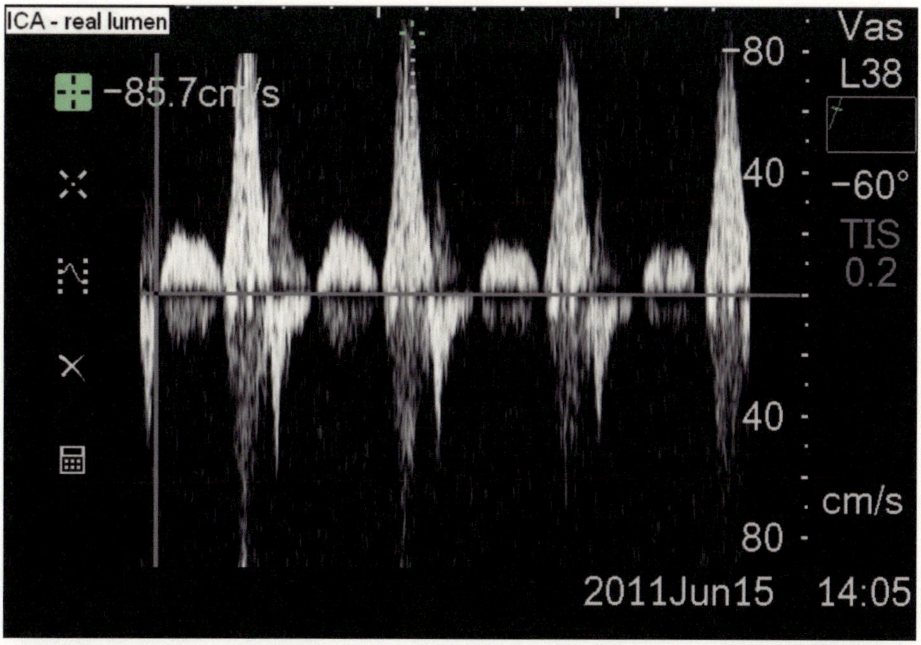

Fig. 13. Reverberating flow in real lumen of internal carotid artery (ICA) as a result of aortic dissection

5.2 Sonographic condition in which false negative findings can be detected

Few years ago, a report of false negative results due to the presence of diastolic flow in intracranial ICA obtained through orbital window in clinically brain dead patients was published (de Freitas GR, et al. J Neurol Sci 2003.). Although not specifically stated in the article, presumably all patients who had ICA flow consistent with cerebral circulatory arrest also had other intracranial arteries demonstrating a similar flow pattern. The authors propose that the ICA should not be routinely studied for confirmation of brain death, except in patients whose transtemporal windows are inadequate, leading to the inability to insonate the MCA. In editorial of the article (Jacobs BS, et al. J Neurol Sci 2003.), reasons for reviewing current criteria for TCD diagnosis of brain death were presented. Beside the de Freitas's (de Freitas GR, et al. J Neurol Sci 2003.) reasons for exclusion of the intracranial ICA insonation, is the suggestion for exlusion examination of the extracranial arteries, which was reviewed and refuted by a recent study (Jacobs BS, et al. J Neurol Sci 20034.). The suggestion (Jacobs BS, et al. J Neurol Sci 2003.) was to be less conservative in the brain death confirmation. Since, no new statement of the NSRG WFN were published, the confirmation of cerebral circulatory arrest using Doppler sonography should be done according to aforementioned criteria (Ducrocq X, et al. J Neurol Sci 1998.). Since the introduction of TCD in brain death confirmation is preferrable, a numerous clinicians addopted its usage. That resulted in a number of publications. Some (Poularas J, et al. Transplant Proc 2006.), reported lower sensitivity than previously reported, but the specificity was 100%. Already mentioned, a meta-analysis of studies assessing the validity of TCD in confirming brain death, was done (Monteiro LM, et al. Intesive Care Med 2006). A systematic review of articles published in English on the diagnosis brain death by TCD, between 1980 and 2004, was performed. TCD oscillating or reverberating flow and systolic spikes, were considered to be compatible with cerebral circulatory arrest. The quality of each study was assessed using standardized methodological criteria. The literature was searched for any article reporting a false-positive result. Two high-quality and eight low-quality studies were included. The high sensitivity 95% (95% CI 92-97%) and high specificity 99% (95% CI 97-100%) for brain death detection using TCD was obtained.

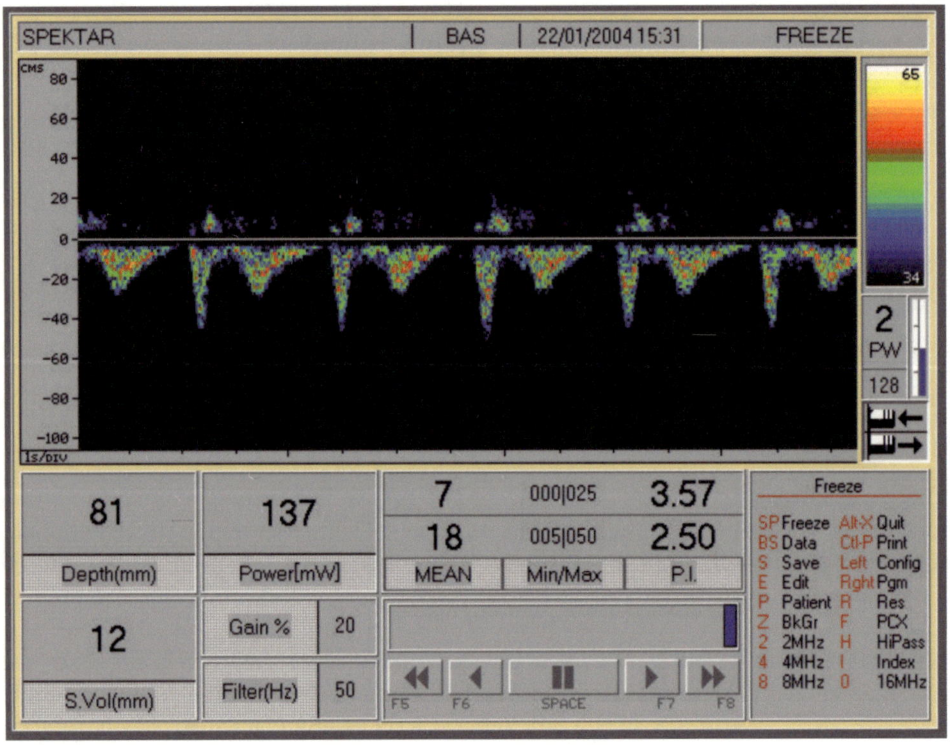

Fig. 14. Reveberating flow in basilar artery due to aortic dissection

6. Advantages and disadvantages of Doppler sonographic evaluation

The greatest advantage of Doppler sonography is the possibility of bedside evaluation, which enables close monitoring and intervention in unstable patient. It must be pointed out, that prerequisits should be fullfiled. No contrast agents are applied, preserving the residual organ function. The recent publication (Lovrencic-Huzjan A, et al. Ultraschall Med/ Europ J Ultrasound 2011.) showed the shortes time to confirm the clinical diagnosis of brain death, and in most paients (61%) cerebral circulatory arrest was confirmed within 2 hours from clinical diagnosis. This is imporatnt since the delay of brain death determination have negative impact on organ donation (Lustbader D, et al. Neurology 2011.), and in study consent for organ donation decreased from 57% to 45% as the brain death declaration interval increased. Conversely, refusal of organ donation increased from 23% to 36% as the brain death interval increased. Also 12% sustained a cardiac arrest between the two examinations or after the second examination.

The disadvantages of TCD is that in up to 20% of individuals the insonation is not possible due to bone hyperostosis. In patients with skull defects or drainage false results can be detected due to inapropriate ICP recording, and therefore the TCD in not a method of choice for brain death confirmation. The blood flow velocities can be affected by marked changes in PCO_2, hematocrit and cardiac output. It cannot be performed in hypotensive patients. Transcranial Doppler ultrasonography requires considerable practice and skill.

7. Conclusion

In comatose patients with absent motor and brainstem reflexes, and evidence of brain damage compatible with the diagnose, brain death is supected. After an observational period repeted examination should be perfomed according to the protocol. Apnea testing should be done, and TCD can be used as an ancillary test for diagnosing cerebral circulatory arrest. It is a preferable test due to noninvasivness, bedside evaluation. Beside it is easy to perform, thus the diagnosis can be confirmed within short time period, mostly in two hours after the clinical diagnosis.

8. Acknowledgment

I thank all the colleagues and staff in Central intensive care unit in Department of Anaesteziology and Neurology intensive care in University Department of Neurology Univeristy Hospital Center "Sestre milosrdnice" in Zagreb, Croatia, where the recording of patients and brain death persons were performed.

I thank DWL for financial support of this chapter.

I thank Marijana Bosnar Puretic, MD, PhD for technical support in preparation of the manuscript.

9. References

Alexandrov, A.V., Sloan, M.A., Tegeler, C.H., Newell, D.N., Lumsden, A., Garami, Z., Levy, C.R., Wong, L.K., Douville, C., Kaps, M. & Tsivgoulis, G.; for the American Society of Neuroimaging Practice Guidelines Committee. Practice Standards for Transcranial Doppler (TCD) Ultrasound. Part II. Clinical Indications and Expected Outcomes. (2010) *J Neuroimaging*, Oct 26. doi: 10.1111/j.1552-6569.2010.00523.x. ISSN 1051-2284

Calleja, S., Tembl, J.I. & Segura, T.; Sociedad Española de Neurosonología. Recommendations of the Use of Transcranial Doppler to Determine the Existence of Cerebral Circulatory Arrest as Diagnostic Support of Brain Death. (2007) *Neurologia, Vol.* 22, No.7, pp. 441-447, ISSN 0213-4853 de Freitas, G.R., Andre, C., Bezerra, M., Nunes, R.G. & Vincent M. Persistence of Isolated Flow in the Internal Carotid Artery in Brain Death. (2003) *J Neurol Sci*, Vol.210, No.1-2, pp.31-34, ISSN 0022-510X

Demarin, V., Lovrencic-Huzjan, A., Vargek-Solter, V., Vukovic, V., Miskov, S., Mikula, I., Peric, M., Gopcevic, A., Kusic, Z., Balenovic, A., Klanfar, Z. & Busic, M. Consensus Opinion on Diagnosing Brain Death - Guidelines for Use of Confirmatory Tests. Report of Croatian Neurovascular Society and University Department of Neurology, Sestre milosrdnice University Hospital, Reference Center for Neurovascular Disorders and the Ministry of Health of Republic of Croatia. (2005) *Acta clin Croat*, Vol.44, No.1, pp.65-79, ISSN 0353-9466

Ducrocq, X., Braun, M., Debouverie, M., Junges, C., Hummer, M. & Vespignani, H. Brain Death and Transcranial Doppler: Experience in 130 Cases of Brain Dead Patients. (1998) *J Neurol Sci*, Vol.160, No.1, pp.41-6, ISSN 0022-510X

Ducrocq, X., Hassler, W., Moritake, K., Newell, D.W., von Reutern, G.M., Shiograi, T. & Smith, R.R. Consensus Opinion on Dignosis of Cerebral Circulatory Arrest Using Doppler Sonography. Task Force Group on Cerebral Death of the Neurosonology Research Group of the World Federation of Neurology. (1998) *J Neurol Sci*, Vol.159, No.2, pp.145-150 ISSN 0022-510X

Eng, C.C., Lam, A.M., Byrd, S., Newell, D.W. The Diagnosis and Management of a Perianesthetic Cerebral Aneurysmal Rupture Aided with Transcranial Doppler Ultrasonography. (1993) *Anesthesiology*, Vol.78, No.1, pp.191-194, ISSN 0003-3022

Grote, E. & Hassler, W. The Critical First Minutes after Subarachnoid Hemorrhage. (1988) *Neurosurgery*, Vol.22, No.4, pp. 654, ISSN 0148-396X

Hadani, M., Bruk, B., Ram, Z., Knoller, N., Spiegelmann, R. & Segal, E. Application of Transcranial Doppler ultrasonography for the Diagnosis of Brain Death. (1999) *Intensive Care Med*, Vol.25, No.8, pp.822-828, ISSN 0342-4642

Hassler, W., Steinmetz, H. & Pirschel, J. Transcranial Doppler Study of Intracranial Circulatory Arrest. (1989) *J Neurosurg* Vol.71, No.2, pp.195-201, ISSN 0022-3085

Jacobs, B.S., Carhuapoma, J.R. & Castellanos, M. Clarifying TCD Criteria for Brain Death – are Some Arteries more equal than Others? (2003) *J Neurol Sci*, Vol.210, No.1-2., pp.3-4, ISSN 0022-510X

Lovrencic-Huzjan, A., Vukovic, V., Gopcevic, A., Vucic, M., Kriksic, V. & Demarin, V. Transcranial Doppler in brain death confirmation in clinical practice. (2011) *Ultraschall Med/Europ J Ultrasound*, Vol.32, No.1, pp.62-66. ISSN 0172-4614

Lovrencic-Huzjan, A., Vukovic, V., Jergovic, K. & Demarin, V. Transcranial Doppler as a Confirmatory Test in Brain Death. (2006) *Acta clin Croat*, Vol. 45, No.4, pp.365-373, ISSN 0353-9466

Lustbader, D., O'Hara, D., Wijdicks, E.F.M., MacLean, L., Tajik, W., Ying, A., Berg, E. & Goldstein, M. Repeat Brain Death Examinations may negatively Impact Organ Donation. (2011) *Neurology*, Vol. 76, No.1, pp.119-124, ISSN 0028-3878

Marinoni, M., Alari, F., Mastronardi, V., Peris, A. & Innocenti, P. The relevance of early TCD Monitoring in the Intensive Care Units for the Confirming of Brain Death Diagnosis. (2011) *Neurol Sci,* Vol.32, No.1, pp.73-77, ISSN 1590-1874

Monteiro, L.M., Bollen, C.W., van Huffelen, A.C., Ackerstaff, R.G., Jansen, N.J. & van Vught, A.J. Transcranial Doppler Ultrasonography to Confirm Brain Death: a Meta-analysis. (2006) *Intensive Care Med,* Vol.32, No.12, pp.1937-1944, ISSN 0342-4642

Poularas, J., Karakitsos, D., Kouraklis, G., Kostakis, A., De Groot, E., Kalogeromitros, A., Bilalis, D., Boletis, J. & Karabinis, A. Comparison between Transcranial Color Doppler Ultrasonography and Angiography in the Confirmation of Brain Death. (2006) *Transplant Proc,* Vol.38, No.5, pp.1213-1217. ISSN 0041-1345

Report of the Ad Hoc Committee of the Harvard Medical School to Examine the Definition of Brain Death. A definition of irreversible coma. (1968) *JAMA,* Vol. 205, No.6 , pp.337-340, ISSN 0098-7484

Report of the Quality Standards Subcommittee of the American Academy of Neurology. Practice Parameters for Determining Brain Death in Adults (Summary statement). (1995) *Neurology,* Vol.45, No.5, pp.1012-1014, ISSN 0028-3878

Segura, T., Calleja, S., Irimia, P. & Tembl, J.I.; Spanish Society of Neurosonology. Recommendations for the Use of Transcranial Doppler Ultrasonography to Determine the Existence of Cerebral Circulatory Arrest as Diagnostic Support for Brain Death. (2009) *Rev Neurosci, Vol.*20, No. pp. 251-9, ISSN 0334-1763

Velthoven van, V. & Calliauw, L. Diagnosis of Brain Death. Transcranial Doppler Sonography as an Additional Method. (1988) *Acta Neurochir (Wien),* Vol.95, No.1-2, pp.57-60, ISSN 0001-6268

Wijdicks, E.F.M. Brain Death Worldwide. Accepted Facts but no Global Consensus in Diagnostic Criteria. (2002) *Neurology,* Vol.58, No.1, pp.20-25, ISSN 0028-3878

Wijdicks, E.F.M. Determining Brain Death in Adults. (1995) *Neurology,* Vol.45, No.5, pp.1003-1011, ISSN 0028-3878

Wijdicks, E.F.M. The Case against Confirmatory Tests for Determining Brain Death in Adults. (2010) *Neurology,* Vol.75, No.1, pp.77-83, ISSN 0028-3878

Wijdicks, E.F.M., Varelas, P.N., Gronseth, G.S. & Greer, D.M. Evidence-Based Guideline Update: Determining Brain Death in Adults: Report of the Quality Standards Subcommittee of the American Academy of Neurology. (2010) *Neurology,* Vol.74, No.23, pp.1911-1918, ISSN 0028-3878

Yoneda, S., Nishimoto, A., Nukada, T., Kuriyama, Y., Katsurada, K. & Abe, H. To- and Fro-Movement and External Escape of Carotid Arterial Blood in Brain Death Cases. A Doppler Ultrasonic Study. (1974) *Stroke,* Vol.5, No.6, pp. 707-13. ISSN 0039-2499

Zurynski, Y., Dorsch, N., Pearson, I. & Choong, R. Transcranial Doppler Ultrasound in Brain Death: Experince in 140 Patients. (1991) *Neurol Res*, Vol.13, No.4, pp.248-52, ISSN 0161-6412